Elasticity in Healthcare Communication

Elastic language is a phenomenon in linguistics that refers to how we stretch the meanings of words depending on the context in which they are used – for example *many, about 20, perhaps, could be.* This study looks specifically at elastic language in the fields of medicine and healthcare, showing how it is used to serve both the patient's and the professional's needs. It explores the pragmatics and metapragmatics of elasticity in the delivery of online medical information as a way of avoiding miscommunication. Based on data from Chinese and English sources, it takes a cross-cultural perspective, to present an account of harmony and disharmony between professional medical websites and their users. Adding exciting new dimensions to the fields of health communication and pragmatics, it is essential reading for scholars and advanced students in semantics, pragmatics, discourse analysis and interactional linguistics, as well as professionals involved in healthcare and communication.

GRACE QIAO ZHANG is Emeritus Professor at Curtin University, Australia. She has published numerous works in the fields of pragmatics and cross-cultural communication, including *Elastic Language* (Cambridge University Press, 2015).

MING-YU TSENG is Professor at National Sun Yat-Sen University, Taiwan. He has published in the *Journal of Pragmatics*, *Pragmatics & Society*, *Pragmatics & Cognition*, *Lingua*, *English for Specific Purposes*, and the *Journal of English for Academic Purposes*.

Elasticity in Healthcare Communication

A Cross-Cultural Perspective

Grace Qiao Zhang

Curtin University, Australia

Ming-Yu Tseng

National Sun Yat-Sen University, Taiwan

CAMBRIDGE
UNIVERSITY PRESS

CAMBRIDGE
UNIVERSITY PRESS

University Printing House, Cambridge CB2 8BS, United Kingdom

One Liberty Plaza, 20th Floor, New York, NY 10006, USA

477 Williamstown Road, Port Melbourne, VIC 3207, Australia

314–321, 3rd Floor, Plot 3, Splendor Forum, Jasola District Centre, New Delhi – 110025, India

103 Penang Road, #05–06/07, Visioncrest Commercial, Singapore 238467

Cambridge University Press is part of the University of Cambridge.

It furthers the University's mission by disseminating knowledge in the pursuit of education, learning, and research at the highest international levels of excellence.

www.cambridge.org
Information on this title: www.cambridge.org/9781108842396
DOI: 10.1017/9781108903134

First published 2022

A catalogue record for this publication is available from the British Library.

ISBN 978-1-108-84239-6 Hardback

Contents

List of Figures *page* viii
List of Tables x
Acknowledgements xii

1 Introduction 1
1.1 Definitions 3
1.2 Purposes of This Study 4
1.3 Concluding Remarks 5

2 Theoretical Foundations 7
2.1 Pragmeme Theory 7
2.2 Integrative Pragmatics 11
2.3 Frame Approach 13
2.4 Elastic/Vague Language and Elasticity Theory 14
2.5 Healthcare Communication 25
2.6 Concluding Remarks 30

3 Methodology 32
3.1 Rationale of the Research Design 32
3.2 Data 34
3.3 Data Analysis 37
3.4 Concluding Remarks 42

4 Elastic Language Used in Chinese 43
4.1 Pragmatic Forms of Elastic Language 43
4.2 Pragmatic Functions of Elastic Language 46
4.3 Frequency Distribution among the Four Categories 58
4.4 Correlations between the Four Categories and Six Diseases 73
4.5 Concluding Remarks 82

5 Elastic Language Used in English 87
5.1 Pragmatic Forms of Elastic Language 87
5.2 Pragmatic Functions of Elastic Language 89
5.3 Correlation between Frequency of Elastic Language and the Six Medical Conditions 100

5.4 Correlations between Pragmatic Forms, Pragmatic Functions and Six Types of Diseases 105
5.5 Concluding Remarks 108

6 Comparison between Chinese and English Regarding Elastic Language Use 109
6.1 Pragmatic Forms of Elastic Language: Top 10 Elastic Expressions in Chinese and English 109
6.2 Pragmatic Functions of Elastic Language 111
6.3 Frequency Distribution among the Four Categories 116
6.4 Correlations between the Four Categories and Six Types of Diseases 120
6.5 Concluding Remarks 122

7 Perceptions of and Attitudes Towards the Use of Elastic Language in Chinese 125
7.1 Responses to Whether Elastic Language Is Difficult to Understand and Why 126
7.2 Responses to Why Elastic Language or Non-elastic Language Is Preferred 132
7.3 Social Factors 152
7.4 Concluding Remarks 157

8 Perceptions of and Attitudes towards the Use of Elastic Language in English 160
8.1 Responses to Whether Elastic Language Is Difficult to Understand and Why 161
8.2 Responses to Why Elastic Language or Non-elastic Language Is Preferred 167
8.3 Social Factors 182
8.4 Concluding Remarks 189

9 Comparison between Chinese and English Regarding Participants' Feedback 191
9.1 Responses to Whether Elastic Language Is Difficult to Understand and Why 191
9.2 Responses to Whether Elastic Language or Non-elastic Language Is Preferred and Why 194
9.3 Social Factors 197
9.4 Concluding Remarks 201

10 General Discussion 204
10.1 Elasticity and Its Framing 204
10.2 Pragmeme and Pragmatic Tolerance Degree of Fitness 205
10.3 Integrated Pragmatic Explanation 209
10.4 Concluding Remarks 211

11 Conclusions and Implications 212
11.1 Conclusions 212
11.2 Applications and Implications 214
11.3 Future Research 218

Appendix 1: English Questionnaire Used in Perth, Australia 220
Appendix 2: Chinese Questionnaire Used in Kaohsiung, Taiwan 229
References 239
Author Index 256
Subject Index 259

Figures

4.1 Top 10 elastic terms in the Chinese corpus *page* 45
4.2 Overall distribution of the four categories of EL in Chinese 59
4.3 Top 10 approximate stretchers in the Chinese corpus 60
4.4 Top 10 general stretchers in the Chinese corpus 63
4.5 Top 10 scalar stretchers in the Chinese corpus 67
4.6 Top 10 epistemic stretchers in the Chinese corpus 69
4.7 Overview of the distribution of the four categories of EL in six disease sub-corpora in the Chinese corpus 74
5.1 Top 10 elastic terms in the English corpus 88
5.2 Overall distribution of the four categories of EL in English 100
5.3 Top 10 approximate stretchers in the English corpus 101
5.4 Top 10 general stretchers in the English corpus 102
5.5 Top 10 scalar stretchers in the English corpus 102
5.6 Top 10 epistemic stretchers in the English corpus 103
5.7 Standardised EL frequency across the six diseases 104
5.8 EL frequency for the six diseases 106
6.1 Top 10 elastic terms in Chinese and English 110
7.1 Summary of answers regarding difficulty in understanding all six excerpts (Chinese data) 126
7.2 Preference for EL/non-EL in six excerpts (Chinese data) 133
7.3 Distribution of six frames (in number; Chinese data) 144
7.4 Most frequently used frames in three cases (Cases 1, 2 and 4) 146
7.5 Coding results of Case 3 148
7.6 Coding results of Case 5 149
7.7 Coding results of Case 6 151
7.8 Male versus female responses to Type A questions 153
7.9 Male versus female responses to Type B questions 154
7.10 Age difference in understanding EL 155
7.11 Age difference in EL/non-EL preference (%) 156
7.12 Age difference in EL/non-EL preference (raw data) 157
8.1 Summary of answers regarding difficulty in understanding all six excerpts (English data) 164

8.13 Indifference frame 178
8.14 Disease-related frame 179
8.15 Top three frames for six diseases 183
9.1 A comparison: Rates of difficulty, numbers of elastic items and diseases 192

Acknowledgements

We would like to express our sincere gratitude to the anonymous reviewers and the copy-editor, Kilmeny MacBride, for their invaluable feedback which has been incorporated into this book. We are extremely grateful to Cambridge University Press editor Helen Barton for her advice and support – it has been an absolute pleasure to work with her. We also owe a debt of gratitude to Laura Simmons, Isabel Collins, Aloysias Thomas and other staff members at Cambridge for their help and patience during the production of this book.

We are truly thankful to James Jing, Hsin-Chin Wang, John Ho, Wei-Ting Hsieh, Shih-Wen Chuang and Xander Huang for their help with data collection, data analysis and data checking (among other things). And we also extend this thanks to Johanna (from The Expert Editor), Stephen Browning and Oliver Drewett for their help with proofreading. Without the willingness of our participants in the data collection, this book would not have been possible. We wholeheartedly thank those who participated in the surveys in Australia and Taiwan.

We acknowledge with gratitude the research grant we received from the Chiang Ching-kuo Foundation for International Scholarly Exchange (Project # RG004-P-16), which enabled us to successfully conduct this research project.

Finally, we extend a thank you to our families for all their love and support during the research for and writing of this book.

Some parts of the publication, Tseng, Ming-Yu and Zhang, Grace (2020) 'Perceptions of and attitudes toward elastic language in online health communication in Chinese', *Lingua* 233: 1–24, https://doi.org/10.1016/j.lingua.2019.102750, are reprinted in this book with kind permission from Elsevier, Amsterdam/London, www.elsevier.com.

Some parts of the publication, Zhang, Grace and Tseng, Ming-Yu (2020) 'Attitudes towards elastic language in Australian online healthcare information', *Internet Pragmatics* 3(1): 34–63, https://doi.org/10.1075/ip.00051.zha, are reprinted in this book with kind permission from John Benjamins Publishing Company, Amsterdam/Philadelphia, www.benjamins.com/catalog/ip.

1 Introduction

Medicine is an applied science and is not always exact. In this context, an ongoing challenge for health professionals is to identify the most appropriate language through which to deliver medical information to a public with varying needs. The core element of health consultation is effective communication between health professionals and their patients (Adolphs et al., 2007; Ainsworth-Vaughn, 1998; Heath, 1986). For example, communication in the health context should enable the delivery of clear and accurate information while also accommodating patients' emotional needs. Doctors are aware of the significant role language plays in this setting, where, for example, using metaphors to refer to cancer (among other illnesses) can help to build rapport between health professionals and their patients (Ordóñez-López and Edo-Marzá, 2016). Elastic language (EL), equipped with its characteristic fluidity, helps to address challenges around health communication (Zhang, 2015). For example, in the statement, 'After the thyroid operation, there may be a need to take some thyroxine', the elastic words 'may' and 'some' are suggestive rather than prescriptive. There is little research on the elasticity of language in health communication, particularly from a cross-cultural perspective. Based on two corpora collected in Taiwan and Australia, the current study is one of few attempts to investigate the information-understanding abilities and preference of the public for EL or non-EL with the aim of determining the effectiveness of medical information disseminated online.

The objective of this study is to illustrate that using EL is integral to effectively imparting medical advice to patients (Adolphs et al., 2007). Having the ability to use EL is an important skill which allows language users to tailor their language to suit the communicative needs of their listeners (Carter and McCarthy, 2006; Channell, 1994; Ediger, 1995). When doctors deliver potentially distressing news to their patients, choosing between a 'tell-it-as-it-is' or a mitigated expression may influence how well the patient copes and cooperates with doctors, and consequently, may affect the success of their medical treatment. Institutional requirements invariably put grey health communication into a black or white box, which may need to be re-evaluated to integrate both precision and imprecision and to strike a balance between straight and mitigated talk. (Adolphs et al., 2007). Precise language cannot replace EL, as EL can function in ways which precise language cannot. Specifically, using EL as opposed to precise language makes it possible to present difficult or sensitive information in an empathetic manner.

Based on online medical data, this study explores how uncertainty is manifested in EL. Uncertainty comes from the limits of medical knowledge itself, as well as from the limits of our own knowledge. Such feelings lead people to consult the Internet to reduce their uncertainty regarding various health matters (Neely, 2014). Put more simply, when people face uncertainty, they may go online to seek information (Bylund et al., 2012; Koehly et al., 2009). This may take the form of gaining knowledge, becoming more educated about risk, receiving professional and emotional support, finding assurance or assisting with decision-making. According to Corrales et al. (2018), approximately half of the gynaecologic-oncology patients in their study consulted the Internet to obtain information about their conditions. But users may not always benefit from seeking information in this way. For example, some people 'may be motivated by inherent personality traits or tendency towards "health anxiety", and unclear or unreliable information may in fact push their anxiety level even higher' (2018: 302). While the Internet is a popular source of health advice for the public (Walther et al., 2018: 57), people may lack the necessary knowledge and skills to assess the credibility of a website's content (Mashiach et al., 2002). One study of online search for health advice for children found that 11% of search results did not give correct information and 49% did not answer the question or gave responses that were unrelated to the question (Davies et al., 2010). Prolific information on the Internet regarding diseases, symptoms, prognoses, treatments and risks may exacerbate readers' anxiety (Miller, 1987; Miller and Mangan, 1983); thus, providers of medical information online need to know how best to effectively present information. Accordingly, there is a need to research language use in online medical information to improve the public's experience of it. This study investigates how EL is perceived and whether it is preferred among online users, which will help to contribute to the successful communication of online medical information.

This study provides an account of how EL works in medical online communication, and its relationship to shared versus culture-specific features in Chinese and English. Several useful studies have been conducted on imprecision in medical language based on spoken data (Adolphs et al., 2007; Ordóñez-López and Edo-Marzá, 2016; Staples, 2015). The current study differs in that it is based on written and online medical data – that is, medical information on various diseases/conditions collected from online professional websites, including medical professional and government agencies in Australia and Taiwan (approximately a quarter of million words each for Chinese and English – half a million in total).

1.1 Definitions

Let us first look at an example. The following is an excerpt from a conversation at a banking royal commission hearing into misconduct in banking. The two interactants, the Commissioner and Commonwealth Bank of Australia (CBA) Boss, were talking about mortgage brokers receiving ongoing commission despite providing no ongoing financial advice.

COMMISSIONER: Are there any ongoing services supplied by a mortgage broker, Mr. Comyn?
CBA BOSS: I think they would be **limited**, Commissioner [audience laughs].
COMMISSIONER: Well . . . uh . . . limited or none.
CBA BOSS: **Much closer to none** [smiles; audience laughs].
COMMISSIONER: I take that as none [smiles; audience laughs].

(Source: Channel 7 Australia 6pm News, November 19, 2018)

Here the words *limited* and *much closer to none* are EL as they are used to avoid giving a definitive answer. The unfolding of the conversation shows that the speaker knows it, the Commissioner knows it, and the listeners know it too. Mr Comyn attempts to mitigate at the start, but the Commissioner points out that the correct answer should be *none* rather than *limited* or *much closer to none*. The audience laugh at every turn in speech during the conversation, suggesting they are aware of what is going on.

The term 'elastic language' is used as a metaphor to describe the ways in which we adjust and modify our utterances to accommodate communicative needs (Zhang, 2011, 2015). According to Zhang (2011, 2015), EL contains a degree of elasticity, which is inherent and unresolvable even with the help of context (fluidity principle); it can be stretched in various directions (stretchability principle); and it can stretch functions to serve communicative needs (strategy principle). In the current study, EL refers to the fluidity, stretchability and strategy of medical communication.

The concept of EL corresponds to elastic (both/and), rather than dichotomous (either/or), thinking. This is because while dichotomous thinking limits us in understanding complex and dynamic phenomena, elastic thinking enables us to deal with complementary, gradual and interdependent phenomena (Munné, 2013). The successful use of elasticity in language appears to result in a high level of interactivity in conversation (Cheng, 2007). Thus, appropriate use of EL is necessary for us to manage the complexity of effective communication.

Haugh and Culpeper (2018) highlight the importance of involving both writer (speaker) and reader (listener) in linguistic research. They argue that 'to analyse pragmatic phenomena, we must go beyond analysing the locally situated understandings of users and embrace observers' understandings' (2018: 235). In this study, both the information provider and the information observer of online medical information are studied to provide a rigorous account of online medical communication through the lens of EL use.

1.2 Purposes of This Study

Whilst the existing literature has shed a useful light on vague language (VL; Channell, 1994; Cutting, 2007; Ruzaitė, 2007), hedging (Hyland, 1998a, 1998b), and imprecision in medical language (Adolphs et al., 2007; Ordóñez-López and Edo-Marzá, 2016; Tseng and Zhang, 2018), there is limited research on the elasticity of language used in healthcare communication, especially from a cross-cultural perspective.[1] The current study attempts to address this gap by focusing on the 'harmony' and 'misfire' (Mey, 2016b: 136) between information on professional medical websites and the potential readers of those sites. Specifically, this study investigates the effectiveness of EL use in healthcare communication based on corpora of online medical information collected in Australia and Taiwan.

There are two major sources of information for the study: language used by the writers of medical websites and feedback (through questionnaires and follow-up interviews) on the language used by participants in this study. By including both the information giver and receiver in the research design, the study provides a rigorous account of how EL is both used and perceived. An investigation into the perceptions of and attitudes around EL among information receivers represents uncharted territory in the existing literature.

Therefore, the four research questions underpinning the study are as follows:

1. What are the pragmatic forms and frequencies of EL?
2. How do these forms perform their pragmatic functions?
3. Are there any protocols concerning EL use? If so, what are they?
4. What are the impacts of context on the use of EL?

The first two questions seek to uncover the pragmatic forms and functions of EL in online healthcare communication and lay the foundation for the last two questions, which reveal patterns of EL and the role of context. Question 3 can be manifested through the perceptions and attitudes of language users (observers) towards the use of language (Haugh and Culpeper, 2018), as the notion of protocols may be used to explain why some interactions are better received than others (Tseng and Zhang, 2018: 42). These protocols may legitimise and guide the use of EL in communication. Question 4 examines the variability of EL behaviours in terms of different contextual conditions (e.g., six diseases) and language/culture (Chinese versus Australian). Hall

[1] The terms 'EL' and 'VL' are used interchangeably in this study.

(1976) points out that Asians are considered to take a less direct approach in communication compared with those from Europeanised cultures. Whether or not this view is exemplified in our data will be explored.

The first two questions uncover the linguistic features of EL, and the last two reveal any (dis)harmony involving the use of EL in medical communication, in turn indicating how such disharmony might be remedied in different cultures according to participants' feedback. By situating research on EL firmly in the health context, we seek to reveal whether medical information is successfully conveyed and what role EL plays in the process. These findings may help to enhance the effectiveness of online healthcare advice and enable better Internet conversations between healthcare professionals and the public.

1.3 Concluding Remarks

The dilemma addressed by the current study is as follows: online medical information providers are required to explain medical issues in a direct way, but, at the same time, they need to ensure their readers can bear their straight talk. On a scale with directness at one end and indirectness at the other, it is difficult to know how much (or how little) to divulge to readers. This project intends to highlight the importance of elastic communication to reveal how EL can both meet institutional needs and match the level of a reader's knowledge and their mental resilience.

Online medical information needs to strike a balance between accuracy and elasticity, a conundrum which this study aims to clarify. Increasingly, the public seek to reduce their uncertainty about various risks through consulting the Internet as an important source of information (Neely, 2014). This is because online medical information involves no cost, no waiting time, no probing, no embarrassment and no need to explain one's circumstances in detail. This study provides timely evidence of how the public view online information in terms of effectiveness.

Medical diagnoses and prognoses are often not clear-cut. Conveying these kinds of vague phenomena is a challenge to health professionals but also a skill they must master. This study analyses real-life medical data to generate communicative patterns and verified strategies that shape the ways in which professionals communicate uncertainty. The resulting findings may help healthcare professionals to deliver medical information in ways that are more accessible to the public.

Elasticity plays an integral part in effectively imparting medical advice to patients in a way that affirms their choices. This study is the first to explore communication effectiveness in healthcare, paying special attention to the role of elasticity in language use and how it performs in an Australia–Taiwan comparison. This research adds a new dimension to the study of health communication and explores better ways to deliver medical information to the public by challenging linear theories in linguistics and promoting non-linear concepts. Language cannot be totally held to a ‘correct’ standard nor used just as one wishes. A ‘one-size-fits-all’ approach for language use does not exist; rather, multiple standards guide our use of it.

2 Theoretical Foundations

This chapter reviews the relevant conceptual frameworks and studies examining health discourse. It is centred on the following: pragmeme theory, integrative pragmatics, frame theory, elastic/vague language and elasticity theory, and healthcare communication. This review lays a theoretical foundation for this study and informs the analysis of the data collected and subsequent discussion.

2.1 Pragmeme Theory

According to Mey (2001: 221), a *pragmeme* is 'a general situational prototype, capable of being executed in the situation'. Treating a situation as a unit of language use, the notion does not regard sentences as necessarily able to perform specific acts irrespective of the situation but, rather, views speech acting as inseparable from a situational context. A pragmeme is actualised through concrete individual pragmatic acts. As Mey (2001: 221) explains, '[t]he instantiated, individual pragmatic acts, the "ipracs" or *practs*, refer to a particular pragmatic pragmeme as its realizations' (emphasis original). As the speaker and listener vary in each situation, the ways in which a pragmeme is realised also vary.

This notion has been elaborated and enriched by subsequent studies. For example, Capone (2005) views a pragmeme as encapsulating the social norms of language use in society. As he puts it, '[a] pragmeme is a situated speech act in which the rules of language and of society synergize in determining meaning, intended as a socially recognized object, sensitive to social expectations about the situation in which the utterance to be interpreted is embedded' (Capone, 2005: 1357). Because each situation is a totality of various factors – including speaker and hearer, their relationship, and the temporal setting – no two practs can be exactly identical. Pragmeme theory, also known as pragmatic act theory, addresses how a range of textual and contextual factors – for example, co-text, reference, metaphor, and shared situation knowledge – collaborate in contributing to the performance of pragmatic acting beyond standard speech act theory (Austin, 1962; Searle, 1975). As Tseng and Zhang (2018: 42) point out, the notion 'is particularly useful in illustrating acts that are understudied yet subtle, situation-bound (Kecskes, 2010), or socio-culturally sensitive'. Previous studies employing pragmeme theory have analysed acts such as evaluating (Blackwell, 2010); referring (Allan, 2010); using proverbs to counsel, assure and/or accuse (Odebunmi, 2006); fishing/phishing for confidential information (Tseng, 2010); insulting (Allan, 2016); prompting social action (e.g., prompting the offer of something; Haugh, 2016); accommodating to the loss of a loved one (Parvaresh and Capone, 2017); interfering with the judiciary system (Capone and Bucca, 2018); and offering online medical consultation (Tseng and Zhang, 2018).

Attempting to move speech act theory beyond lexico-grammatical accounts, pragmeme theory firmly situates speech acting in the social context. As Mey (2016c: 139) articulates it, a pragmeme encapsulates 'a *function* from user to user, from user to the world, and vice versa' (emphasis original). This offers at least three insights relevant to this study. First, delivering health information to the general public via the Internet is a type of social activity and, therefore, a pragmeme. Viewing the social activity as a pragmeme provides a fresh perspective on the writing. As Mey (2016a: 245) continues, 'human knowledge is more properly seen as an *adaptation* to, [rather] than a "representation" of, reality' (emphasis original). Such *adaptation* 'evolves across space and time, in a localized *situation* and a temporal *sequence*' (Mey, 2016a: 245, emphasis original; see also Mey, 2013). This perspective has a significant implication for this study: health information, even when it concerns the same disease, may be delivered in a different manner across languages and cultures. This study investigates the use of EL in the online delivery of health information to the general public. Of special interest are issues such as which particular Chinese and English elastic terms are used in health information regarding the same health condition, how they are distributed, whether possible connections exist between the information surrounding the disease and the use of EL, and how speakers of Chinese and speakers of English respond to EL in Chinese and English health excerpts, respectively. These issues are examined based on the collected Chinese and English corpora, and a cross-linguistic and cultural comparison is also made. Second, with its emphasis on the situation, pragmeme theory stipulates that the choice of an utterance is affected by the affordances of the situation where the social activity takes place. The situation covers who speaks to whom, the participants' relationship, and their common ground, among other things. Thirdly, the situation has its affordances and constraints, and language can be used in ways that adapt to the situation to maximise potential affordances and minimise constraints. Of particular relevance to our study of EL are affordances and adaptability, each of which is discussed in more detail below.

2.1.1 *Affordance*

In pragmeme theory a situation is not understood as a physical environment where communication takes place; rather, it is a communication context charged with affordances and constraints that make speech acting possible or impossible. The concept of affordance was originally developed by psychologist Gibson (1986) in his ecological account of visual perception, a view that emphasises humans' interaction with the environment. As animals live in environments that nourish them (i.e., those places that afford them the opportunity to continue living), so too do humans. As Gibson (1986: 127) writes, '[t]he affordances of the environment are what it offers the animal, what it provides or furnishes, either for good or ill'. The same applies to humans, who 'interact to attain specific goals, according to situational affordances as institutionally constrained and culturally filtered' (Vasilescu, 2016: 307). In other words, affordances are possible actions that an environment allows one to take.

Extending the notion of affordance to language use, Mey (2001: 219) states that a speech situation is 'the environment in which both speaker and hearer find their affordances, such that the entire situation is brought to bear on what can be said in the situation, as well as what is actually being said'. The addressee's uptake – that is, their willingness to participate in and understand the utterance as intended by the addresser – crucially impacts how the performance of the pragmatic act is received (Mey, 2001). Pragmeme theory, owing to the equal attention it pays to the addresser and the addressee co-producing meaning, considers both how a participant utilises the affordances of a situation and how affordances are exercised and received. In light of this, we can treat the use of EL as providing affordances in online health information as it enables the health professional to deliver health information in a flexible manner, as well as to cope with the constraints of the online environment and a variety of potential readers in the general public. As EL is the main focus of this study, we seek to investigate what EL can do (see Sections 4.2 and 5.2) and whether it necessarily facilitates the reception of health information (see Chapters 7 and 8).

2.1.2 *Adaptability*

According to Verschueren (1999: 61), adaptability 'is the property of language which enables human beings to make negotiable linguistic choices from a variable range of possibilities in such a way as to approach points of satisfaction for communicative needs'. This adaptability perspective has been used to characterise pragmatics of language use (Verschueren, 1999; Verschueren and Brisard, 2009). Mey also uses it to characterise pragmatic acts. As he puts it, 'a pragmatic act is an instance of adapting oneself to a context, as well as (on the basis of past situations and looking ahead to future situations) adapting the context to oneself' (Mey, 2001: 227). Pragmatic acting is viewed as 'contextualized adaptive behavior' (Mey, 2001: 227). Based on Mey (2001, 2016b) and Verschueren (1999), this study treats adaptability as the property of language and the language user's ability to adapt to the situation. In online health communication, adaptability is manifested in how health information (including advice) is delivered in a way that is accessible and acceptable to the public. Previous studies that examined how different demographic groups respond to health information also shed light on how adaptability can be more firmly utilised (Delorme et al., 2006; Southwell, 2010).

As language use and situational affordances are tightly intertwined, it is unnecessary to attribute a given feature of discourse to language or a situation alone. Therefore, in this section, we address the stretching of affordances and of language in an integrated manner. More specifically, we explore how elasticity (the stretching of language; Zhang, 2011, 2015) contributes to adaptability. At least five factors pertain to health professionals' adaptability: the health issue, intended reader (i.e., laypeople), online setting, socio-institutional considerations (e.g., social activity, healthcare organisation and medical knowledge) and the purpose of the health communication. These are different aspects of online health communication but are all connected to each other in one way or another because they are part and parcel of the discourse (cf. Johnstone, 2018). One question that the current study addresses is whether the use of EL correlates to the type of health information being delivered (cf. Sections 4.4, 5.4 and 6.4).

The aspects of adaptability affect language use. For example, according to Tseng and Zhang (2018), a striking feature of language use in online medical consultation cases rated satisfactory by enquirers is the appropriate use of elasticity. It is found that EL (e.g., *sometimes*, *many*) is used to help combat a series of dilemmas that face the doctor in the online environment. These cover various predicaments, such as having insufficient information about the patient and yet having to deliver medical advice; not being able to conduct a medical diagnosis and yet needing to help the patient; and exercising caution around the information given – which could be misinterpreted – and yet feeling obligated to offer help to those in need. By making meaning more elastic, the trap of having to say something precise when uncertainty exists can be circumvented. Given the constraints of the online context, appropriately using EL enables doctors to stretch language. As such, strategic elasticity helps serve communicative goals such as answering a medical query in an online context where a proper diagnostic assessment cannot be conducted.

This investigation into EL echoes and extends previous studies examining VL in the context of health communication. Hedging has been found frequently used in medical discourse to adjust the communication need of expressing uncertainty and to represent medical knowledge (Prince et al., 1982). The delivery of medical diagnoses and prognoses renders it helpful to use VL (Nicholson-Perry and Burgess, 2002). Vagueness in language use eases the tension between professional requirements and interpersonal considerations, and different medical situations may require different levels of vagueness (Adolphs et al., 2007).

We treat strategic elasticity and adaptability as connected in three aspects (Tseng and Zhang, 2018: 43–44). First, the use of elasticity is shaped by interconnected factors of discourse such as the availability of knowledge, writer-reader relationship, and situation and purpose, all of which also affect adaptability. Second, elasticity is a manifestation of adaptability at the micro level inasmuch as it realises how the addresser uses VL (Channell, 1994) to write about a specific health condition for the general public – who are not homogeneous in nature. Third, the pragmatic functions that elastic expressions serve may subtly add extra pragmatic meaning to the overall pragmatic force of online health communication, thereby contributing to enhanced adaptability because they enable the health professional to shift on a series of continua between firm and flexible, and between cooperative and uncooperative (Zhang, 2011). Take, for instance, the elastic expression *often* in 'People in general *often* attribute anxiety disorders to "psychological stress", and this is wrong.' The pragmatic functions of using the stretcher do not seem to be restricted to merely qualifying the statement. This is because, in the context of online health communication, the elastic term also allows the doctor to correct a misconception without making the tone personal, thereby serving the function of correcting a misconception widely held in the public. Embedded, as it is, within the performance of speech acts (e.g., advice and explaining a health issue), the function may go unnoticed, but it is nevertheless suggestive of adaptability at work.

2.2 Integrative Pragmatics

The central tenet of integrative pragmatics (Culpeper and Haugh, 2014; Haugh and Culpeper, 2018) is that pragmatic meaning must be constructed by both users and observers, and how observers interpret the utterance is just as important as whatever users may have intended. According to Haugh and Culpeper (2018: 235), a 'potential fruitful way forward' is to focus on analysing both user and observer perspectives on pragmatic phenomena, because 'in order to fully explicate the understandings of users themselves, we very often need to draw from the understandings of observers as well'. They insist that only by taking this broad perspective can a nuanced and complex linguistic theory be achieved. This is the approach adopted in this study: a holistic approach to look at both the online information providers' use of language as well as the information receivers' evaluation of the language used.

This study adopts Haugh and Culpeper's (2018) definitions of pragmatic form, function and context. A pragmatic form refers to 'any linguistic or non-linguistic unit that is understood as interlinked with a particular pragmatic function'; a pragmatic function refers to 'some purpose or activity for which that form is fitted, employed or understood to accomplish'; and a pragmatic context refers to 'social or discourse information that users orient to as licensing the recognition of particular forms as indexical of particular functions, or as inferable from those forms in that context' (Haugh and Culpeper, 2018: 221). They also add that this kind of context is by its nature dynamic, which shapes and is shaped using language itself.

Integrative pragmatics emphasises two strengths: strong empirical orientation and a combination of pragmatic and metapragmatic perspectives. A pragmatic perspective refers to pragmatic meaning drawn on the relationship and interconnection between pragmatic forms, functions and context. Metapragmatics refers to interactional meaning based on interaction between users and observers and is commonly defined as a systematic study of both the users themselves and observers' reflexive awareness about the use of language (Verschueren, 1999). One of the advantages of integrative pragmatics is to examine a broad range of meanings in dynamic fashion, including pragmatic meaning, pragmatic acting and interpersonal relations/attitudes. Pragmatic meaning comes from the speaker's utterance, adhering to Grice's (1975) Cooperative Principle and Sperber and Wilson's (1995 [1986]) relevance correlations (e.g., labour and effect), among others. Pragmatic acting considers meaning as action, manifested through a pragmatic act. A pragmatic act is a situated speech act, interpreted not primarily based on the linguistic form but more on social situations (e.g., participant responses and social activities; Mey, 2001). Interpersonal relations refer to 'power, intimacy, roles, and rights and obligations' (Culpeper and Haugh, 2014: 197), and interpersonal attitudes include generosity, sympathy and anger.

The relevance of integrative pragmatics for this study is that the study adopts its principles in drawing on authentic written health communication corpora and real-life readers' understandings and perceptions of such data. This study also explores the interactional meaning emphasised by integrated pragmatics through looking at what EL health professionals select in delivering health information online and how readers react to a particular health information item. Readers' feedback on EL use is part of metalanguage, which conveys the reflective awareness of users' language use (Culpeper and Haugh, 2014: 240). This study supports the points made by Tseng and Zhang (2020: 3), that 'understanding how elastic terms are perceived and interpreted contributes to revealing aspects of the metapragmatics of elasticity. Such understanding complements and enriches an analysis of language purely from the analyst's viewpoint and can shed light on how public health communication may improve due to its being empirical'. In this way, we investigate EL use from a broad view to provide an in-depth and rigorous account of EL use in online health communication.

2.3 Frame Approach

Goffman (1974: 10–11) defined frames as 'principles of organization which govern [social] events . . . and our subjective involvement in them'.[1] A frame implements a perspective from which to understand a social interaction. In health communication studies (Akl et al., 2011; Hong, 2012; O'Keefe and Jensen, 2007; Rothman and Salovey, 1997; Rothman et al., 2006), framing has been developed using prospect theory (Kahneman and Tversky, 1979; Tversky and Kahneman, 1981), which contends that, when making a decision, people are generally averse to risk when they target potential gains, and they embrace risk when they inspect potential losses associated with their decision. Often the gain-versus-loss frame is adopted when examining whether health information concerned with the benefits (gains) or the risks (losses) of health issues will make a stronger impact on recipients (Cho and Sands, 2011; Hwang et al., 2012). A gain-framed message emphasises the pros of conforming to the advocated view, while a loss-framed message highlights the cons of not complying with it.

The framing adopted in the delivery of health information shapes how health advice is delivered (e.g., by encouraging or warning against certain behaviours or lifestyles). The reader's perception of health information may also be shaped by a frame activated when reading it – one not necessarily the same as the frame used by the writer – as health experience varies individually. An inquiry into which frames are frequently activated when people read EL can help us better understand how health information and advice using EL may be better delivered. Therefore, the notion of framing is useful in explaining the governing principles that underlie participants' attitudes towards EL. What frames were activated can be identified based on their written feedback. According to Gamson and Modigliani (1989: 3), there are five framing devices employed in news discourse: metaphor, catchphrases, exemplars, depictions and visual images. These devices are applicable to news discourse, which usually contains a few paragraphs. Nevertheless, the data collected from participants' written comments on health information tended to be straightforward and relatively short, ranging from only a few words to one or several sentences. As such, it is sometimes difficult to

[1] An earlier version of Section 2.3 appears in Tseng and Zhang (2020).

determine which frame is used when a comment is read on its own, but it is the case that the more such comments are juxtaposed, the more a frame composed of related parts and elements emerges. Following the study of Tseng and Zhang (2020), we identify a frame using the notion of thematic structure, which was proposed by van Dijk (1988: 30–48) in his analysis of news discourse. The theme of a news report is succinctly expressed in its headline and lead, and the rest of the report serves to provide details. We treat participants' comments as revealing part of their knowledge structure and beliefs and as forming aspects of themes that constitute frames (cf. Pan and Kosicki, 1993: 60–61). A theme becomes identifiable when comments connected by aspects pertaining to it are juxtaposed. For example, comments mentioning *clear*, *unclear*, *informative enough* and *too trivial* are grouped as representing aspects or subthemes of a theme concerning communication. This modified notion of thematic structures facilitates the identification of frames.

2.4 Elastic/Vague Language and Elasticity Theory

Whilst it is a common assumption that language is (or should be) precise, the reality is that vagueness is pervasive in language (Channell, 1994; Hyland, 1998b; Ruzaitė, 2007; Zhang, 2015) and is used regularly in daily life (Jucker et al., 2003). Precise language is not necessarily better than VL, as VL 'may carry more relevant contextual implications than would a precise expression' (Jucker et al., 2003: 1737). VL is desirable and often good enough for the purpose in hand, as too much precision may cause time-wasting and inflexibility (Williamson, 1994: 4869). VL can be more effective than precise language (Stubbs, 1981: 1) due to its versatile nature and fluidity.

Conventionally, VL is discouraged and direct language is required in health communication (Sontag, 1991). While medical information is often expected to be precise (Jucker et al., 2003: 1738), it is common to find uncertainty in medical diagnoses and prognoses (Nicholson-Perry and Burgess, 2002). Drawing on spoken healthcare data, Adolphs et al. (2007) argue that the language of healthcare professionals must necessarily reflect scientific uncertainty using VL. VL also appears in written medical research (Varttala, 1999). Both spoken and written medical discourse includes VL as part of their make-up. Studies reveal that VL is an indispensable part of health communication and plays an important role in medical advice negotiation and in affirming patient choice (Adolphs et al., 2004). VL can solve the dilemma between professional requirements (tell it as it is) and interpersonal needs (it is not too alarming) (Adolphs et al., 2007), as VL can mitigate imposition, decrease social distance, build rapport and boost solidarity and politeness (Adolphs et al., 2007; Channell, 1994; Holmes, 1984). A real-life example of vague language used in a medical setting is presented by Adolphs et al. (2007: 69), as follows:

NURSE: Cos we have to **kind of** un . . . we . . . we always do **like** the worst case scenario and work downwards.
PATIENT: All right. [laughs]. Okay.
NURSE: We always like look at **the meningitis type symptoms** first.
PATIENT: Yeah.
NURSE: Okay and then we work downwards. So just bear with me.

The conversation between nurse and patient is about meningitis symptoms, which could indicate serious disease. The nurse needs to find a way to deliver the medical information without causing unnecessary distress to the patient. VL comes to the rescue here. The terms *kind of*, *like*, and *meningitis-type symptoms* work together to mitigate the alarming nature of the news while the disease is being described. Adolphs et al. (2007) point out that VL, used as a softening device, can calm the patient, while the nurse then carefully introduces the 'worst-case scenario' in detail after the patient is prepared for it. They found that VL enables healthcare professionals to carry out their institutional duty as well as establish an interpersonal relationship with a patient; therefore, 'the language of the healthcare professional must necessarily reflect this degree of scientific uncertainty' (Adolphs et al., 2007: 64). It can become problematic when uncertainty is conveyed using precise language; it seems much better to resort to VL.

Communicative styles, a hedged or blunt language/manner, impact the effectiveness within healthcare communication (Staples, 2015). Staples examined two groups of nurses, one whose members were educated in the United States and the other whose members were educated internationally (mostly in Asian countries). They found the two nursing groups employed different communicative styles when interacting with patients due to their different sociopragmatic and pragmalinguistic approaches (2015: 124–125). The international group spoke to patients in a blunt manner, while the US group used a more hedged manner. The US group was rated higher than the international group by patients, showing that hedged language led to more successful health communication. Staples's findings are tested in this study to determine whether they are applicable in a different discourse.

This section provided a review of categories and functions of EL/VL, and elasticity theory. For more such reviews, see Zhang (2015) and Ruzaitė (2007), among others.

2.4.1 Elastic/Vague Language Categories

A similar term to EL is the term 'vague language' (VL). VL, often chosen deliberately, refers to a linguistic phenomenon that expresses intrinsic uncertainty by rendering the same proposition with more than one expression (Sadock, 1977, cited in Channell, 1994: 20). Folkman et al. (1979: 276) define uncertainty as 'a person's mental confusion' about the meaning of information.

VL consists of 'words or phrases with very general meanings which deliberately refer to people and things in a non-specific, imprecise way' (Carter and McCarthy, 2006: 928). For example, in the sentence, 'She has **a few** friends', *a few* refers to a fluid continuum rather than a specific number – it could be three, five or some other number. VL is pervasive in our language (Channell, 1994; Cutting, 2007; Hyland, 1998b; Ruzaitė, 2007) and is also a typical feature of healthcare interactions (Bryant and Norman, 1979; Prince et al., 1982). Knowing how to appropriately use VL can improve the effectiveness of medical and non-medical communication.

VL consists of two characteristics: context dependability (the interpretation of VL depends on context) and the unresolvability of vagueness, even with the help of context (Cheng, 2007; Cheng and Warren, 2003; Zhang, 2011). These are further confirmed by Parvaresh (2018: 169), who states that VL includes 'expressions whose meaning is negotiable by the interactants (i.e., context-dependable) but which do not lose their vague status (i.e., unresolvable)'. EL has a similar characteristic, where the elasticity of language cannot be contextually resolved. VL is 'inherently and intentionally imprecise', which is a fundamental element of everyday language (spoken and written) and a central aspect of one's communicative competence (Cutting, 2007: 4–5). Jucker et al. (2003: 1738) assert that communicative competence includes a speaker's ability to vary the precision of utterances and to use them in appropriate contexts. Ediger states that 'the ability to use appropriately VL in certain situations . . . allows speakers and writers to tailor their language more suitably to a particular context or situation' (1995: 127). VL plays an important role in communication, one that is unmatched by precise language. Accordingly, the nature of VL enables language users to interpret it in greater detail (Ruzaitė, 2007).

The term 'EL' is promoted for its positive image (Zhang, 2011, 2015), as there are some negative connotations associated with the term 'VL' (Channell, 1994; Cutting, 2007). Negative attitudes towards the use of VL are also reported in Cutting (2015), as its use is associated with indifference, laziness, incompetence, unreliability and the uneducated. In this study, the term 'EL' is adopted, but the term 'VL' is also used where needed – for example, in the literature reviews.

VL is classified using two general approaches: open set and closed set, or in Zhang's (2015: 35) terms, liberal and conservative approaches, respectively. The first one considers VL as an unlimited category, and any utterances contextually underspecified can be regarded as VL (Parvaresh, 2018), including vague nouns (e.g., *bush*), verbs (e.g., *run*) and adjectives (e.g., *red*). The closed set puts a limit on the VL category and excludes vague nouns, verbs and adjectives (Cheng, 2007). Most researchers adopt a closed set, or conservative approach, in their works. Zhang (2015), for example, classifies EL into the following four categories: approximate stretchers, general stretchers, scalar stretchers, and epistemic stretchers.

Approximate stretchers refer to imprecise numbers and quantities and are used when exact numbers are unavailable, unimportant or unnecessary (Zhang, 2015: 29). There are two subcategories: approximators (e.g., *about 10, 20 or 30*) and quantifiers (e.g., *several, a little*). The numerals that partially make up approximators tend to be round numbers (Sigurd, 1988: 243), which refer to numerical amounts, times, or dates (Koester, 2007: 52). Words such as *about* and *or* are termed 'vague additives' (Channell, 1994: 18) because they can be added to a number to make approximation. Words such as *more than* (10) and *less than* (10) are called 'partial specifiers' (Channell, 1994: 62) because they have an exact number at one end (e.g., 10) as their lower or upper limit, and only the other end is vague. Quantifiers, on the other hand, refer to non-numerical quantities. Unlike approximators, quantifiers convey implicature (Channell, 1994) – for example, *many* can indicate popularity (Jucker et al., 2003) and also represents a different attention focus (Moxey and Sanford, 1993). As Ruzaitė (2007: 38) states, '[t]he meaning of quantifiers frequently encodes some evaluative content concerning the significance of a quantity'. Quantifiers tend to have a more complex usage than approximators.

General stretchers create global meaning. There are two subcategories: general nouns (e.g., *someone, sometime*) and general extenders (e.g., *things like that, or something like that*). General nouns are 'totally vague' without much referential content (Crystal and Davy, 1979: 112). They enable the speaker 'to refer to an entity or a person without knowing exactly which "name" would be the best word to use' (Yule, 1996: 18). Thus, it is the hearer who needs to work out the referent (Clark and Wilkes-Gibbs, 1986: 112). General nouns also include 'placeholder', which refers to a noun or name – for example, *whatshisname, thingy,* and *what-do-you-call-it* (Channell, 1994: 158–161). Placeholders perform 'a highly significant role mainly in oral communication when the aim is to avoid derogatory, offensive, pretentious or forgotten words' (Ruzaitė, 2007: 45). General nouns can 'help the conversation go smoothly' using their 'open-ended' semantic referents (Shirato and Stapleton, 2007: 396). They can be used to avoid specifying someone to avoid impoliteness and create solidarity (Zhang, 2015: 32). Often it is problematic to work out whether a placeholder is used out of necessity or on purpose.

The term 'general nouns' in this study is defined as a closed set of words versus an open set. Cutting (2012) considers general nouns with a much wider range, including words such as *people* and *results*. Based on a conference abstracts corpus, the author found that the functions of such general nouns include 'courtesy', 'modesty', 'caution' 'textual cohesion', 'convenience', 'self-defence', 'power', 'anticipation' and that they 'disguise the incompleteness' (2012: 285–286). The current study does not adopt the open set definition as it would make it unmanageable.

General extenders (Overstreet and Yule, 1997) are also referred to as vague category indicators (Zhang, 2015: 30), which vaguely refer to a particular category. Conjunctive (*and*) and disjunctive (*or*) are two basic forms of this, as in 'I bought apples, oranges **and/or things like that**'. Cutting (2015: 109) states that a conjunctive general extender implies 'more could be said', which adheres to Grice's (1975) Maxim of Quantity, and disjunctive general extenders imply that what has been said is possibly imprecise, which adheres to Grice's cooperative maxim of quality. The use of general extenders suggests that a full list of items is unnecessary, and if the listener wants to know more details, they can choose to ask more. General extenders come with implicature, based on shared knowledge, experience and conceptual schemes. According to Overstreet (1999: 68), the implicature of using a general extender is, 'I do not need to be explicit; you will be able to supply whatever unstated understandings are required to make sense of the utterance'. For example, the hearer is supposed to be able to work out the meaning of 'and things like that' when the speaker says, 'I went to shops and bought bread, milk, **and things like that**'. The category loosely pertains to a category exemplified by *bread* and *milk*, which are prototypical of this category. The use of general extenders enhances the efficiency of language used by avoiding a long list, which is often unnecessary or impossible to do. General extenders are co-constructed formulaic expressions (Simpson, 2004), where shared common background and knowledge are needed (Aijmer, 2002: 248). The two-way understanding between speaker and hearer is key for general extenders to work. General extenders were used more by working- than middle-class Australian native speakers of English (Dines, 1980). The former also used more *and that*, while the latter used more *and stuff* and *and things* (Cheshire, 2007). This suggests that social class may influence the use of general extenders.

Scalar stretchers can increase (intensifier) or decrease (softener) the strength of an utterance in an unspecific way (Cheng, 2007). An intensifier is normally a relative adjective or adverb (Cruse, 2006: 89), typically exemplified by *very* and *extremely*. Intensifiers are 'linguistic devices that boost the meaning of a property upwards from an assumed norm' (Quirk et al., 1985). There has been debate about whether intensifiers are vague. While some do not consider they are (e.g., Channell, 1994), others do. For example, Cheng argues that 'all items constituting scalar implicature are vague and only understood within an assumed shared understanding of approximate parameters in a particular context' (2007: 167). Intensifiers emphasise the tone of the utterance (Zhang, 2011), thus maximising the language user's attitudinal visibility (Hyland, 2005). A persona of assertiveness and a sense of conviction can be performed by an intensifier (Hyland, 1998b, 2000). As opposed to intensifiers, the strength of utterance can be decreased by adding a softener, exemplified by *sort of* and *kind of* (Holmes, 1990). Softeners deliver uncertainty (Kay, 2004: 700), mitigation and politeness.

Epistemic stretchers express possibility without the speaker's commitment to what they assert, (e.g., *maybe*, *sort of*, *I think*, *according to*). Epistemic stretchers 'express the speaker's judgement about the certainty, reliability, and limitations of the proposition; they can also comment on the source of the information' (Biber et al., 2010: 854). The speaker's judgement here is a subjective opinion that is not necessarily a fact (e.g., *I think*) but, rather 'a means of offering an idea without the obligation of commitment to its truth' (Rowland, 2007: 86). Epistemic stretchers 'qualify the speaker's confidence in the truth of a preposition' (Hyland, 1996: 477). They also indicate 'there is an intended concept, which she cannot explain precisely or for which she knows of no adequate word' (Holmes, 1988: 96). For example, in the sentence, 'he is **sort of** nice', the speaker is saying that 'he' is not exactly nice, but they cannot find a better word and, therefore, use *sort of* to indicate that 'he' does not fall into the 'standard' nice but close to it. Epistemic stretchers make speech less authoritative and less assertive (Carter, 2003: 11) to shield the speaker from being wrong. Self-protection is among the major purposes when epistemic stretchers are used (Zhang, 2015: 35). Speakers are careful in not committing firmly to what they utter to avoid getting into trouble.

This study adopts a closed-book approach and Zhang's four categories of elastic expressions (see Section 3.3 for details).

2.4.2 Elastic/Vague Language Functions

There are various pragmatic functions of EL/VL discussed in the existing literature. VL is versatile, conveying uncertainty, cooperation (Andersen, 2010) and evasiveness (Zhang, 2011), among others. Jucker et al. (2003: 1765–1766) identify the following functions that VL performs. First, it conveys propositional attitudes such as newsworthiness (I know **a lot of** colleagues in this university), expectedness of a statement (She **often** laughs) and evaluative meaning (She looks **very** unhappy today). Second, it conveys social function such as politeness (I am **kind of** not interested), softening complaints and criticisms (This dish is **a bit** salty) and establishing a social bond (I bought apples, bananas, **and things like that**). Third, it conveys significance (**Many** students like this lecturer). Finally, it conveys procedural (not conceptual) meaning (I was **like** surprised). In this section, we review six commonly recognised functions, primarily based on the works of Channell (1994),

Ruzaitė (2007) and Zhang (2011, 2015). All functions are enabled by the tentativeness of EL/ VL.

Delivering the right amount of information: EL/VL can convey just a good enough amount of information through tailoring its vagueness to suit the communicative needs in context, when precise information is not needed or unavailable (Channell, 1994; Zhang, 2015). This function adheres to Grice's (1975) Maxim of Quantity: providing an appropriate amount of information as required, no more and no less. For example, when Gabby is asked what time it is, and she thinks it is about 2 pm but does not know the exact time, she replies, 'it is **about 2 pm**'. The approximator *about 2 pm* serves to provide not too much and not too little information, given what Gabby knows. More specifically, Gabby can communicate the right amount of information with the help of VL. The hearers tend not to be aware of vagueness in language (Channell, 1994), and the vast majority of them are not bothered by EL/VL (Zhang and Tseng, 2020). These factors are important in terms of EL/VL and can be an integral part of our everyday communication.

Mitigation: EL/VL is used to soften the tone of speech and 'minimise imposition and attenuate negative discursive moves, such as complaint or criticism' (Zhang, 2011: 576). EL/VL serves as a politeness strategy (Stubbs, 1986), as the most efficient form of polite communication (Jucker et al., 2003), as a way to avoid impoliteness (Caffi, 1999; Fraser, 1980), to resolve conflicts and strategically manage tensions (Trappes-Lomax, 2007) and to reduce the force of a confrontation (Terraschke and Holmes, 2007). VL also contributes to shaping three face-saving orientations – towards self, towards others and mutual interaction (Trappes-Lomax, 2007). VL is used as a softener to ease the over-directness or 'unduly authoritative or assertive' mode in expressions used (Carter and McCarthy, 2006: 202). Thus, VL can play an important role in maintaining interpersonal relationships, as discussed next.

Solidarity: EL/VL shows solidarity between interlocutors (Brown and Levinson, 1987) and builds rapport, informality and intimacy (Cutting, 2007; Terraschke and Holmes, 2007; Zhang, 2015). VL is a marker of in-groupness (Carter and McCarthy, 2006; Cutting, 2000). By using VL, the speaker indicates social group similarity (Aijmer, 2013), where a 'social group sharing interests and knowledge employs non-specificity in talking about their shared interest' (Channell, 1994: 193). For example, in a supervisor–PhD-student meeting, the supervisor says, 'please add more reviews on VL used in different discourses, healthcare, academic, **and things like that**'. The supervisor uses a general extender here, as she expects that the student, as an in-group member of the academic group, can infer more discourses (e.g., business and public speech) so that she does not need to provide more on the list. This example suggests that when VL is used, shared common knowledge is assumed, and it also indicates solidarity. Shared background is a prerequisite for VL performed as a solidarity marker (Channell, 1994; Koester, 2007; Terraschke and Holmes, 2007) and is essential for the addressee to interpret VL (Spencer-Oatey, 2000). The functions of solidarity and rapport-building reveal the collaborative nature of VL (Evison et al., 2007). Often VL gains informality to maintain a cooperative tone (Cheng and Warren, 2001). These findings are in line with a positive correlation. Cutting (2007) reports that the longer the friendship, the more VL is used. The logical correlation is that closer friendship leads to a more informal atmosphere and, therefore, greater use of VL. VL is associated with 'the natural and informal, convergent tenor of everyday talk' (McCarthy, 1998: 108). EL/VL is therefore a good tool in establishing interpersonal relationships.

Strengthening: EL/VL can 'strengthen the claim of an utterance or the intensity of an argument' (Zhang, 2015: 44). Intensifiers (mostly adverbs), such as *extremely* and *very*, tend to perform this function (Parvaresh and Zhang, 2019: 49). For example, in 'He is **extremely** good with children', if we remove *extremely*, the illocutionary force of the utterance is significantly weakened. This means that *extremely* enhances the illocutionary force of VL (Zhang, 2011: 575). With its forceful manner, the strengthening function is a marker of certainty (Hyland, 2005), assertiveness and persuasion (Channell, 1994; Hyland, 1998a). In addition to adverbs, multal quantifiers can also function in the same way, such as *a lot* and *many*. These quantifiers 'do not simply refer to a number of certain objects, but put a special emphasis on the hugeness of the amount under discussion' (Ruzaitė, 2007: 87). As opposed to the strengthening function, VL is primarily used to soften the tone of speech (mitigation function). This function is more widely recognised than the strengthening function, however both functions are equally useful in their own right.

Self-protection: VL is used to guard against the speaker being blamed, by allowing something to be stated with a degree of elasticity. VL can avoid the speaker being on the record as wrong. It is preferred over precise language, as the latter cannot be 'unsaid' and 'backs the speaker into a corner' (Zhang, 2015: 42). Vague expressions 'express a cautious and uncommitted attitude to a claim the speaker makes, to shield self from vulnerability and being wrong' (Zhang, 2015: 44). An example is 'She is the one who raised the question, **I think**'; without *I think*, the statement has the speaker's commitment. However, once *I think* is added, the statement no longer contains the speaker's commitment. When positioned at the end of an utterance, *I think* tends to be a vague marker (Zhang and Sabet, 2016) that protects the speaker from liability if the utterance turns out to be incorrect (Matthews, 1997). As a defensive device, VL indicates a lesser degree of assertiveness, which means that the speaker is less likely to be challenged and/or refuted (Jucker et al., 2003). Self-protection is called self-distancing in Ruzaitė's work, where the speaker distances him- or herself from the commitment to the truth of what is being claimed (2007: 158). The difference between self-protection and mitigation functions is that the former focuses on the speaker only, while the latter could include the listener as well.

Withholding information: VL can be used as a tool to deliberately withhold information (Channell, 1994: 4), and people want to 'manipulate the amount of information they provide' using VL (Ruzaitė, 2007: 48). As Zhang (2015: 43) states, 'VL functions as a device to evade some sort of unfavourable situation the speakers find themselves in'. Cheng and Warren (2001: 98) find that although people know exact information, they still tend to use VL, which means that, for some reason, they do not disclose what they know. There are two reasons for withholding information, one which is appropriate and one which is not. An example of appropriately withholding information is on social occasions, where people may be reluctant to disclose their age for various reasons – for example, they may say 'I'm in my **30s**'. The elastic expression used here is a way of avoiding giving out personal information. An example of inappropriately withholding information is a real-estate agent evading telling his clients the truth by failing to tell them that the house they are about to purchase has some major defects. Evasive language (e.g., lying) is considered a non bona-fide mode of communication (Verschueren, 2017: 324). Channell notes that VL 'is part of our taken-for-granted world, and that normally we do not notice it unless it appears inappropriate – for example, when someone seems to be deliberately withholding information' (1994: 4). When VL causes confusion, it tends to be challenged (Zhang, 2020). The function of withholding information using VL is a strategic part of language use, which is overlooked in the existing literature. The important issue is that when EL is used for withholding information, miscommunication needs to be avoided. Constructing a message resorts to both linguistic conventions (e.g., the form) and communicative competence (e.g., social norms), and lacking either can cause miscommunication (Wong, 2010; Capone, 2018). This means that both language and sociocultural competences are crucial in effectively conveying information.

The above six functions of EL/VL are not a complete list. There are more functions. For example, vagueness helps interlocutors to find the right words in real-time stressful situations (Metsä-Ketelä, 2016). VL can also fill in knowledge gaps (i.e., lexical and conceptual gaps) and carry out language modification to accommodate each other strategically (Cheng and Warren, 2001). Three general functions of vagueness in written academic discourse are hedging ('courtesy', 'modesty' and 'caution'), non-hedging ('convenience', 'self-defense', 'power' and 'anticipation') and disguise Cutting, 2012).

An elastic expression is not limited to performing only one function; it can perform multiple functions to suit the given context. Wu et al. (2010) find that *I think* in the context of English as a second language can serve to mitigate, to strengthen, to turn-take, to delay turn-taking (in search for the proper word) and to self-repair (among others). Ruzaitė's (2007) study on the functions of vague quantifiers in teacher–student interactions finds that they can mitigate, allow one to save face and help make apologies, promises and self-justifications. These show that EL may serve opposite purposes: mitigating (collaborative) and withholding information (competitive). EL also has different orientations: information-based (e.g., providing the right amount of information) and relationship-based (e.g., solidarity). This shows that EL is multi-faceted and essential to make communication effective and efficient.

There have been studies regarding how EL functions in different languages. For example, the particle *ba* in Mandarin Chinese is used to soften a threat (Ran, 2010; Zhang, 2016). General extenders are used for hedging and politeness in German (Cutting, 2015: 112). It is expected that there would be commonalities and differences in terms of EL functions across different languages.

2.4.3 *Elasticity Theory*

While VL has been studied from a linguistic perspective for some years, there is a lack of theorisation and systematicity specifically for VL (Ruzaitė, 2007: 13). Elasticity theory has been developed by Zhang (2011, 2015) to explain the operation of EL. The elasticity framework makes 'a great contribution to the field by filling a significant theoretical gap' (Parvaresh, 2017b: 115). It is a step in the right direction, from where the conceptualisation of EL can be developed further.

Elasticity theory considers language as a piece of elastic (metaphor), which can be stretched to fit moment-to-moment communicative needs. How far and in which direction it stretches depend on the situation at the time of speaking. EL is defined as something whose interpretation can be 'stretched or shrunk according to the strategic needs of communication' (Zhang, 2013: 88). Such elastic use of language has been described as 'fluid, dynamic and multidimensional' (Parvaresh, 2018: 187). The theory is developed and tested based on the corpora of officer–passenger encounters in Australian customs, confirming that people stretch EL in different ways to accomplish different communicative goals. The success of EL communication rests on the co-construction of the pragmatic meanings among the interlocutors (Zhang, 2011: 573), which means that the stretching of EL needs to be understood by the listener to ensure both speaker and listener share the intended message through the use of EL.

At an earlier stage of the elasticity theory development, Zhang (2011: 578–579) proposed four maxims: go just-right ('provide the right amount of information'), go general ('speak in general terms'), go hypothetical ('speak in hypothetical terms') and go subjective ('speak in subjective terms'). Here, the 'go just-right' maxim is taken as an example. Suppose you are asked what time you are planning to attend a party, which will be held at 2 pm, and you reply with 'about 2 pm'. This should represent an appropriate answer, because the factor of traffic (among other things) may impact your arrival time. If you say '2:03 pm', it may sound odd, because in a casual context like this, time tends to be described as a round number. It is also likely that you cannot get there at 2:03 pm precisely, so choosing precise language is unnecessary and you may back yourself into a corner. Therefore, using a vague expression like *about 2 pm* provides the right amount of information and is better than using a precise expression.

The initial four maxims have been replaced by a main maxim and four specific maxims (Zhang, 2015). The following is the main maxim: stretch language elastically in discursive negotiations to achieve communicative goals. The four specific maxims are go approximate (elasticise in approximate form, exemplified by *about 10* and *quite a few*), go general (elasticise in general form, exemplified by *someone*, *things* and *things like that*), go scalar (elasticise in scalar form, exemplified by *most*, *extremely*, *some* and *a bit*) and go epistemic (elasticise in hypothetical and subjective form, exemplified by *may*, *probably* and *I guess*) (Zhang, 2015: 63). The updated maxim versions contain less overlap between maxims and are less general (e.g., the previous maxim of 'provide the right amount of information' is perhaps too general to implement in practice). While the four updated maxims are distinctive enough to be their own category, they are guidelines only, not rules.

Glinert (2010) presents an intriguing analysis based on his interview data in relation to cross-national political negotiations (China and USA) during the two Sino-American crises of 1999 and 2001. Glinert argues that elasticity led to peace in the end, meeting the face-saving requirements of both sides in the diplomatic face-off (2010: 61–62). He finds that it is useful to stretch the words, and the use of elastic expressions in Chinese–English translation 'stretched the "rubber band" between West and East cultures' and helped to reach a resolution (2010: 57–58). It shows that EL offers a link between people, languages and cultures. Based on institutional data (encounters between Australian customs officers and passengers), Zhang (2015) finds that EL can stretch between two ends of a continuum of polarities (soft and tough, firm and flexible, cooperative and competitive).

There are three principles in the elasticity theory: fluidity (a matter of degree, overlap and context-dependence), stretchability (stretching upwards, downwards and sideways to meet communicative needs) and strategy (serving strategic purposes). These three principles point to the typical feature of EL, that it is 'inherently, purposely, and strategically fluid and stretchable' (Zhang, 2015: 57). The three principles are complementary to each other: foundation (fluidity), means (stretchability) and ends (strategy; Zhang, 2015). Without the fluidity of EL, the other two (means and ends) would not be realised. EL should only be stretched to an appropriate level and should not be overdone. If stretched too far, it may lead to deception (Zhang and Sabet, 2016), which would be considered an inappropriate use of language.

Based on her data, Zhang (2015) generates four pragmatic forms and six pragmatic functions to represent the linguistic realisation and usage of EL. The four lexical categories are as follows: approximate stretcher, general stretcher, scalar stretcher and epistemic stretcher. The six pragmatic functions are just-right elastic, mitigating elastic, rapport elastic, intensifying elastic, self-protection elastic and evasive elastic. These classifications are used in this study for data analysis.

2.5 Healthcare Communication

The review of health communication in this section is conducted in the context of spoken, written and online healthcare discourses.

2.5.1 Spoken versus Written Discourse

Many studies on health communication have drawn on spoken data from day-to-day healthcare, as diagnosis and treatment, for example, usually involve conversational interactions. Various types of spoken discourse were examined, for example, doctor–patient conversations (Ainsworth-Vaughn, 1998; Heritage and Maynard, 2006a, 2006b; Peräkylä et al., 2008), nurse–patient interactions (Staples, 2015), phone calls in medical contexts (Fele, 2014; Heritage and Raymond, 2005; Zimmerman, 1992) and discussions about a severe health condition among family members (Beach, 2002). Many of the previous studies on medical discourse adopt conversation analysis; therefore, their findings reveal insights into the structure, organisation and construction of meaning in medical discourse. Some pioneering work on VL has appeared in studies of conversations that took place in clinical settings (e.g., Prince et al., 1982).

Compared with spoken medical discourse, written health discourse has received relatively less attention. Written health communication covers a wide range of genres. As Clerehan (2014: 216) observes, some are produced primarily for patients in general (e.g., dietary information, patient education brochures and consent forms), others are written mainly for disease-specific patients (e.g., medication information and patient decision aids), and still others are designed largely for another health provider, organisations or people who are not patients (e.g., prescriptions, sick notes and referral letters). Written health discourse serves functions that spoken medical discourse cannot fulfil, as the former creates a permanent record and may have an official status when issued by a hospital or signed by a physician. Among the issues that have received reasonable attention are the readability of written health documents (Crouch et al., 1990; Payne et al., 2000) and ways of evaluating the quality of such texts (Clerehan and Buchbinder, 2006; Clerehan et al., 2005, 2009). However, as Clerehan (2014: 215) points out, the focus of much research on written patient communication has been non-linguistic. By addressing EL in online written disease-specific health information, this study extends the line of language-based research into written health discourse.

2.5.2 Online Discourse

The Internet serves as a useful tool that promotes health information (Cocco et al., 2018; des Bordes, 2017; Fiksdal et al., 2014). Online health information can be represented in various modes and across media: text, speeches, images, graphics, audio and video (among others). Indeed, online health information has provided a rich source of data for health communication studies and has also created new ways of disseminating health information to the public beyond physical constraints. Among the various issues raised in such studies are aspects of the users, such as their sociodemographic background (e.g., gender; Haluza et al., 2017; Lumpkins et al., 2017), information behaviours (e.g., forwarding information or clicking likes; Yan et al., 2018), anxiety level, doctor–patient relationship (Lee and Zuercher, 2017; Zummo, 2015) and their trust or credibility perceptions of health information. How users react to aspects of information has also been investigated: mode (e.g., visual, auditory or both; Nguyen et al., 2018), message framing (Borah and Xiao, 2018), information-carrier-related factors (e.g., trustworthiness of information; Basnyat et al. 2018), online media and platforms (Corrales et al., 2018; Ruck et al., 2017; Strekalova and Krieger, 2017) and language features (e.g., technical versus non-technical). For example, Thon and Jucks (2017) revealed that while medical information seekers considered information provided by authors with medical credentials more reliable, technical-language use hindered the credibility of their health information. Paige et al. (2017) found that different sociodemographic groups differed in their perceptions of trustworthiness towards online health information from various sources and channels. For example, while African Americans with high eHealth literacy placed more trust in government and religious organisation sites, those with low eHealth literacy trusted information from YouTube and Twitter more.

Bennett and Glasgow (2009: 274) define Internet interventions as 'systematic treatment/prevention programs, usually addressing one or more determinants of health (frequent health behaviors), delivered largely via the Internet (although not necessarily exclusively web-based), and interfacing with an end user'. Such programs are designed to elicit information about the user's health situation and to provide tailor-made help and advice in response to the user's health problem (Ritterband, 2003). They are interactive and usually enhanced by graphics, animations and/or other audio-visual aids. An increasing number of studies have addressed Internet interventions aiming to promote good health or to change health behaviour (Han et al., 2017; Hennemann et al., 2017; Maertens et al., 2017). Studies dealing with Internet interventions offer valuable insights into the implementation of treatment or prevention programs that provide online support to patients.

What roles online communities play is also a significant area that has received attention, whether the communities mainly comprise health professionals or patients with similar health problems. Rising et al. (2017) call for collaboration among patients, clinicians and online community administrators to design online interventions that meet social support needs. Walther et al. (2018) suggest that consensus user-generated ratings by laypeople who are members of the online community significantly affect the evaluation of health advice. Willis and Royne (2017) reported that online communities consisting of laypeople with the same chronic disease contributed to educating advice seekers with the same health problem and positively changing their health behaviour. Beck et al. (2017) examined the extent to which task messages (information sharing, suggestions, opinions and asking questions) and relational messages (showing solidarity and friendliness) contributed to generating emotional support in the exchange of messages within such groups. Although relational messages seem pertinent to developing emotional support, task messages substantially facilitated the creation of such support when uncertainty experienced by patients with depression was alleviated by group members' provision of information (cf. Britt, 2017).

Also under scrutiny are topics concerning uncertainty management (Arribas-Ayllon et al., 2011; Zayts et al., 2016) and the communication challenges facing precision medicine (i.e., tailor-made treatment based on 'individual variability in genes, environment, and lifestyle for each person').[2] Rauscher (2017: 900) examined how individuals diagnosed with a genetic variant managed uncertainty related to health issues (e.g., genetic cancer risk) and found that 'experiencing an emotional reaction to one's genetic variant impacts information

[2] The definition of 'precision medicine' was retrieved from the site of National Institutes of Health at https://ghr.nlm.nih.gov/primer/precisionmedicine/definition (accessed on 16 September 2018).

seeking in different ways than one's emotional reaction to uncertainty discrepancy'. One implication is that genetic counsellors should pay attention to how patients feel and should help patients express their emotional responses and communicate those responses. Han et al. investigated how to communicate scientific uncertainty about public health threats and suggested the need 'to convey scientific uncertainty in a way that avoids the extremes of both overconfidence and underconfidence and that ensures thoughtful, deliberative decision-making' (2018: 443). In a study proposing the type of communication scholars can investigate as precision medicine develops, Scherr et al. (2017) suggested identifying effective ways for communicating risk information and expediting decision-making based on up-to-date information. As Scherr et al. (2017: 843) put it, 'conveying complex, and at times uncertain, scientific information while ensuring comprehension are challenges' facing communication scholars even in precision medicine.

Uncertainty has been a significant issue in health communication. Babrow et al. (1998) examined the meanings of uncertainty in the studies cast in three broad traditions. One covers individual-psychological models, which address uncertainty in relation to making clinical decisions, coping with illnesses and explaining causes for illness. The second one consists of linguistic and discourse analyses that focus on hedging devices used in doctor–patient conversations. The third adopts sociocultural and historical perspectives on uncertainty in illness, which attend to uncertainty management and/or recognise medical practices as characterised by uncertainty (Bursztajn et al., 1990). Babrow et al. (1998) synthesise the three traditions and propose a tentative typology of various meanings of uncertainty consisting of five types: complexity (e.g., contingency, multicausality and unpredictability), information qualities (e.g., regarding degrees of clarity or accuracy), probability, information structure (e.g., order of information) and lay epistemology. They call for a further development of their account to facilitate the good practice of health communication. We believe the examination of uncertainty in illness can be further advanced by closely analysing health-related texts, and, by doing so, we can discuss the issue in a relatively concrete manner. By analysing elastic terms in actual health communication discourse, the current study is also aimed at offering practical advice on effective communication in a culturally sensitive way.

It has been shown that specific patterns of language use in online or offline contexts may generate particular effects. For example, Samuelsson et al. (2014) demonstrated that, when interacting with patients with language impairments and helping improve their speech, language pathologists would do a better job if they implemented defusing practices (i.e., reducing any unwelcome discomfort and face threat) by using figurative language and collective pronouns (*we*), as well as referring to well-known phenomena rather than explicitly pointing out speech problems. Major (2018) explored the effect of gain- or loss-framing that organises stories about depression on audiences' support for health policies. The result showed that '[t]he loss frame stories seemed to spark the desire in individuals to engage in civic activities that could make a difference' (Major, 2018: 58). Sharkey et al. investigated how a protective stance was taken in an online group supporting young people who self-harm, and they found that using mitigation devices as face-work may 'help to build rapport, minimise imposition and stay online' (2012: 78). Pounds and De Pablos-Ortega (2015) analysed data from online medical consultations and suggested that expressions of empathy (e.g., *The hardship that you've had to face in recent times*) contributed to patient-centred communication. Crawford et al. (2018) showed that in nurse–patient conversations, when the nurse displayed empathy, the patient tended to elaborate on their concerns and, thus, developed rapport and trust. Based on video recordings of doctor–patient interactions, Bigi (2011) identified different persuasive strategies that physicians used to construct their professional ethos. For example, when the patient referred to an alternative medical opinion, the physician could cite an evidence-based opinion (e.g., *There are studies based on controlled trials showing that* . . . ; Bigi, 2011: 70).

The studies under review offer valuable insights into multifaceted health communication, particularly in the online environment. As a whole, health communication studies tend to address communication behaviours in diverse medical or health-related contexts (Thompson et al., 2011). Nuance of language is not their main concern. By contrast, another line of research into health communication addresses issues of language use and is situated within applied linguistics (Candlin and Candlin, 2003; Sarangi, 2004). As Jones (2013: 18) observes, applied linguistics offers the resources to understand 'how people make meanings around health and risk' and 'how people "do" health through daily embodied and discursive practice' (Paugh and Izquierdo, 2009: 188; as cited in Jones, 2013:18). An applied linguistic perspective puts language use at the centre of enquiries and is aimed at enriching our understanding of language structure and function and revealing how language use affects health communication. Hamilton and Chou (2014a) endorse this view and encourage theoretical and methodological diversity in the pursuit of achieving the goal of health by drawing on insights from research on the role of language in health communication (cf. Hamilton and Chou, 2014b).

Babrow and Mattson (2011) reappropriate Craig's (1999) account of communication theory in the context of health communication and state that studies of health communication emphasise different aspects and types of the identified tensions that characterise health communication. For example, the rhetorical tradition, which stresses the persuasive nature of discourse, is associated with scientific–humanistic tensions and uncertainty–value tensions because the rhetorical tradition regards efficacy of communication as significant and is keen to investigate how the target audience of a text may react to scientific knowledge (Kline, 2007; Segal, 2005). Among other traditions of communication theory are the cybernetic tradition (i.e., communication as information processing), the sociopsychological tradition (i.e., human behaviours expressing psychological traits), and the sociocultural tradition (i.e., communication made possible by shared systems of beliefs, values and language). Particularly pertinent to the current study is the tension between science and humanism and that between uncertainty and actual values. The scientific–humanistic tension is exemplified 'in debates about biomedical vs. biopsychological models, disease vs. illness, technique vs. meaning, conflicts about alternative therapies, and medical ethics' (Babrow and Mattson, 2011: 21). We suggest that scientific, accurate language versus vague/elastic language can be added to the list. The tension regarding uncertainty versus values (e.g., expectations) is intertwined with scientific and humanistic tension because the accurate communication of knowledge and uncertainty in illness inevitably co-exists in health communication (2011: 23). As Babrow and Mattson (2011: 24) put it, 'the meaning of uncertainty in general (i.e., in any of its particular forms) is profoundly dependent on the value at stake' (cf. Babrow et al., 1998). Specifically, our evaluation of what is significant, desirable, or valuable is subject to 'how we formulate uncertainty or make sense of what we know' (Babrow and Mattson, 2011: 24).

Building on the studies under review and taking them as a point of departure, the current study examines how EL is used in online health information concerning specific health conditions. By paying close attention to language use and examining how EL is perceived, it provides a detailed pragmatic account of such information and addresses the configuration of EL manifested in the datasets about these diseases.

2.6 Concluding Remarks

The above literature review provides the reader with a useful understanding of the background for this study. There will be strategic differences between writing a newspaper article and having a conversation with a friend, where the former does not have the opportunity to clarify things with the reader as the latter would have (Capone, 2018: 93). This study is based on written and online healthcare data that differs, therefore, from the existing findings, which are primarily based on spoken data. Whilst there has been growing interest in the use of vagueness in medical discourse, there is little research from cross-cultural perspectives, and this study is a step in filling the gap.

The four theoretical frameworks reviewed here are relevant to the conceptualisation of EL: pragmeme theory, integrative pragmatics, frame theory and elasticity theory. They are adopted as a guide through the research of EL in the present study. These four all focus on pragmatic meanings grounded in context and complement each other for the benefit of this study. Pragmeme theory states that a pragmeme refers to a situation or an act that captures the goal of the situation (e.g., online healthcare information dissemination). This study expects there to be regular patterns or protocols of EL use that are manifested in the pragmeme of delivering online health information using EL. The EL pragmeme can be realised in different situations, which can manifest, according to integrative pragmatics, in the pragmatic behaviours of online website writers and observers' evaluations. The two focuses highlighted in integrative pragmatics are empirical evidence and the importance of observers' participation (metapragmatics), both of which are adopted in this study. Frame theory helps guide the investigation of participants' perceptions of and attitudes towards the use of EL undertaken by this study. We look at how observers frame their reasons in terms of choosing EL or non-EL. Finally, the principles and classifications proposed in elasticity theory govern the data analysis performed in this study.

3 Methodology

This study investigates how EL is used and perceived. The research questions are addressed through the analysis of the corpus of medical information from professional websites (hospitals, government agencies and specialists) in Australia and Taiwan. There were two parts to data collection in this study: (1) the language used by the writers of the websites (focusing on the use of EL), and (2) the evaluation of the use of EL by the observers recruited for this study. The instruments for the latter were questionnaires and follow-up interviews. Particular EL co-occurs with particular context types, which amount to types of protocol or regularity and enable us to deploy quantitative as well as qualitative methodologies (Haugh and Culpeper, 2018: 230). A mixed-methods (i.e., quantitative and qualitative) approach was adopted in this study to provide an account of the use of EL in healthcare discourse.

3.1 Rationale of the Research Design

This study adheres to the principles of integrative pragmatics (Haugh and Culpeper, 2018), which state that both user and observer perspectives on pragmatic phenomena should be considered. There are two parties in meaning construction: writer and reader. We need to adopt an integrated approach combining both the user's and observer's views. This is consistent with what Kecskes (2010: 289) calls 'a holistic interpretation of utterance from both the perspective of the speaker and the perspective of the hearer', an approach which can provide a rich account of language and communication. While most studies have focused on speakers, the present study also considers observers' feedback to determine what they think about the use of EL.

This study is based on naturally occurring online data as well as metapragmatic data. The triangulation of data from different sources reduces the risk of being overly reliant on any single source (Patton, 1990). The choice of online health information is because the Internet has become a primary and popular source of health information and advice for the public (Walther et al., 2018). The common purposes for using the Internet are to improve knowledge of a medical condition and to reduce anxiety (Neelapala et al., 2008). Compared with reading pamphlets and other printed material containing medical information or going to see a doctor, many people find searching online more convenient, more accessible and less expensive (Westerman et al., 2012). It is important to know how online medical information is interpreted to ensure health information communicated to the public is effective.

Participant comments in this study were collected via questionnaires and follow-up interviews. A questionnaire is a common instrument to explore people's opinions of a certain phenomenon (Muijs, 2011). The advantage is cost effectiveness, namely the low cost of preparing and administering a survey that can be delivered to a large sample in a short period (Bryman, 2012; Muijs, 2011). The disadvantages include participants' limitations (e.g., under- or over-reporting; Bryman, 2012), potential social desirability bias and the possibility that the de-contextualised content might lead to superficial judgements (Layder, 2013). These concerns could be reduced by (1) ensuring the anonymity of participants (Krosnick and Presser, 2010) and (2) giving participants the opportunity to answer open-ended questions (Tseng and Zhang, 2020). Follow-up interviews enable participants to elaborate on their choices and provide further explanation.

The research questions for this study (see Section 1.2 for details) require that it adopts a combination of quantitative and qualitative methods to triangulate the data analysed for convergence or divergence (Jick, 1979; Tashakkori and Teddlie, 2009). This combination is an asset that could lend itself to a richer explanation of the phenomenon under study (Jick, 1979). The 'pluralistic approach' (Creswell, 2009: 10) aims to enhance the validity of the study and provide a more rigorous account of EL behaviours. This mixed-research method can explore, explain and incorporate the use of EL by maximising the best part of the quantitative (e.g., general patterns, typical frequency) and qualitative (e.g., detailed and contextual analysis, typical function) approaches (Creswell and Plano Clark, 2011: 73). Triangulating data can reveal trends as well as in-depth language use in context allowing the development of a multifaceted investigation.

This study uses written discourse because most studies of EL in healthcare communication focus on spoken interactions, such as phone-in medical services or hospital face-to-face encounters. Different modes of communication may require EL that belongs to one data set rather than the other. Adolphs et al. (2007) find that phone-in medical services attract more VL use than hospital chaplain–patient face-to-face interactions and speculate that this is an effect of the physical distance between the speakers. Contrary to dialogues, online medical communication in this study occurs through a written medium and without spoken interaction, which includes turn features, interruptions and overlap, false starts, and corrections (Uhlirovà, 1994). It is therefore important to study online medical information as a largely one-way form of written health communication, as it may differ from that in more dialogic health communication settings. It is useful to recognise the differences between various settings to disseminate online medical information effectively.

3.2 Data

For the current study, two online medical corpora were collected in Australia (English) and Taiwan (traditional Chinese) using websites, questionnaires and interviews. The in-depth interviews and discussions provided high-quality raw data (Patton, 1990), and the open-ended responses in the questionnaires captured nuances. This study is observer-focused and develops a 'data-informed understanding of patterns and contexts of language use' (Cheng and O'Keeffe, 2015: 376). Ethics approval from one researcher's institution and consent from participants were sought before the data were collected. Anonymity and privacy have been maintained throughout the research. The data-collection procedures used for both the Australian and Chinese context are comparable.

3.2.1 Websites

Websites were sought from professional medical bodies in Australia or Taiwan, primarily on 7 September 2017 and 14 March 2018. The websites provide health information to members of the public who are seeking reliable health information online. The official status of the websites ensures the authenticity of the data. The information is asynchronous and open for public access, which made data collection less problematic.

The websites were selected based on three criteria. (1) They were credible websites, belonging to three types of health institutions: professional medical bodies/foundations, government, private and public hospitals. (2) They communicated information about one of six diseases/ conditions: the common cold, influenza, pancreatic cancer, thyroid cancer, anxiety, and schizophrenia – which enable a comparison of data in terms of sensitivity and severity. (3) The content of the websites contained at least 1.8% EL, as this study focuses on the investigation of EL. Two examples were the English website of Cancer Council of Western Australia (https://www.cancerwa.asn.au) and Formosa Cancer Foundation in Taiwan (台灣癌症基金會 https://www.canceraway.org.tw).

For each website, only the main text was included in the corpora, excluding references and promotional information about specific hospitals or organisations, contact details and so on.

3.2.2 Respondents

There were altogether 1,057 participants in this study, 541 recruited in an Australian university in Perth and 516 in a Taiwanese university in Kaohsiung. Most participants were in their 20s and their first language was either English (Australia) or Mandarin Chinese (Taiwan). The students primarily studied humanities and health-science subjects.

There are associations between Internet searching and being of a younger age (Fox and Duggan, 2013; Russell and Ward, 2011). Therefore, young university students were selected for this study, as they are e-health literate and most likely use the Internet for medical information. They are representative of educated people in understanding such online information.

In this study, purposive sampling (Creswell, 2009) was used, particularly homogeneous case sampling (Morse, 2003; Patton, 1990). Purposive sampling is a form of non-probability sampling, also termed judgemental, selective, or subjective sampling. Researchers rely on their own judgement to produce a sample that can be logically assumed to be representative of the population. Homogenous sampling involves selecting similar groups or cases to investigate a phenomenon. In this study, researchers determined that young and educated university students were the most suited for the purpose of this research – that is, they were deemed savvy users of the Internet.

The procedure used to recruit participants involved the researchers asking their colleagues (lecturers) for permission to allow the research assistants to go to classrooms and talk to students either before or after class to encourage them to participate in the research questionnaire.

3.2.3 Questionnaire and Interview

The feedback from participants on the use of EL was investigated through questionnaires and interviews. The questionnaire was designed using Oppenheim's descriptive model to analyse respondents' perceptions and attitudes. This model 'is essentially fact-finding and descriptive – although the data collected are also often used to make predictions' (Oppenheim, 1992: 12). Questionnaires in Chinese or English were piloted in Perth (Australia) and Kaohsiung (Taiwan) with no need for revision. There were altogether 1,057 questionnaires and 202 interviews: 541 questionnaires and 112 interviews (approximately 17 hours of recordings) in English, and 516 questionnaires and 90 interviews (approximately 11 hours 30 minutes of recordings) in Chinese.

The content of the questionnaire consisted of both closed- and open-ended questions so that the participants could elaborate on their views, through which perceptions of and attitudes to the use of EL could be examined. Open-ended questions elicit 'the points of view' (Patton, 1990: 24) that may not be forthcoming from the pre-determined and closed-ended questions in a survey. The comments showed how successfully (or otherwise) online medical information was conveyed, particularly the public's capability of interpreting EL. In the questionnaire, there were six naturally occurring excerpts directly taken from the corpora of online medical information. Each of the six excerpts contained several elastic expressions, which were put in bold and underlined. Participants were asked two types of questions: (a) whether they had difficulty understanding the EL in the excerpt, and (b) whether they preferred EL or non-EL (multiple choices allowed). Participants were encouraged to comment on the choices made. What follows is an example of the excerpts taken from the questionnaires given to respondents (for a full version of the questionnaire, please see Appendix).

Excerpt: **Many** people today have ultrasounds and other scans for totally unrelated health issues, and those tests **sometimes** end up picking up **very** small thyroid nodules. Even if they turn out to be cancerous, **many** of these are **so** tiny and slow-growing that they **might** not ever cause problems during your lifetime.

a. Do you have difficulty understanding the paragraph presented above as a result of the underlined expressions?
   - □ Yes
   - □ No
b. Which of the following expressions do you prefer (multiple choices allowed)?
   - □ Many of these are so tiny and slow-growing that they **might** not ever cause problems during your lifetime.
   - □ Many of these are so tiny and slow-growing that they will never cause problems during your lifetime.

Please briefly explain why you prefer such expression/s:

As shown, each question has two options. For the Type B question, one choice was cited from the excerpt verbatim (the first one in this case), and the other was an invented sentence with a meaning that matched the original one, except that the first one used EL (*might*) and the second was changed to incorporate non-EL (*will*). For the six excerpts, we alternated the order of the two choices (with EL or non-EL) of Type B to minimise the potential bias of the ordering.

The criteria for selecting the excerpts were as follows. Each of the six excerpts contained three or more elastic expressions, which were bolded and underlined[1]. Each excerpt had to contain one or more types of the four categories of EL (see Section 2.2.3 for details), and the six excerpts altogether covered all four categories. Selecting these four types of EL provided a wide

[1] There was some different feedback from the participants on the formatting: some liked the highlighting of elastic expressions in the excerpt, but some felt the highlighting somehow made reading less smooth.

range of elastic expressions to ensure the excerpts were representative and to minimise the potential for bias in the EL types. Another criterion is that the excerpts needed to convey medical information about the following three general disease/condition categories and six specific diseases/conditions: common diseases (influenza and cold), cancer (thyroid cancer and pancreatic cancer) and mental health conditions (anxiety and schizophrenia).

Participants were involved in one or two stages of the study, the initial questionnaire (stage 1) and follow-up interview (stage 2); both were entirely voluntary. In English, all questionnaires and interviews were administrated by one person to minimise response bias (Lavrakas, 2008). The questionnaires were primarily distributed in classrooms towards the end of class. The administrator (research assistant) first explained the voluntary survey and encouraged students to ask questions to ensure that everyone was clear about what to do. Volunteers completed the questionnaires before they left the classroom. A small number of questionnaires were filled in after class and returned to the lecturers later. It took approximately 10 minutes to complete the questionnaire. The questionnaires were collected in person – not online – for reliability purposes. The Chinese questionnaire data collection followed a similar procedure to that of the English one.

The recruitment of participants for the interviews was conducted via the inclusion of a request in the questionnaire so that the volunteers could be contacted afterwards. On average, interviews were conducted for 8–9 minutes each. Some interviews were conducted right after the questionnaire session and others were conducted on a separate occasion, with chocolates being given as a token of appreciation. The follow-up interviews were audio-recorded and professionally transcribed. The participants were asked to comment on two aspects of the identified EL used in the six excerpts: (1) why they did or did not have a problem understanding the EL; and (2) why they preferred the use of EL/non-EL. Typical questions were 'why did you tick this . . . ?', and 'what do you mean by saying . . . ?'. Questions were asked in English or Chinese in accordance with the location.

3.3 Data Analysis

The overarching approach for the data analysis is data-driven, to identify tendencies in the corpora. This approach also enabled the researchers to reveal differences between Chinese and English data. The qualitative part of the study adopts frame analysis drawn from the data, which provides triangulation to validate the quantitative data (Bernard, 2011). The questionnaire and interview data were both analysed following Auerbach and Silverstein's (2003) procedure for identifying patterns and frames: (1) identify relevant reasons regarding why

EL was/was not problematic to understand or why EL was/was not preferred, (2) filter repeated reasons, and (3) group repeated reasons to form frames.

In terms of validity with respect to the coding in this study (be it in Chinese or English), two well-trained research assistants performed the initial coding, with ongoing discussions with the two authors to refine the coding for clarity and explicitness. The initial coding was checked by the authors, and in borderline cases, agreement was reached through discussions between members of the research team.

With the aim of responding to the four research questions set out in Section 1.2, the data analysis consisted of four parts: lexical analysis (website data), pragmatic function analysis (website data), frame analysis (questionnaire/interview data) and comparative analysis (Chinese and English data).

3.3.1 Lexical Level (Quantitative Analysis, Addressing Research Question 1)

The lexical items were identified for the investigation of Research Question 1 (What are the pragmatic forms and frequencies of EL?). The data revealed four categories of EL forms consisting of approximate stretcher, general stretcher, scalar stretcher and epidemic stretcher (Zhang, 2015). These are discussed in Section 2.4.1 in detail to establish the terms of reference for this study. Examples of these four categories selected from the data are listed in Table 3.1 and Table 3.2.

3.3.2 Pragmatic Level (Qualitative Analysis, Addressing Research Question 2)

This level of analysis concerns pragmatic functions, answering the second research question (How does EL perform its pragmatic functions?). The pragmatic function refers to phenomena pertaining to the area of communicative intentions, goals, and exterior circumstances of use (Vasilescu, 2016: 315). Elastic words were analysed in terms of their pragmatic functions, rather than merely their semantic meaning. This approach echoes the view of EL as a pragmatic phenomenon, instead of an inherent property of lexical items (Parvaresh and Tayebi, 2014; Parvaresh, 2018). The functions drawn on the data are listed in Table 3.3.

As Table 3.3 shows, the functions that were identified in the data of this study are situated firmly in the context of online health information. Eleven functions identified are further divided into two groupings: first-order and second-order. They operate on two different levels of signification. A first-order function (the first six) is enacted on the lexico-grammatical level as it is

Table 3.1 *Examples of elastic expressions in Chinese by category*

Category	Example
Approximate stretcher (vague quantity)	約/大約 ('about')、少許 ('a little')、少量 ('a little/a few')、少數 ('minority')、大多數 ('majority')、大多 ('most')、大量 ('many/much')、將近/近 ('close to')、幾(種) /數(個) ('several')、許多 ('many/much')、很多 ('many') 、一點/點 ('a bit/a little')、些/一些/些許/有些 ('some')、多 ('over')、少於 ('less than/fewer than')、不少 ('not a small number')、多於 ('more than')、部分 ('part of')、大部分/大部份('majority/a large part')、多半 ('most')、上 ('about/over')、以上 (over')、以下 ('under/less than')、左右 ('or so')、幾乎 ('almost')、近乎('nearly')、超過 ('over')、部份 ('part of')
General stretcher (less specific words with broad meaning)	General terms: 東西 ('thing') 、事情 ('matter/stuff/ thing')、某人 ('someone')、有人 ('someone')、有時 ('sometimes')、有的/某些/某 ('some')、某種 ('some sort')、或多或少/多多少少/多少 ('more or less')、其餘 ('the rest')、不等 ('somewhere between')、一段 ('a period/some time')
	General extenders: 等等 ('and so forth')、等 ('etc./and so on')、各種/各種各樣/各式各樣 ('all sorts of ')、種種 ('things like that')
Scalar stretcher (increase or decrease the strength of a claim)	通常 ('usually')、極 (extremely')、經常/常/時常/往往 ('often')、多 ('frequently')、相當 ('quite')、十分 ('extremely/very much')、極/極度 ('extremely')、少 ('rarely/ infrequently')、很 ('very')、更 ('more/ even')、遠遠/遠 ('far')、太 ('too') 、頗 ('rather')、過度 ('too')、大大/大幅 ('considerably')、這麼/那麼 ('so')、不少 ('not a little bit'), 輕微 ('a bit/slightly')、有點 ('a little bit/sort of')、一點 ('a little bit')、略 ('slightly')、少之又少 ('rarely').
Epistemic stretcher (hypothetical and subjective)	可能 ('may/possibly/possible')、似乎 ('seem')、好(發) ('most likely')、也許/或許 ('perhaps')、可望 ('can be expected')、(我)相信 ('I believe')、(我)覺得 ('I think') 、有機會 ('likely')、好像 ('seem like')、彷彿/看似/像似 ('look like')、不一定 ('may not/not necessarily')

signified mainly by the meaning of the elastic term. For example, *about 20* conveys an approximation. When one (or more) first-order functions are operationalised on the discourse level, it may enact a second-order function (the bottom five). This distinction shows the versatile nature of EL, functioning at both the lexico-grammatical level and higher-level/discourse signification.

Table 3.2 *Examples of elastic expressions in English by category*

Category	Example
Approximate stretcher	Many, a few, about 20, around 20, approximately 20, 10 or 20, 20 or so, nearly 20, almost 20, more than 20, less than 20, over 20, lots of, a lot of, a bit, a little bit, bit, loads, tons of, a great deal of, a number of, thousands, millions, like (5 months)
General stretcher	Some, something, someone, somewhere, sometimes, and stuff/things like that, thing, things, stuff, anything, or something, and all that, or whatever, all sorts of things, all that sort of thing, or anything, and the rest, (and) etc., and so on, and so forth
Scalar stretcher	Very, somewhat, few, much, more, too (good to be true), so, extremely, quite, often, frequently, rarely, pretty (good), too much, really, just, a fair bit
Epistemic stretcher	Possible, could, might, probably, sort of, could be, maybe, might be, kind of, I think, I guess, I suppose, I/we believe, likely, look like, seem, appear, perhaps, may

Table 3.3 *Pragmatic function categories of EL*

Function	Example (excerpts from our corpora)
	First-order function
1. Softening Soften the certainty of health information, with a self-protective and defensive tone.	'Anxiety disorders are thought to be caused by a combination of factors. Most anxious people are **probably** born with a genetic vulnerability to develop an anxiety disorder.'
2. Intensifying Intensify the degree of a medical phenomenon, an aspect of health information or the strength of a health claim.	'Nothing helps with schizophrenia **more than** uninterrupted, long-term treatment.'
3. Deintensifying Lessen the degree or extent of a medical phenomenon, such as a symptom, severity.	'Schizophrenia can appear to be **somewhat** different in different people.'
4. Approximating Make the quantitative health information containing a specific number more flexible.	'In Australia, it is thought that **around** 14% of adults are affected by the condition every year.'
5. Avoiding Using general terms to avoid the mention of specific and complex technical health information, unnecessary information, sensitive and undesirable topics, or items with different interpretations.	'People with anxiety disorders may be unable to stop worrying about seemingly unimportant **things**.'
6. Shortening Highlight exemplary health items from a long list.	'Surgery is particularly advantageous in younger patients, those with eye disease, those with suspicion for cancer, those with large glands with pressure symptoms (difficulty in breathing, swallowing, **etc**.), or in whom medical management is difficult or not tolerated.'

Table 3.3 (*cont.*)

Function	Example (excerpts from our corpora)
	Second-order function
7. Tendency Describe a common clinical scenario or a medical tendency using EL without involving any specific number. This type presents factual information, no added tones such as a defensive tone.	'Treatment for thyroid cancer **usually** includes surgery, thyroid hormone replacement therapy and radioactive iodine treatment. Some people also need external radiotherapy or chemotherapy.'
8. Reporting Report others' medical findings, evidence-based research.	'**Some** studies have suggested that people with schizophrenia develop enlarged ventricles, natural connected spaces in between the folds of the brain that carry cerebral spinal fluid, but this finding is not present in all people with schizophrenia.'
9. Correcting Assist in introducing a common medical misconception that is to be dismissed.	'The term "common cold" refers to a set of symptoms, rather than a specific disease. Mild influenza may have similar symptoms to the common cold. Mild "strep throat", which is caused by bacteria, **may** be incorrectly classified as a common cold, though usually it is easy for a doctor to distinguish between the two.'
10. Advising gently Make the delivery of health advice less strict.	'You **might** feel overwhelmed, scared, anxious or upset if you have been diagnosed with cancer – these are all normal feelings. It's **very** important to have support from family, friends, health professionals or other services to help you cope with cancer.'
11. Supporting emotionally This function is to provide emotional support to the patients using EL.	'If thyroid cancer is suspected, your doctor may order a number of tests. The tests you may have depend on your specific situation. Waiting for the test results can be a stressful time. It **may** help to talk to a friend, family member or health professional.'

3.3.3 *Perceptions and Attitudes of the Participants (Qualitative Analysis, Addressing Research Question 3)*

This level of data analysis answers the third research question of this study: 'Are there any protocols concerning EL use? If there are, what are they?' The instruments used here to determine the participants' perceptions of and attitudes towards the use of ES were questionnaires and interviews.

The Chinese data produced the following frames: communication frame (clear, fluent, effective and others), folk–idiosyncratic frame, trust–scepticism frame, voluntary–involuntary frame, lay–professional frame and the difference–indifference frame (see Section 7.2 for more details on frames in the Chinese data). Based on the English data, three groupings of frames were identified: language-focused, language-user-focused and disease-focused. There is a total of 12 frames in the English corpus, and seven frames are similar to that of the Chinese data (see Section 8.2.2 for more details on frames in the English data).

3.3.4 Comparison of the Above Three Analyses (Qualitative Analysis, Addressing Research Question 4)

The final research question is 'What are the impacts of contexts on the use of EL?'. The contexts here refer to the different languages and different medical conditions. Through comparing the findings in relation to the abovementioned three research questions, the similarities and differences among different diseases and languages can be revealed. Underpinning sociocultural factors are also discussed. For example, Australians, who are commonly perceived as more overt than Taiwanese, may use EL less often and may possess less favourable attitudes towards EL.

3.4 Concluding Remarks

The methodology used in this study is data-driven and evidence-based. This approach strengthens the credibility of findings drawn out of the two corpora in Chinese and English. Most medical discourse studies focus primarily on spoken data, but this study focuses on written data, and the online data is the first written corpus of its kind. New findings regarding shared and culture-specific features of EL shed light on how and why language users stretch their words to increase the efficiency of health communication. This study not only contributes to the conceptualisation of EL in healthcare discourse but also offers methodological insights into cross-cultural research on health communication.

One of the goals of this study is to identify solutions to communication breakdowns between health professionals and the public. This study can help people better understand each other and interact more effectively to reduce miscommunication. By examining pragmatic variations in the use of EL, we can develop strategies for improving communication in healthcare discourse. The findings also benefit the public by showing healthcare professionals how medical information may best be communicated through EL. The new insights and resources may also inform policymaking by highlighting EL use as an important skill for healthcare professionals.

4 Elastic Language Used in Chinese

The Chinese corpus comprises 249,037 characters. It consists of six sub-corpora: anxiety (46,058, 18.49%), schizophrenia (44,737, 17.96%), cold (41,249, 16.56%), flu (40,531, 16.28%), thyroid cancer (38,923, 15.63%), and pancreatic cancer (37,539, 15.07%).

This chapter first introduces the forms of EL in the Chinese data. Then, we identify a range of functions served by EL, followed by a discussion of the frequency distribution of each category of EL. We also investigate whether correlations exist between the four categories of EL and specific health conditions.

4.1 Pragmatic Forms of Elastic Language

VL in Chinese has received increasing attention (see R. H. Zhang, 2010 for a review). Nevertheless, little research into Chinese VL in the health context has been conducted (Tseng and Zhang, 2018, 2020). Zhang and Feng (2013) provided a classification of six categories of VL using Mandarin conversational data: approximator and vague quantifier (e.g., *san, siqian* 三、四千 'three or four thousand', *zuoyiou* 左右 'about'), possibility and plausibility indicator (Jucker et al., 2003; e.g., *keneng* 可能 'may/ possibly'), vague category identifier (e.g., *(shucai a) shenmede* [蔬菜呀)什麼的 '(vegetables or) whatever'), intensifier (e.g., *hen* 很 'very'), deintensifier (e.g., *youdian* 有點 'a bit') and subjectiviser (e.g., *wuojuede* 我覺得 'I think') – the last of these is similar to what Prince et al. (1982) called *shield*. The classification was developed by Zhang (2015), whose more concise reclassification is adopted as it is well suited to the data collected for this study. However, we observed that written health information does not use some of the common vague expressions in conversational data, e.g., *shenmede* (什麼的 'whatever') and *wanyi* (玩意 'stuff').

Approximate stretchers (AQ) consist of approximators and quantifiers (cf. Channel, 1994; Ruzaitė, 2007). Approximators in Chinese include *(da)yue* ([大]約 'about'), *shang* (上 'about/over') and *shaoyu* (少於 'less than'), all of which are followed by a rough number; and *yishang* (以上 'over') and *yixia* (以下 'under/less than'), both of which follow a number. Elastic quantifiers in

Chinese include *xuduo* (許多 'many/much'), *duo* (多 'many/much'), *yixie* (一些 'some') and *ji* (幾 'several') and *yidian* (一點 'a little').

General stretchers (GE) are expressions with general, non-specific meaning and consist of two subcategories: (1) general terms referring to things, people and time; and (2) general extenders. In our Chinese data, we pay special attention to general expressions such as *dongxi* (東西 'thing'), *shiqing* (事情 'matter/stuff/thing') and to those with *mou* (某) or *you* (有) in the initial position of the general expression, both of which are similar to the qualitative 'some' (e.g., *mouren* 某人 'someone', *mouxie* 某些 qualitative 'some', *youren* 有人 'someone', *youshi* 有時 'sometimes' and *youde* 有的 qualitative 'some').[1] General extenders elicit a loose category without providing an exhaustive list of items (Channel, 1994; Overstreet, 1999; Overstreet and Yule, 1997). The forms and functions of general extenders in English have received increasing attention, as some of them (e.g., *and stuff like that*) are regarded as pragmatic markers in spoken interaction (Aijmer, 2015; Overstreet, 2014; Parvaresh et al., 2012). However, general extenders in Chinese have not extensively been discussed. Hsieh (2019) investigated the Chinese general extender *zhelei(de)* (這類的 'of that kind') based on spoken and written corpora of Chinese and found there were differences in the form and function of the extender between the spoken and written data. Based on our Chinese data, general extenders include *deng* (等 'etc./and so on'), *dengdeng* (等等 'and so forth') and *gezhong* (各種 'all sorts of').

Scalar stretchers (SC) tone up or down the force of an utterance in terms of the scale, strength or extent of a feature or an action. The term 'boosters' is often used to refer to intensifiers that scale up the degree (Quirk et al., 1985: 445). Chinese high-end scalar stretchers, that is, those that scale the degree upwards, include *ji* (極 'extremely'), *hen* (很 'very'), *chang* (常 'often'), *tongchang* (通常 'usually'), *duo* (多 'frequently') and *geng* (更 'more'). By contrast, low-end scalar stretchers scale the degree downwards, e.g., *shao* (少 'rarely/infrequently') and *qingwei* (輕微 'slightly'). Lim and Hong (2012: 18) point out that several Chinese intensifiers are significantly correlated with specific genres; one example is *hen*, which occurs much more frequently in press editorials than in press reports. As editorials are a genre characterised by the writer's view and evaluation, *hen* contributes to providing expression or opinion and, therefore, it is used more frequently in editorials than in news reports, which are more oriented towards events than personal views. This reinforces the theory that the intensifier is a resource for expressing attitude, that is, 'the feelings and values that are negotiated with readers' (Martin and Rose, 2003: 17).

[1] According to Tsai (2003), *you* (有) in Chinese forms an existential construction, and, in syntactic terms, it has three different properties: presentational *you* (e.g., *youren* 有人 'someone'), partitive *you* (e.g., *yude ren* 有的人 'some of the people') and specific plural *you* (e.g., *youxie ren* 有些人 'some people'). However, in discourse-pragmatic terms, an expression starting with *you* can be a general stretcher (e.g., *youren* 有人 'someone'; *yude* 有的 qualitative 'some'), an approximate stretcher (*youxie* 有些 quantitative 'some'), an epistemic stretcher when followed by *keneng* (可能 'may/possibly'), or a scalar stretcher (e.g., *youdian* 有點 'a bit').

Epistemic stretchers (EP) concern the speaker's evaluation of and attitude towards the statement being made in terms of possibility. Epistemic stance markers are employed 'to present speaker comments on the status of information in a proposition' (Biber et al., 1999: 972). In Chinese, epistemic stretchers, used to hedge or mitigate statements, include *keneng* (可能 'likely/ possibly/may'), *sihu* (似乎 'seem'), *(wo)xiangxin* ([我]相信 'I believe'), *wojuede* (我覺得 'I think'), *huoxu* (或許 'perhaps') and *haoxiang* (好像 'seem like'). Focusing on how *wojuede* ('I think') was used in eight telephone conversations between native speakers of Chinese, Lim (2011: 296) argues that the epistemic expression may express not only the speaker's subjective stance but also 'possible next-turn objections from the recipient', a highly intersubjective phenomenon.

Figure 4.1 demonstrates the top 10 stretchers in the Chinese corpus. As can be seen, they cover the four categories. The most used elastic expression is the general stretcher *deng* (等 'and so on'), a result that is somewhat surprising as it is expected that health information is explicit without too much 'assumed' information (see Section 4.3.2 for further discussion). The second EL item is the epistemic stretcher *keneng* (可能 'likely/possibly/may'), the only stretcher of its kind on the top-10 list. All the other stretchers on the list (Figure 4.1) are scalar (e.g., *chang* 常 'often', *hen* 很 'very', *duo* 多 'frequently/much', *geng* 更 'more' and *tongchang* 通常 'usually') and approximate (e.g., *yue* 約 'about', *duo* 多 'many/much/over' and *xuduo* 許多 'many/ much').[2] As this chapter unfolds, the significance of the

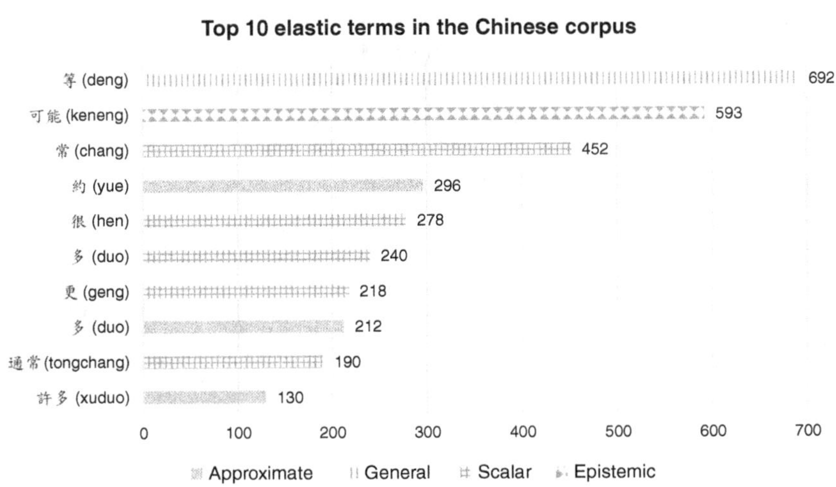

Figure 4.1 Top 10 elastic terms in the Chinese corpus

[2] When *duo* (多) is an adjective, it is treated as an approximate stretcher expressing quantity. When used as an adverb, it is regarded as a scalar stretcher. See Sections 4.3.1 and 4.3.3 for further discussion.

stretchers on the top-10 list is further illustrated with examples from health information, and other stretchers beyond the list are also introduced. We turn next to the functions of EL in the health context.

4.2 Pragmatic Functions of Elastic Language

Some studies investigating Chinese VL point out the pragmatic functions of fuzzy language, either in everyday or online contexts – that is, to increase communication efficiency (due to the right amount of information and less processing time), and to enhance interpersonal relationships (e.g., politeness; Wang, 2003; Zhou and Zhang, 2018). Nevertheless, these functions are rather general and seem to apply to VL irrespective of the context. In this study, we situate the use of EL firmly in the context of online health information. By adopting a data-driven approach, we identify eleven functions of EL in the Chinese corpus, which are further divided into two groupings as they operate on two different levels of signification: first- and second-order. A first-order function is enacted on the lexico-grammatical level as it is mainly signified by the meaning of the elastic term. For example, a high-end scalar (e.g., *hen* 很 'very') intensifies the quality that it modifies whilst a low-end scalar (e.g., *youdian* 有點 'a bit') deintensifies a feature placed after it. A first-order function, when operationalised on the discourse level and/or combined with another first-order function in a specific health context, may enact a second-order function. In the following functional account of EL, the first six functions are first-order (see Sections 4.2.1–4.2.6), while the seventh to the eleventh functions are second-order (see Sections 4.2.7–4.2.11). This distinction is useful in that it informs us of how the functions of EL on the lexico-grammatical level are re-utilised in the higher-level signification (i.e., in the context of online health communication). Each of the functions is illustrated below with several examples.

4.2.1 Softening

The first function of EL is to soften a statement. It is typically performed through the use of one or more epistemic stretchers as Excerpts 4.1–4.3 show. Such stretchers cover *keneng* (可能 'likely/ probably/may'), *sihu* (似乎 'seem'), *yexu* (也許 'maybe'), *huoxu* (或許 'perhaps'), *fangfu* (彷彿 'look like'), *haoxiang* (好像 'seem like'), *buyiding* (不一定 'may not/not necessarily') and *kewang* (可望 'can be expected'). By making the given information not absolutely certain, these stretchers allow health professionals to provide useful health information without having to make a full commitment to it, as is the case with epistemic modality (cf. Palmer, 1986: 51). However, in health contexts, this is not necessarily motivated by health professionals' lack of medical knowledge but, rather, by their knowledge that patients vary in their symptoms (e.g., 4.1) and that a medical issue is not always a black-and-white matter (e.g., 4.3). The use of an epistemic stretcher may also be due to the consideration of expressing a view without making it sound like a strong imposition (e.g., 4.2).

4.1 患者可能伴隨下列症狀:容易疲倦、靜不下來、難保持專心、肌肉緊繃、易怒或睡眠障礙等。

'Patients **may** have the following symptoms: constant fatigue, inability to calm down, difficulty in maintaining concentration, muscle tightness, irritability, sleep disturbance, etc.'
(www.kmuh.org.tw/www/kmcj/data/9608/7.htm)[3]

4.2 當我們努力推動「憂鬱症防治」時， 似乎不應忘了同樣重要的「焦慮疾患」。

'When we work hard to promote 'depression prevention', it **seems** that we should not forget the equally important "anxiety disorders".'
(www1.cgmh.org.tw/intr/intr2/c3360/E_LCY(anxiety).htm)

4.3 免疫功能就像我們的國防武力一樣, 主要的功能是防範外界一些細菌或病毒入侵, 維持身體的完整。但問題是外來的東西不一定是不好的[...]。

'The function of the immune system is like that of national defence: to prevent the invasion by some bacteria or viruses from the outside world and to maintain the integrity of the body. But the problem is that things from the outside are **not necessarily** bad [...].'
(www.kmuh.org.tw/www/kmcj/images/10404/page/p07.htm)

4.2.2 *Intensifying*

The second function of EL is to intensify aspects of health information, for example, the safety and effectiveness of medicine, prospect of prognosis and results of comparisons. As the highlighted elastic terms in Excerpts 4.4–4.6 demonstrate, this function is fulfilled by high-end scalar stretchers that maximise or tone up the extent or scale of a phenomenon (cf. Zhang, 2015: 97–98). They are typically placed before an adjective, which often has a positive or negative valence. Such elastic terms highlight the features of the health information being delivered, thereby accentuating the intensified aspects of that information. For example, *hen* (很 'very'), *ji* (極 'extremely'), *xiangdang* (相當 'quite'), *geng* (更 'more'), *yuan* (遠 'far') and *tai* (太 'too') may intensify a positive or negative feature. Other high-end stretchers such as *guo* (過 'over') and *guodu* (過度 'too') tend to

[3] We have made every effort to ensure that the websites from which the cited excerpts were taken are available at the copy-editing stage. Nevertheless, websites are constantly updated, and some online information, which was available at the time of writing this book, may subsequently have been changed or even removed. This is beyond our control.

collocate with certain adjectives that express undesirable features, for example, *guo pang* 過胖 'overfat/obese', *guo zhong* 過重 'overweight', and *guodu jiaolü* 過度焦慮 'too anxious'. Whether heightening a positive or negative property, they contribute to amplifying the degree of the feature being described.

4.4 一般而言, [減少粘膜血管充血藥]雖然都算是安全性相當高的藥物, 不會有特別的副作用[. . .]。

'Generally speaking, although [medicines for reducing mucosal vascular congestion] are considered to be **quite** safe and do not have particular side effects [. . .].'
(www.sinlau.org.tw/mode05_02.asp?num=20100129143959)

4.5 胰臟癌已邁入國人十大癌症死因之列, 但因早期診斷不易, 以致胰臟癌的預後仍然很差。

'Pancreatic cancer has become one of the top ten causes of cancer death in the country, but the prognosis of the cancer is still **very** poor due to the difficulty of early diagnosis.'
(https://dept.edah.org.tw/gi/commond10.php)

4.6 要扮演多重角色, 且責任心強、追求完美的女性尤其容易比男性更會操心, 承受更大的壓力, 往往變得身心俱疲。不論國外或台灣的臨床報告都發現, 焦慮或憂鬱症女性患者都遠高於男性。

'Women who have to play multiple roles, have a strong sense of responsibility and pursue perfection are especially prone to worry **more** and withstand pressure **more** than men, thus often becoming physically and mentally exhausted. Both foreign and Taiwanese clinical reports have found that there are **far** more women with anxiety disorders or depression than men.'
(www.commonhealth.com.tw/article/62208)

4.2.3 Deintensifying

In contrast to the second function, the third function of EL is to deintensify, or to lessen, the perception of the scope or extent of a medical phenomenon being described. As Excerpts 4.7–4.9 show, this function is served by lower-end scalar stretchers that tone down the degree of a common feature being introduced (cf. Zhang, 2015: 98), for example, *shaowei* (稍微 'slightly'), *qingwei* (輕微 'a bit') and *youdian* (有點 'a little bit/sort of'). The function of deintensifying aligns with the function of mitigation served by VL. As Zhang (2019: 79) argues, *youdian* (有點) and *youyidian* (有一點) are pragmatic markers in verbal interactions and can serve different purposes in different contexts as they are 'used less for information provision and more for maintaining interpersonal relationships'. In the health context, the function of deintensifying assists in alerting the reader to the results of medical or clinical comparisons or contrasts in a less alarming manner. When referring to a negative or undesirable aspect of a health phenomenon (e.g., in Excerpt 4.8, a group more at a risk of a type of schizophrenia), the function of deintensifying is useful as its presence creates less of a panic than the mention of the risk, without toning it down.

4.7 良性腫瘤比較軟，平滑且有點彈性，然而堅硬不平滑的腫塊則要考慮癌症的可能。

'A benign tumour is soft, smooth and a **bit** elastic, but for a hard and unsmooth lump, the possibility of cancer will need to be considered.'
(www.canceraway.org.tw/page.asp?IDno=2167)

4.8 情感性思覺失調症女性稍微比男性多, 尤其是婚後的女性[...]。

'There are **slightly** more women with schizoaffective disorder than men, especially married women [...].'
(https://bit.ly/3JfziNE)

4.9 **大部份**的時候，喝完薑湯稍微流汗，發燒惡寒、鼻水滴不停的狀況就會好一點[...]。

'**Most** of the time, after having a ginger drink, you will sweat **slightly** and your fever and chills and runny nose will ease **a little bit** [...].'
(www.sinlau.org.tw/01_news_page.asp?num=20160729093857)

4.2.4 Approximating

The fourth function, approximating, contributes the element of quantity or quantification to health information as it is typically identified by the use of an approximate term with or without a number, as Excerpts 4.10–4.11 indicate. Approximate stretchers not followed by a number include, for example, *henduo* (很多 'many'), *bufen* (部份 'part of'), and *youxie* (有些 'some'). The approximate stretchers that co-occur with a number comprise *yue* (約 'about'), *dayue* (大約 'about'), *chaoguo* (超過 'more than'), *yishang* (以上 'over'), *yixia* (以下 'under/less than') and *zuoyou* (左右 'or so'). *Duo* (多) is sometimes preceded by a rough number (e.g., *yibai duo zhong* 100 多種 'over 100 types'). The function of using these stretchers exemplifies the tension between professional medical research and laypeople's expectation of accessible health information, as a number rounded up or down is presumably based on research, and the approximate stretcher used without the number is commonly used in everyday contexts. Although the sources of statistics are not normally given in online health information and the figures are not precise, the given numbers nevertheless offer a clearer picture of the health information being conveyed than would otherwise be the case. For example, in Excerpt 4.11, were the phrase *can be as high as over 90%* to be replaced by *can be high*, the message would be less clear. In reliable health information, the number that goes with an approximate stretcher is presumably cited from research based on clinical data, thus rendering the given health information credible. Quantification is based on data and samples, which vary in size, and as Potter et al. (1991: 333) put it, 'a range of calculation, fractionation, aggregation and presentational practices can be selectively drawn on to form the scaffolding of contrasting versions'. Yet in certain situations (e.g., survival and death rates), health seekers need quantification in order to make a medical decision.

4.10 廣泛性焦慮症的一年盛行率約為 3%, 而終身盛行率約為 5%, 在焦慮症門診, 大約 12%患者屬於廣泛焦慮症疾患。

'The one-year prevalence rate of generalized anxiety disorder is **about** 3%, and the lifetime prevalence rate is **about** 5%. In the anxiety clinic, **about** 12% of patients suffer from generalized anxiety disorder.'
(www1.cgmh.org.tw/intr/intr2/c3360/E_HsuSJ.htm)

4.11 大部分的甲狀腺癌病人, 經由手術及放射性碘治療的預後都很好, 十年存活率可達 90%以上。如果罹患時的年齡在 45 歲以下, 那麼預後會更好 [...]。

'**Most** patients with thyroid cancer have a **very** good prognosis after surgery and radioactive iodine treatment, with a 10-year survival rate of **more than** 90%. If the age at the time when one has the cancer is **under** 45, the prognosis will be **even** better [...].'
(https://public.mch.org.tw/index.php?action=publications_edm_in&id=1916)

4.2.5 Avoiding

The fifth function of EL is to avoid mentioning sensitive or complicated information. The function is typically fulfilled by using such general terms as *mouxie* (某些 'some'), *mouzhong* (某種 'some sort') and *youren* (有人 'someone'), especially when the information to be given is negative, harmful, undesirable or doubtful, as Excerpts 4.12–4.15 show. The use of these stretchers in the health context differs from their use in non-health contexts. For example, in political contexts, when using *youren*, the speaker, though possibly having a specific person in mind, does not want to name the person in order to avoid any confrontation or controversy. In other words, VL enables the speaker to observe politeness and/or self-protection by reducing tension (Trappes-Lomax, 2007). By contrast, in the health context, the motivation for using it is not so much a question of politeness but relates more to the undesirability of the topic or to the unnecessary mention of the person. Furthermore, in the Chinese corpus, when *mouzhong* or *mouxie* ('some') is used, one or two items which the general terms cover are sometimes offered (e.g.,

Excerpts 4.12 and 4.13). This a somewhat paradoxical phenomenon – the use of a general stretcher serving the function of avoiding negative information being followed by an example – exists because the nature of the health information requires the writer to explain, not evade, information useful to the public unless no mention of any example does not hinder communication (e.g., 4.14). Excerpt 4.15 is interesting in that, although it purports to report a view widely held by Western scientists, *mouxie* collocates with the ingredients in chicken soup. The use of the stretcher casts the introduced view in doubt, and this is reinforced by citing a view from a Taiwanese professor of medicine, who is not convinced that chicken soup has a healing effect on people with a cold.

4.12 畏懼症患者會出現對某種物體或情境的害怕(例如怕蜘蛛、怕坐電梯) [. . .]。

'People with phobias are afraid of **some sort** of object or situation (for example, fear of spiders, fear of riding in elevators) [. . .].'
(https://health99.hpa.gov.tw/material/3231)

4.13 某些牽涉到性、猥褻、自殺、傷人等等令人不悅的強迫意念, 即使沒有引發強迫行為, 但如已造成強烈痛苦, 也算是強迫症。

'If **some** unpleasant compulsive thoughts involving sex, indecency, suicide, wounding and so forth, have generated intensive distress, they are considered to indicate obsessive-compulsive disorder even if they do not trigger compulsive behaviour,.'
(https://health99.hpa.gov.tw/material/3231)

4.14 當家族中有人患有髓質癌(MTC)時 (不管有沒有帶有 MEN 2), 做基因篩檢是必須的[. . .]。

'When **someone** in the family has medullary carcinoma (MTC) (with or without MEN 2), doing a genetic screening is necessary [. . .].'
(https://kelwww.cgmh-mi.com/examnm/exampet/petthyroid)

4.15 西方科學家認為雞湯中某些成分可以抑制中性白血球活動, 幫助身體免疫系統對發炎產生反應, 但黃立民認為, 還需要更多研究證實此論點。

'Western scientists believe that **some** ingredients in chicken soup can curb the activity of neutrophils [a type of white blood cell] and help the body's immune system respond to inflammation, but [Dr.] Limin Huang believes more research is needed to confirm this claim.'
(www.commonhealth.com.tw/article/62597?from=search)

4.2.6 *Shortening*

The sixth function involves the use of general extenders such as *gezhong* (各種 'all sorts'), *zhongzhong* (種種 'things like that'), *deng* (等 'etc.') and *dengdeng* (等等

'and so forth') in order to shorten a list of items related to a health issue. Each of these stretchers co-occurs with a list of one or more items. As Excerpts 4.16–4.18 demonstrate, they are a useful means of making manageable a potential long list of symptoms, complications, prevention methods or virus types, as these stretchers are used to conveniently introduce a list and yet do not require it be exhaustive. As such, they make it possible for the health professional to offer several representative items without having to produce a potentially long list, a factor that contributes to achieving conciseness in communication (cf. Grice, 1975).

4.16 A型流感病毒區分成各種亞型,到目前為止,一共發現了15種HA與9種NA。人類身上所分離出的病毒株以H1、H2、H3與N1、N2為主。

'Type A influenza viruses are divided into **all sorts** of subtypes. So far, 15 subtypes of HA and 9 subtypes of NA have been identified. The virus strains isolated from humans are mainly H1, H2, H3 and N1, N2.' (https://bit.ly/3JfD75s)

4.17 面對焦慮症最好的預防與治療方式是「充足的睡眠、適當且持續的運動、經常深呼吸練習放鬆、良好的壓力管理、足夠的人際支持與情緒宣洩」, 上述種種說來容易做來難[...]。

'The best ways to prevent and treat anxiety disorders are "enough sleep, proper and regular exercise, constant practice of deep breathing to relax, good stress management and adequate interpersonal support and emotional release". **Things like that** are easier said than done.' (www.smh.org.tw/mag1/44/44windows.htm)

4.18 流感的症狀多為突發性的,包括高燒、畏寒、頭痛、肌肉疼痛、乾咳等等,至於咽喉炎、鼻炎等普通感冒(common cold)常見的症狀則很少見。

'The symptoms of flu are **often** sudden outbursts, including high fever, chills, headaches, muscle pains, a dry cough **and so forth**. The common cold symptoms, e.g., pharyngitis, rhinitis etc. are very rarely found [among patients of flu].' (https://bit.ly/3jed0kI)

4.2.7 Describing Tendency

The seventh function of EL is to describe a medical tendency. This function may be regarded as an inherent function of EL, especially when elastic terms are combined, as health information for the public inevitably describes common, known health situations or conditions, that is, what has happened in clinical scenarios and in medicine. Unlike the first to sixth functions, which are fulfilled by specific types of EL, the function of describing tendency can be performed by all four categories of stretchers: approximate (e.g., *henduo* 很多 'many'; *bufeng* 部份 'part of'; *youxie* 有些 'some'), general (*youshi* 有時 'sometimes'), scalar (*chang* 常 'often'; *hao(fa)* 好(發) 'most likely (to happen)/mostly'; *duo* 多

'frequently/much') and epistemic (*keneng* 可能 'may/possibly'). Although this function can be served by one elastic expression (e.g., 4.20), it is often the case that the co-use of more than one elastic term in the same sentence contributes to describing a medical tendency, as 4.19 and 4.21–4.23 show.

4.19 大部分胰臟癌長在體部或尾部的病患，發現時大多很晚期，已無法進行手術切除。

'**Most** patients whose pancreatic cancer grows on the body or tail of the pancreas are **mostly** found at a **very** late stage, and it cannot be surgically removed.' (http://web.tccf.org.tw/lib/project/books/book02.php)

4.20 流感除了會引起厲害的全身性不適症狀外，有時會引起併發症，甚至導致死亡。

'In addition to causing severe systemic symptoms, flu **sometimes** causes complications and even death.'
(www.cdc.gov.tw/Bulletin/Detail/I0ZrKHkxewPfCOSVOyHRqg?typeid=9)

4.21 當然每種水果的涼性不同，所產生的影響也不一樣，有些吃完可能微咳，有些就會劇烈的咳嗽。

'Of course, the cooling properties of each fruit are different, and each creates a different effect. **Some may** cause one to cough **slightly** after eating, and **some** cause severe coughing.'
(www.tcm.tw/articleview.php?id=2589)

4.22 談到精神分裂症，可能很多人仍覺得陌生、不相關、或是害怕，典型的印象多半認為患者外觀看起來就不正常，會有幻覺、妄想，行為混亂衝動，最常被形容為不定時炸彈[...]。

'When it comes to schizophrenia, **many** people **may** still find it unfamiliar, irrelevant or frightening. **Most** people have the typical impression that the patient looks abnormal in appearance, has hallucinations and delusions and behaves impulsively; the patient is most **often** described as a 'walking time bomb' [...].'
(https://health.ntuh.gov.tw/health/new/6023.htm)

4.23 [感冒]任何季節都可能發生，但好發於秋季至初春。治療方式多以舒緩症狀為主，多休息及均衡飲食，就能儘速復原。

'[A common cold] **may** happen in any season, but it is **likely** to occur between autumn and early spring. The treatment is **mostly** aimed at relieving symptoms. Getting as **much** rest as possible and having a balanced diet will help you achieve a speedy recovery.'
(https://health.udn.com/disease/sole/177)

4.2.8 Reporting (Medical Research)

The eighth function highlights the research-based quality of health information, that is, to report medical research. Online health information for the public may explicitly point out a research finding by attributing it to medical research. As

Excerpts 4.24–4.25 show, approximate stretchers such as *xuduo* (許多 'many/much'), *youxie* (有些 'some'), and *shu(ge)* (數[個] 'several') participate in adding a research-based quality to the general health information. When performing this function, the stretcher is typically followed by a noun (e.g., *yanjiu* 研究 'research') or noun phrase (*linchuang yanjiu* 臨床研究 'clinical research'), indicating some academic base for the medical evidence. Nevertheless, the exact source of the research or finding is not usually named.

4.24 目前仍有許多臨床研究正在進行中, 期許未來這些療法可以使胰臟癌病患的整體存活期更加延長[. . .]。

'There are still **many** clinical studies in progress, and it is anticipated that in the future, treatments will be able to prolong the overall survival of pancreatic cancer patients [. . .].'
(http://web.tccf.org.tw/lib/project/books/book02.php)

4.25 **數**個研究指出, 經常服用維他命 C 無法降低得到感冒的頻率。也有些研究認為, 每天至少攝取 200 毫克維他命 C 可將成人感冒病程**稍微**短一些。

'**Several** studies have pointed out that regular intake of vitamin C cannot reduce the frequency of catching colds. **Some** other studies believe that taking at least 200 mg of vitamin C a day can **slightly** shorten the course of a cold in adults.'
(www.kmuh.org.tw/www/kmcj/data/10409/7.htm)

4.2.9 Correcting

The ninth function of EL is to correct misconceptions of health information. The function is typically performed by deploying *xuduo* (許多 'many'), *henduo* (很多 'many') or *chang* (常 'often') to introduce a behaviour adopted by many patients or a 'treatment' accepted by members of the public, before the spurious belief is rejected as counterproductive (see Excerpts 4.26–4.28). Other stretchers that also serve this pragmatic function include non-number approximate stretchers such as *yixie* (一些 'some') and *bushao* (不少 'not a small number'). Using the approximate and scalar stretchers helps the health professional deliver a health misconception without being personal as no specific persons are named, thus causing no offence or embarrassment to anyone. The reader tacitly checks if s/he believes the misconception to be true.

4.26 很多焦慮症患者以為自己只是失眠或「好操煩」問題, 所以只是一直服用安眠藥或鎮靜劑, 沒有針對焦慮症作根本治療而導致藥物越吃越多或身體出狀況。

'**Many** patients suffering from anxiety disorders think that they just have insomnia or "worry too much", so they just take sleeping pills or tranquilizers

all the time and fail to receive proper treatment for the anxiety disorder, thus leading to taking more and more drugs or causing more physical problems.'
(www.kmuh.org.tw/www/kmcj/data/9906/4.htm)

4.27 長庚醫院中醫內科部主任楊賢鴻指出，常聽到有人吃抗病毒的藥材，如黃連、大青葉、板藍根、牛蒡子，以為能增強抵抗力預防感冒，其實，反而適得其反。

'As Yang Xianhong, director of the Department of Internal Chinese Medicine of Chang Gung Memorial Hospital, pointed out, it is **often** heard that people eating antiviral herbs, such as *huanglian* [*Coptis chinensis*], *daqingye* [indigowoad root], *banlangen* [Isatis indigotica], and burdock seed [*Arctii fructus*], think that they can boost their immune system and prevent colds. In fact, these practices are counterproductive.'
(www.commonhealth.com.tw/article/62597)

4.28 許多人卻誤以為精神分裂症完全是表面上的一些誘發因素所致， 如:聯考失敗、感情受挫、婚姻或家庭衝突，如果只處理這些問題，則往往徒勞無功、也延誤了治療。

'**Many** people mistakenly believe that schizophrenia is exclusively caused by **some** obvious factors, such as failing an entrance exam, relationship break-ups, marital problems or family conflicts. If you only deal with these problems, **often** your efforts end in frustration and also cause a delay in treatment.'
(https://bit.ly/3JbG8Ua)

4.2.10 Advising Gently

The tenth function of EL is to gently advise the reader on a health issue, a function that corresponds to the ultimate goal of online health communication, that is, to provide the public with correct, useful health information so that they know how to cope better with health problems. The health professional may advise the reader to do something (Excerpts 4.29–4.30, 4.32–4.33) or not to do it (4.31). An imperative in Chinese may have an adverbial scalar stretcher – for example, *duo* 多 'frequently' (4.29), *shao* 少 'infrequently/rarely' (4.29) and *jinchang* 經常 'often' (4.30) – placed before a verb, thus forming advice. Advice may be expressed by an imperative containing a scalar stretcher (e.g., *guo* 過 'too'; *guodu* 過度 'too') followed by an approximate stretcher (e.g., *duo* 多 'much') plus an undesirable phenomenon (e.g., stress; see 4.31). Advice may also be expressed by a negative imperative construction initiated by *buyao* (不要 'don't') or a not-to-do verb (e.g., *bimian* 避免 'avoid') followed by a phrase containing a scalar stretcher (e.g., 4.31). A general term (e.g., 4.33) or an approximate stretcher (e.g., 4.32) may also be used in advice. All the elastic terms make the advice flexible and, at the same time, less pushy, as they do not make the advice sound like an absolute order.

4.29 有感冒症狀時多休息, 多喝開水, 多進食些清淡好吸收的飲食, 少出入公共場所[. . .]。

'When you have cold symptoms, rest **frequently**, drink boiled water **frequently**, and eat light and easy-to-absorb food **regularly** but visit public places **infrequently** [. . .].'
(https://wd.vghtpe.gov.tw/obgy/Fpage.action?fid=4252)

4.30 經常洗手, 有效降低感冒風險。

'Wash your hands **frequently**, as this effectively reduces the risk of getting a cold.'
(https://health.udn.com/disease/sole/177)

4.31 避免給病人過多的壓力, 或是生活過度的緊張

'Avoid putting **too much** pressure on [schizophrenia] patients or causing them **too much** stress in life [. . .].'
(www.jushan.com.tw/area2.asp?all=yesandsn=1000h)

4.32 鼻塞、流鼻水、喉嚨痛、咳嗽是感冒常見的呼吸道症狀, 雖不致影響腸胃道消化功能, 但會讓食慾變差 [. . .] 蒸蛋時加一點點香菇丁和肉末就成了茶碗蒸, 這都是在少份量食物中增加熱量的方法。

'Nasal congestion, a runny nose, a sore throat, and coughing are common respiratory symptoms of a cold. Although it does not affect the digestive function of the gastrointestinal tract, having a cold will reduce the appetite [. . .]. When steaming eggs, add a **little** shiitake mushroom and minced meat, to make chawanmushi [a Japanese dish]. This is a way to increase calories in a small amount of food.'
(www.commonhealth.com.tw/article/66820)

4.33 鼓勵孩子討論他的畏懼, 有時將想法感覺化為文字可以減輕焦慮。

'Encouraging your child to discuss his fears, and **sometimes** turning thoughts into words can reduce anxiety.'
(https://health99.hpa.gov.tw/material/3231)

4.2.11 Supporting Emotionally

Previous studies of VL in conversation have highlighted that VL assumes shared knowledge and may be used to mark in-group membership, thus contributing to building rapport (Carter and McCarthy, 2006: 202; Cutting, 2000; Evison et al., 2007). For example, using an expression such as *and things like that* in verbal interaction may appeal to shared understanding and common ground (Terraschke and Holmes, 2007: 214; Zhang, 2015: 131–133). However, in online written health communication, the use of EL does not seem to involve a strong rapport-building presence as found in spoken dialogues. This may be due to the relatively non-interactive discourse style of written health information.

We identified a function coterminous with, but different from, rapport building, as it relates less to politeness or solidarity than to the emotive and affective dimension of language use: to support the target reader emotionally, which is the eleventh function of EL in the health context. It reassures and/or empathises with the reader either as the patient or a family member of the patient. In Tseng and Zhang's (2018) study of online medical consultation in Chinese, reassuring and empathising are psychological acts among the features that contribute to high-rated online medical consultations. Despite being non-conversational, online written health information can be produced with the emotionally supportive function being fulfilled. This function is enacted when the writer shows a strong, shared understanding of the feeling – shock, pain, fear or worry – experienced by the reader, who may be the patient (Excerpts 4.36–4.37) or a close relation of his/hers (4.34–4.35).

Some of these examples might purport to be describing tendency; however, the subtle function of emotional support outweighs the offer of hard facts. As can be seen, high-end stretchers (e.g., *hen* 很'very'; *guodu* 過度 'too much'; *chang* 常 'often') or approximate stretchers indicating a large quantity (*xuduo* 許多'many') are frequently used to articulate emotional support to the target reader. In this phenomenon, the use of the stretchers signifying a large number or maximal extent corresponds to the intensity of overwhelming emotions, which the patients and their close relations must have felt. As such, they subtly assist in conveying emotional support to the reader who has experienced the described emotions. They lend themselves to fulfilling the emotive-affective dimension of online health communication as they are used to evaluate the extent and volume of negative emotions felt by patients and their families and to respond to such emotions in a positive manner.

Thibault (2011: 212) characterises language as 'languaging': 'Human language is seen more and more as a suite of flexible and adaptive behaviors that are based upon a naturalistically grounded intersubjective sensitivity to the bodily dynamics (movement) of others and the sensorimotor coupling relations between persons and their worlds that result from this in the intersubjective matrix'. According to Jensen (2014: 6), this view regards language as 'intimately tied to affective attunement' – that is, as affect-based and intersubjective. Our examples show that EL helps substantiate this affective view of language as EL is stretchable to serve purposes, including lending emotional support to patients and their families (see Excerpts 4.34–4.37).

4.34 對於家中有精神疾病病人的家屬而言，照顧是一條漫長的路，期間難免會有許多無法控制的情緒出現而愛恨交織，因此家屬如何保持平衡是很重要的。

'For people who have a family member suffering from a mental condition, it is a long-term commitment looking after her or him. In the process, **many**

uncontrollable emotions will inevitably appear, with love coupled with hate. Therefore, how family members maintain a balance is **very** important.'
(www.vhyl.gov.tw/code_upload/HealthInfo/file1_452_2327421.doc)

4.35 一般人碰到家人發病都會驚慌失措, 其實家屬的支持對病人的幫助很大[. . .]。

'People generally panic when their family members are falling ill [with schizophrenia]. In fact, the support of family members is **very** helpful to the patient [. . .].'
(www2.mohwpaper.tw/inside.php?offset=1andcid=203andtype=history)

4.36 甲狀腺癌病人除了在於頸部多了一條疤痕之外, 生活上其實跟一般人完全一樣, 不必過度擔心甲狀腺癌影響到你的生命, 不要讓甲狀腺癌影響到你的生活, 應該將甲狀腺癌當成是與你共存的朋友。

'Except for a scar on the neck, the life of thyroid cancer patients is exactly the same as that of others. Don't worry **too much** that your life would be affected by thyroid cancer. Don't let thyroid cancer affect your life. Thyroid cancer should be regarded as a friend co-existing with you.'
(https://public.mch.org.tw/index.php?action=publications_edm_in&id=1916)

4.37 甲狀腺結節有 5%是惡性的甲狀腺癌, 但有些結節無法明確辨認是良性或惡性, 需做進一步的細針穿刺檢查, 不少人為了要不要進行侵入性的細針穿刺, [. . .]要不要進一步切除甲狀腺左右為難, 常可以感受到病人的焦慮。

'Five percent of thyroid nodules are malignant thyroid cancer, but some nodules cannot be clearly identified as benign or malignant, and fine-needle biopsy is required. **Plenty** of people are torn between having invasive fine-needle biopsy and not having it, between having the thyroid gland removed and not having it done. The patient's anxiety can **often** be sensed.'
(https://health.tvbs.com.tw/medical/305939)

4.3 Frequency Distribution among the Four Categories

In Sections 4.3.1–4.3.4, the top 10 elastic items from each of the four categories of EL are provided. It is useful to know which elastic items from each category are most frequently used in the Chinese health corpus. Due to the limitations of space, our discussion of each category is selective and focused on two elastic terms, but a range of examples illustrating the top five elastic terms from each category are provided in order to briefly showcase what aspects of health information are stretched by EL.

The overall distribution of the four categories of EL in the Chinese corpus is shown in Figure 4.2. The most used items of EL are scalar stretchers, followed by approximate and general stretchers, with epistemic stretchers far behind.

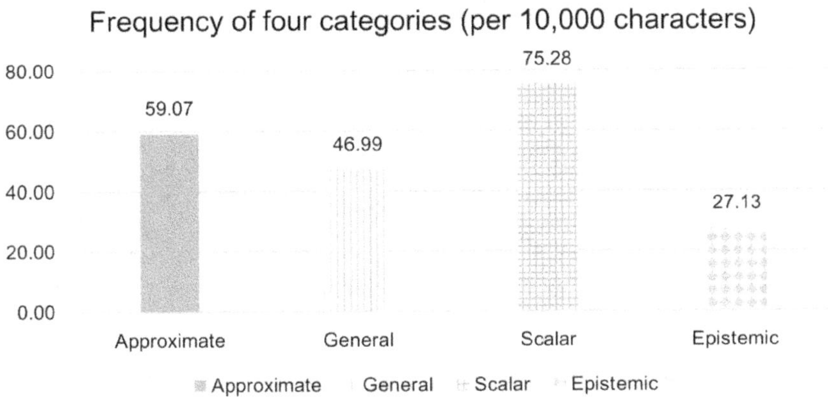

Figure 4.2 Overall distribution of the four categories of EL in Chinese

Scalar stretchers are the most frequently used per 10,000 characters. This is possibly because, in addition to the first-order functions of intensifying and deintensifying, scalar stretchers can serve almost all the second-order functions. Furthermore, according to Pullen et al., expressions of sympathy coupled with intensifiers in the health context are better received than otherwise would have been the case because '[v]erbal intensifiers augment simple statements' (2012: 348–349). Scalar stretchers are particularly adaptive to the task of augmenting health information, including the delivery of emotional support. The lowest normalised frequency of epistemic stretchers in the Chinese corpus suggests that the function of softening health information is not intensively performed in the Chinese corpus. More importantly, the contrast in frequency count suggests that health professionals, when delivering medical information in Chinese, place intensification, commonalities and comparisons as the priority whilst they attend least to the uncertainty of medicine (cf. Adolphs et al., 2007; Sarangi and Clarke, 2002). However, whether the frequency distribution pattern has a cultural value remains unclear until a cross-cultural comparison is made (cf. Chapter 6).

4.3.1 Approximate Stretchers

Figure 4.3 lists the 10 most frequently used approximate stretchers in the Chinese corpus. As can be seen, they occur approximately between 40 and 300 times in this corpus. They play a key role in contributing to the quantification of health information. In the corpus, *yue* and *yishang* typically co-occur with a phrase containing a number. *Duo* may also be used with a number (e.g.,

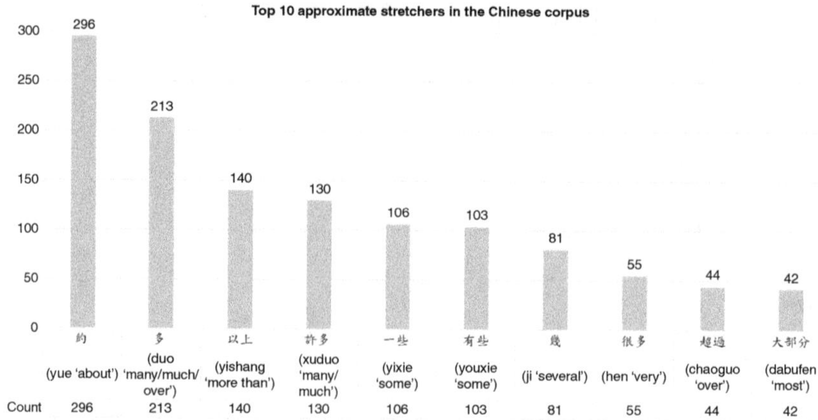

Figure 4.3 Top 10 approximate stretchers in the Chinese corpus

yibai duo zhong 100 多種 'over 100 types') and is also used in a comparative construction (e.g., *jiaoduo* 較多 'many more', *bi . . . duo* 比 . . . 多 'many more than'). *Xuduo* and *yixie* do not co-occur with a number but assist in making generalisations about how a relatively large number or medium-sized group of people or things behave.

Generally, *yue* is used to refer to an approximate quantity relating to people, time and rates of various sorts. More specifically, in medical contexts, it is used to deliver aspects of health information in a flexible, quantitative manner. We divide the use of *yue* into four health-specific contexts: patient demographics (i.e., statistics related to patient population; e.g., Excerpt 4.38); time related to a health issue (4.39–4.40); the description of a specific disease, including the cause, the organ involved and the pathology (e.g., virus; 4.41) and histology (e.g., structure of tissues and cells; 4.42); and aspects of treatment (e.g., a measure of the effectiveness of a diagnostic test; 4.43).

4.38 精神分裂症的盛行率約 1%, 換句話說, 一百個人就有一個人會得精神分裂症。

'The prevalence rate of schizophrenia is **about** 1%. In other words, one in 100 people will develop schizophrenia.'
(www1.cgmh.org.tw/intr/intr2/c3360/E_LYH(Schizo).htm)

4.39 普通感冒的症狀較為輕微, 於病毒感染後 1-3 天發作, 病程約持續 1-2 週。

'The symptoms of the common cold are relatively mild, with an onset of tell-tale signs 1–3 days after the viral infection, and the course of the illness lasts **about** 1–2 weeks.'
(https://epaper.ntuh.gov.tw/health/201012/project_1_1.html)

4.40 精神分裂症，是一種嚴重的精神疾病，它的發病約在青春期前後與成人早期。

'Schizophrenia is a serious mental illness. Its onset is **around** adolescence and early adulthood.'
(www1.cgmh.org.tw/intr/intr2/c3360/E_CCM(Schizophrenia).htm)

4.41 流感病毒屬於正黏液病毒 (orthomyxovirus), 它們的直徑約 80-120 奈米[. . .]。

'Influenza viruses are orthomyxoviruses, and their diameter is **about** 80–120 nanometers [. . .].'
(https://bit.ly/3NKMKwm)

4.42 [甲狀腺癌]組織病理上一般分為(1)分化良好型癌—約佔所有甲狀腺癌 90%。(2)髓質癌—約佔 5%[. . .]。

'[Thyroid cancer] is generally divided into (1) well-differentiated cancers – **about** 90% of all thyroid cancers; (2) medullary carcinoma – **about** 5% [. . .].'
(www.canceraway.org.tw/page.php?IDno=)

4.43 甲狀腺[癌]症狀會出現腫瘤，血液中並不一定會顯示出甲狀腺荷爾蒙異常，唯一會被注意到的是頸部上的腫瘤。超音波檢測約 15 分鐘左右便可測出[. . .]。

'Thyroid cancer has the symptom of a tumour. The blood does **not necessarily** show thyroid hormone abnormalities. The only sign that will be noticed is the tumour on the neck. Ultrasonic detection can check it out in **about** 15 minutes **or so** [. . .].'[4]
(http://org.vghks.gov.tw/ent/a_details.asp?newsid=60)

As can be seen from the examples given above, *yue* is almost always followed by a phrase containing a rough number or range of numbers although it can also precede a prepositional phrase indicating a time period (e.g., *from early puberty to early adulthood*; see 4.40). More importantly, the highest frequency of *yue* ('about') among all the approximate stretchers in the Chinese corpus implies that the statistics using *yue* in health communication are significant, as the statistics provide the reader with a general picture of a specific aspect of a health issue in quantitative terms. On the other hand, they suggest the information given is research-based, although the scales of the source samples remain unknown. The second most frequently used approximate stretcher is *duo* (多), generally meaning 'many' or 'much'. It can function as an adjective or adverb. It is treated as an approximate stretcher when used as an adjective. Its use as an adverb is treated as a scalar stretcher (see Section 4.3.3). *Duo* is often preceded by a scalar stretcher such as *jiao* (較 'more'), *tai* (太 'too') or *geng* (更 'more'; cf. Section 4.3.3) and followed by

[4] In the cited excerpts in Sections 4.3.1–4.3.4, elastic terms that do not fall into the particular category of EL being discussed are emboldened but not underlined.

a noun (e.g., *calories*, *nutrients*). It can also form a comparative construction in the structure 'noun + *bi* . . . *duo*' ('*more* + noun + *than* . . . '; 4.44). It can also be used in conjunction with a relatively large number when a verb such as *chaoguo* (超過 'exceed') or *gaoda* (高達 'be as high as') precedes the number (e.g., 引發感冒的病毒超過 200 多種 'the number of virus types that cause a cold exceeds 200').

Apart from signifying quantity, one interesting phenomenon regarding *duo* as an approximate stretcher is that the heightened amount signified by it and intensified by a high-end scalar stretcher sometimes has a cautionary or hortative connotation in the health context. For example, in Excerpt 4.44, the use of *duo* as an approximate stretcher is couched in the advice of having an intake of sufficient energy given to people with a cold. Excerpt 4.45 sustains the suggestion regarding surgery timing by aligning it with extensive research. Excerpt 4.46 casts doubt over the view that chicken soup boosts the body's immune system by saying many more studies need yet to confirm it, and Excerpt 4.47 warns against possible intake of too many antibiotics.

4.44 [感冒時]在缺乏食慾或味覺苦澀的情況下, 多攝取身體所需能量, 如濃湯所含的熱量及營養素就比清湯多 [. . .]。

'In the case of having a lack of appetite or of food tasting bitter, take in **regularly** the energy that is required by the body. For example, thick soup contains **more** calories and nutrients than clear soup [. . .].'
(www.commonhealth.com.tw/article/66820)

4.45 較多的研究報告建議, 若非緊急的手術, 建議在感冒症狀緩解後 4 個禮拜以上, 再安排手術。

'**More** research reports suggest that if it is not an emergency situation, surgery should not be conducted when one has a cold but be postponed by **more than** 4 weeks after the symptoms of the cold have passed.'
(www.kmuh.org.tw/www/kmcj/data/9610/5.htm)

4.46 西方科學家認為雞湯中某些成分可以抑制中性白血球活動, 幫助身體免疫系統對發炎產生反應, 但黃立民認為, 還需要更多研究證實此論點。

'Western scientists believe that **some** ingredients in chicken soup can curb the activity of neutrophils [a type of white blood cell] and help the body's immune system respond to inflammation, but [Dr.] Limin Huang believes **more** research is needed to confirm this claim.'
(www.commonhealth.com.tw/article/62597?from=search)

4.47 在父母拼命希望孩子感冒快快好起來的同時, 可能也讓孩子吃下太多的感冒藥甚至抗生素,

'While parents desperately hope that their children's colds will get better soon, they **may** also allow their children to take **too much** cold medicine or even antibiotics.'
(www.femh.org.tw/epaperadmin/viewarticle.aspx?ID=4426)

Our count of *duo* as an approximate stretcher excludes the counts of other similar approximators also containing the character *duo* – for example, *xuduo* (許多 'many/much'), *henduo* (很多 'many/much'), *duoban* (多半 'most') and *duoshu* (多數 'majority') – as these are lexical units and, therefore, are counted separately. If they were all counted within the use of *duo*, then the total would exceed that of *yue*. This suggests that references to quantity are very significant in online health information for the public. *Duo* differs from *yue* in that it is not necessarily followed by a number. *Yue* and *duo*, together with other stretchers of the same category, serve the function of approximating quantity of items that affect health, thereby contributing towards the enrichment of the quantitative dimension in health information. The use of approximate stretchers in combination with other categories of EL may also fulfil second-order functions such as describing tendency, correcting a misconception and gently advising (see Section 4.2).

4.3.2 General Stretchers

The 10 most common general stretchers in the Chinese corpus, together with their raw frequency counts, are listed in Figure 4.4. As can be seen, the general extender *deng* (等 'etc./and so on') occurred far more frequently than all the other general stretchers, about 8–40 times the number of any of the other general stretchers on the list. *Deng* is not only the most frequently used general stretcher in each of the six Chinese sub-corpora but is also the most frequent elastic term in the whole Chinese corpus (see Figure 4.1). Other general extenders are *dengdeng* (等等 'and so forth'), ranked third and meaning the same as *deng* (though used much less frequently), and *gezhong* (各種 'all sorts of'), ranked eighth.

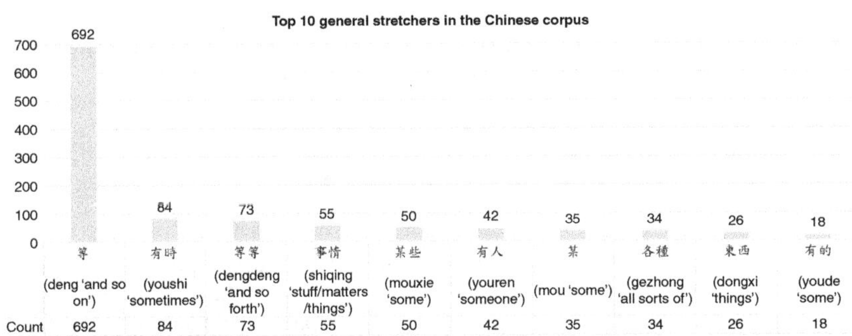

Figure 4.4 Top 10 general stretchers in the Chinese corpus

Deng is used immediately after a list of two or more items. Although *deng* may occasionally be followed by an ellipsis (Excerpt 4.48), most of its examples are not. It is a general stretcher placed at the end of a list and suggests the list is incomplete. It is extensively used when a list of health-related items is introduced, whether it relates to treatment methods (4.48), symptoms (4.49), spread of a cancer to other organs (4.50), factors that worsen a health condition (4.51), side effects (4.52), examples to support a point being made (4.53) or something else. The general stretcher allows the health professional to provide a short list of health-related items without making it too complicated. It is a convenient term that showcases the complexity of a health condition and/or a range of options in a manageable way by listing only several prototypical issues or items. The stretcher performs the function of shortening a list of items.

4.48 放射性同位素碘 131 對乳突性或濾泡性甲狀腺癌早期之遠端轉移可達到治癒之效果, 臨床更可依其所需採用不同或搭配之治療方式 (手術、電療、化療 ... 等) 以獲最大之療效與最小之副作用。

'The radioactive isotope iodine 131 can achieve a cure for early distant metastasis from mastoid or follicular thyroid cancer. Clinically, different or combined treatment methods (surgery, electrotherapy, chemotherapy **and so on**) can be **very much** adopted according to need in order to ensure the biggest curative effect and the smallest side effect.'
(https://web.tccf.org.tw/lib/addon.php?act=post&id=1316)

4.49 若甲狀腺癌轉移到骨頭及肺部, 可能會影起疼痛、咳嗽、呼吸困難等症狀。

'If thyroid cancer spreads to the bones and lungs, it **may** cause symptoms such as pain, coughing, difficulty breathing **and so on**.'
(web.tccf.org.tw/lib/addon.php?act=post&id=4027)

4.50 髓質癌 (Medullary cancer) [...]可藉由腺內淋巴轉移到腺內其他部位或局部淋巴結, 也可藉由血流而轉移至遠處如肺、骨骼及肝臟等。

'Medullary cancer [...] can be metastasized by intraglandular lymph to other parts of the gland or local lymph nodes and can also be metastasized by blood flow to distant places such as the lungs, bones, liver **and so on**.'
(www.cmuh.cmu.edu.tw/HealthEdus/Detail?no=5134)

4.51 長期有焦慮症或恐慌症的病人, 可能因為癌症的診斷、癌症藥物治療的副作用、身體不適的症狀或住院治療的環境等加重其原本的焦慮症狀。

'The original anxiety symptoms of patients with long-term anxiety or panic disorder **may** be aggravated by the diagnosis of cancer, the side effects of cancer drug treatments, physical discomfort or the hospital environment **and so on**.'
(http://web.tccf.org.tw/lifetype/index.php?op=ViewArticleandarticleId=1835andblogId=1) .

4.52 接受放射線治療的患者常出現焦慮、無助感、坐立不安、惡夢及失眠等。

'Patients receiving radiation therapy often experience anxiety, helplessness, restlessness, nightmares, insomnia **and so on**.'
(http://web.tccf.org.tw/lifetype/index.php?op=ViewArticleandarticleId=1835andblogId=1)

4.53 精神病患家屬的壓力調適: [...]尋求支持與協助, 如社區復建中心及康復之支協會等。

'How family members of metal patients adjust to the pressure: [...] Seek support and assistance from, for example, community rehabilitation centres, rehabilitation support associations **and so on**.'
(http://taipei.tzuchi.com.tw/wp-content/uploads/2020/06/PSY-E18.pdf)

As well as general extenders, general stretchers also cover general expressions for time (*youshi* 有時 'sometimes'; Excerpt 4.54), things (*shiqing* 事情 'stuff/matter/thing', *dongx i* 東西 'thing'; Excerpt 4.55), qualitatively-oriented use of *some* (*mouxie* 某些, *youde* 有的; 4.56–4.59), and a person whose identity is anonymous (*youren* 有人 'someone'; 4.56). While *youshi* (有時 'sometimes') assists in performing the function of describing tendency, *youren* (有人 'someone') helps to avoid mentioning sensitive, complicated or unnecessary content when health information is communicated.

4.54 民眾有時服用醫師開立的感冒藥一、二帖沒有好, 就急著換醫師, 結果是多吃了一堆不必要的藥。

'People **sometimes** take the first or second cold medicine prescribed by the doctor and are in a hurry to change doctors. As a result, they take **a lot of** unnecessary medicine.'
(www.hch.gov.tw/hch/MedicalTeams/PrintNew.aspx?MNO=C087andID=7588)

4.55 精神分裂症最麻煩的不是幻聽、妄想, 而是「退化」。病人可能會越來越缺乏動機, 或因為許多事情漸漸做不來乾脆放棄。

'What is the most troublesome about schizophrenia is not auditory hallucinations and delusions, but "degeneration". The patient **may** become less and less motivated or simply give up because **many things** are gradually becoming difficult to do.'
(https://health.businessweekly.com.tw/AArticle.aspx?id=ARTL000022323)

4.56 有人不斷扔工作給妳[精神分裂症患者], 或家人事事都依賴妳來解決時, 要適度說「不」。

'[If you are diagnosed as having an anxiety disorder], when **someone** keeps giving you work to do or when family members rely on you for everything, do say "no" where appropriate.'
(www.commonhealth.com.tw/article/62208?from=search)

4.57 某些特殊的疾病, 像是甲狀腺機能亢進、腎上腺腫瘤、心臟疾患等, 會引起相關神經傳導異常的, 都可能併發焦慮症。

> '**Some** particular diseases, such as hyperthyroidism, adrenal tumours, heart disease **and so on**, can cause nerve conduction abnormalities related to them, and anxiety disorders **may** co-occur.'
> (https://health.udn.com/disease/sole/176)

4.58 停止服用甲狀腺素後, 身體會處在甲狀腺功能不足的狀況, 可能出現疲倦、增胖、易抽筋、胃口不佳、嗜睡、記憶力較差、水腫等暫時性不適, 有的病患可接受, 有的病患卻很不舒服[...]。

> 'After ceasing to take thyroxine, the body will be in a state of insufficient thyroid function, and you **may** experience temporary discomfort such as fatigue, weight gain, cramping, poor appetite, lethargy, poor memory, oedema **and so on**. While **some** patients can tolerate it, **some** patients feel very uncomfortable [...].'
> (https://bit.ly/3NOSTYx)

4.59 某些日常生活飲食或習慣如香菸, 乃是確定與胰臟癌最有關的危險因子[...]。

> '**Some** aspects of diet or habits, such as smoking, are the most relevant risk factors for pancreatic cancer [...].'
> (wwwv.tsgh.ndmctsgh.edu.tw/unit/10021/20000)

In English, the vague/elastic expression *some* is highly complicated, as it covers different meanings and functions (Le and Zhang, 2018). In Chinese, at least three terms are available to distinguish two aspects of *some* in English. While *yixie* (一些) and *youxie* (有些) are quantitatively focused (see Section 4.3.1), *mouxie* (某些) is qualitatively oriented in that it often has a more-negative-than-positive valence attached to it. In everyday contexts, using *mouxie* immediately before a noun or noun phrase allows the speaker not to name the specific persons or issues being referred to, thus covering up the explicit identity of the person or item involved and making the statement less personal. In the medical context, the use of this vague expression is often coupled with a short list of examples related to the 'unnamed' items that the general stretcher originally purports to introduce (e.g., Excerpts 4.57 and 4.59). More specifically, in the medical context, it is not necessarily used in order to hide specific information the writer already has in mind but due to the complexity and/or uncertainty of the health information being delivered. Furthermore, usually, a negative valence is attached to it. As Excerpts 4.57 and 4.59 suggest, *mouxie* is usually used to introduce a statement containing a health issue that raises concern.

4.3.3 Scalar Stretchers

Figure 4.5 demonstrates the top 10 scalar stretchers in the Chinese corpus. Two striking features can be found. First and foremost, the raw counts of the top five

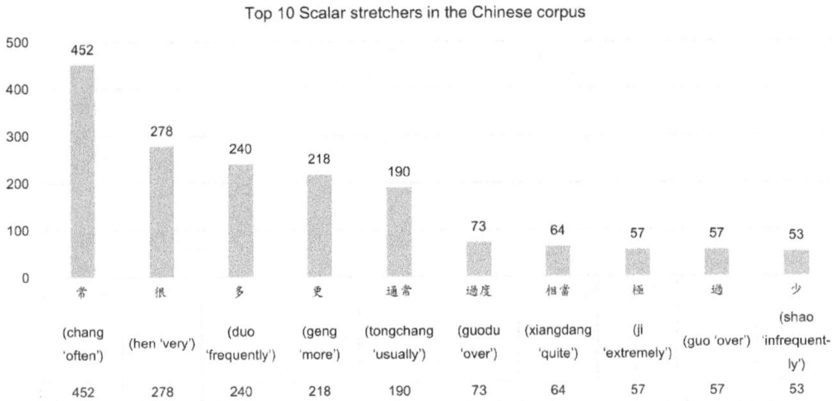

Figure 4.5 Top 10 scalar stretchers in the Chinese corpus

scalar stretchers are quite high, ranging between approximately 200 and 450, a number not seen at all in the other three categories of EL. This suggests that the collected online health information in Chinese relies most heavily on scalar stretchers. Second, all the top nine scalar stretchers are high-end and the only low-end stretcher is *shao* (少 'rarely/infrequently'), ranked tenth.

Why do high-end stretchers appear much more frequently in the Chinese corpus than low-end stretchers? A glimpse into the use of *chang* (常 'often/usually'), consistently the most frequent scalar term in each of the six disease-specific subcorpora, sheds light on possible answers. The term's frequency suggests a rhetorical feature of online health communication in Chinese: by depicting what is commonly seen (Excerpt 4.60), often heard (4.61), frequently used (4.62), constantly needed (4.63) and so forth, health professionals can present health information assumed to be familiar to the health professional and expected to be known to the general public. As such, health writers adapt the information to what the general public need to know and pave the way for the delivery of health information/advice, whether the 'common' phenomenon being described is a reinforcement of accurate health information or the correction of a health misconception. The frequent use of this scalar stretcher reinforces the practice that healthcare information for the public focuses more on what is often the case with a condition rather than on exceptions. On the other hand, the high frequency is possibly motivated by the various functions *chang* (常) may serve, for example, to describe tendency (e.g., Excerpt 4.60), correct a health misconception (e.g., 4.61), give advice gently (e.g., 4.30) and emotionally support the target reader (e.g., 4.37).

The second most frequent scalar stretcher is *hen* (很 'very'). It is an intensifier heightening the features associated with aspects of health information (e.g., Excerpts 4.64–4.65). In addition to intensifying, *hen* or its combination with other stretchers (e.g., 4.34–4.35) may also perform the function of proffering emotional support to the target reader of health information. As the intensifier raises the interpersonal force of an evaluative statement (Martin, 2000; Martin and White, 2005), it is suited to striking a chord with the reader, particularly when the statement touches on a feeling shared by the reader (e.g., 4.65).

4.60 鼻塞、流鼻水、喉嚨痛、咳嗽是感冒常見的呼吸道症狀。

'Stuffy nose, runny nose, sore throat and coughing are **often**-seen respiratory symptoms of a cold.'
(www.dgnet.com.tw/articleview.php?article_id=19653andissue_id=3850)

4.61 常聽到有人吃抗病毒的藥材, 如黃連、大青葉、板藍根、牛蒡子, 以為能增強抵抗力預防感冒, 其實, 反而適得其反。

'It is **often** heard that people taking antiviral herbs, such as *huanglian* [*Coptis chinensis*], *daqingye* [indigowoad roots], *banlangen* [Isatis indigotica], and burdock seed [*Arctii fructus*], think that they can boost their immune system and prevent colds. In fact, these practices are counter-productive.'
(www.commonhealth.com.tw/article/62597?from=search)

4.62 大家太常用這個臆斷, 稍有頭痛或喉嚨不適甚至嚴重咳嗽合併高燒都算是感冒 [. . .]。

'People use this assumption **too often**, and a **somewhat** mild headache or sore throat or even a severe cough combined with a high fever is considered to be a cold [. . .].'
(https://wd.vghtpe.gov.tw/obgy/Fpage.action?fid=4252)

4.63 約有 70%的胰臟癌病人會有疼痛問題發生, 而疼痛控制是一個相當大的問題, 常須要使用嗎啡才能控制疼痛。

'**About** 70% of pancreatic cancer patients have pain issues, and pain control is **quite** a big problem. Morphine is **often** needed to control pain.'
(https://www.cgb.com.tw/j2j0/cus/cus1/hel/hel2/20017.jsp)

4.64 流感剛開始全身的症狀很明顯, 包括高燒、全身肌肉痠痛、虛弱無力、食慾減少。

'The symptoms of flu are **very** obvious at the beginning; they include a fever, systemic muscle pain, lack of energy, and reduced appetite.'
(https://health.ntuh.gov.tw/health/new/6010.htm)

4.65 對一些焦慮精神官能症的患者而言, 家庭的一些問題 (如經濟問題、子女教育問題) 很可能帶給他們心理上的極大的壓力、情緒的不安、緊張、過份的焦慮 [. . .]。

'For **some** patients with an anxiety disorder, **some** of their family problems (such as financial problems, children's educational problems) are **very** likely to bring them **extremely** heavy psychological pressure, emotional insecurity, tension and **a fair bit** of anxiety [. . .].'
(www.auh.org.tw/NewsInfo/HealthEducationInfo?docid=1639)

4.3.4 *Epistemic Stretchers*

In semantics, epistemic modality refers to modal expressions that convey the speaker's commitment to the truth of the proposition (Palmer, 1986: 51; Lyons, 1977: 797–809). While recognising the widely accepted view of epistemic modality, this study recasts it in terms of epistemic stretchers, defined as epistemic stance markers, because the interactional meaning of stance well captures the communicative property of language use (Conrad and Biber, 2000; Jaffe, 2009). Epistemic stance markers express the addresser's evaluation of the proposition being expressed in terms of possibility. This study does not cover assertive expressions of high certainty (e.g., *biding* 必定 'surely', *yiding* 一定 'certainly') but the epistemic stretchers with a relatively uncertain valence (e.g., *keneng* 可能 'likely/possibly/ may'). This is owing to the significant issue of uncertainty in health communication (see Section 2.5.2). Figure 4.6 lists the top 10 epistemic stretchers in the Chinese corpus.

As is clearly shown, *keneng* was used disproportionately more frequently than any other epistemic stretcher. According to Li and Thompson (1981: 179), *keneng* is 'an adjectival verb', not an auxiliary verb, because it can be modified by *hen* ('very') and *geng* ('more'), but 'auxiliary verbs cannot be modified by intensifiers' (1981: 180). Despite its grammatical status not being the same as an auxiliary verb, *keneng* can express meanings covered by a few lexical items in English, for example, *may*, *could*, *might*, *likely*, and *possibly*. The current study is concerned with what *keneng* can pragmatically do in health discourse. The stretcher was used almost 40 times more than *sihu* (似乎 'seem'), ranked second on the list of epistemic stretchers. The main reason is that *keneng* allows the health professional to stretch the meaning that lies between

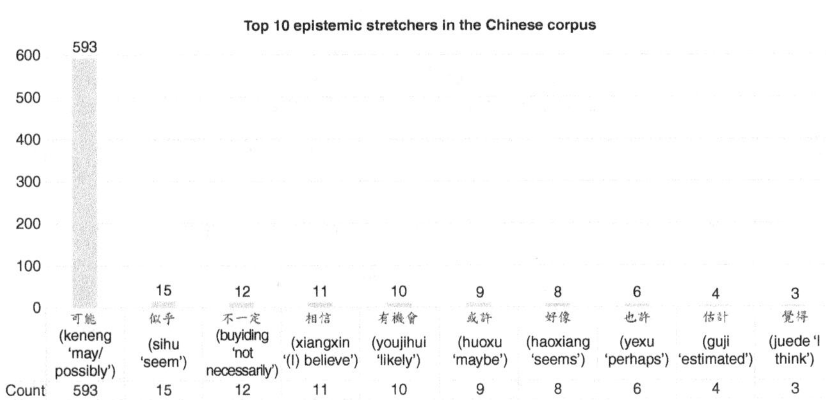

Figure 4.6 Top 10 epistemic stretchers in the Chinese corpus

knowing and not knowing in all manner of situations. *Keneng* can be used to soften aspects of health information, ranging from health advice (Excerpts 4.68, 4.69), through symptoms (4.66), to side effects (4.67), and from recovery (4.73), through risk evaluations (4.70–4.71), to estimated life expectancy (4.72). More importantly, when used to describe a desirable situation (e.g., recovery), it has a promising prospect. When employed to articulate an unwanted phenomenon, it can be interpreted as merely a 'possibility' that will not necessarily happen. It can be like a thick cloud signalling a cautionary effect but also a faint light offering something hopeful in times of darkness. It is this stretching of meaning in between that makes *keneng* an all-time favourite in the Chinese corpus. The use of *keneng* serves the function of softening the statement and, amongst other functions, also assists in delivering health advice in a less dictatorial manner (Excerpt 4.68).

4.66 若甲狀腺癌轉移到骨頭及肺部，可能會[引]起疼痛、咳嗽、呼吸困難等症狀。

'If thyroid cancer spreads to the bones and lungs, it **may** [cause] symptoms such as pain, coughing, difficulty in breathing **and so on**.'
(https://web.tccf.org.tw/lib/addon.php?act=post&id=4027)

4.67 此類藥品可能引起嗜睡、口乾、頭昏、視力模糊及胃部不適等副作用。

'Such drugs **may** cause side effects such as drowsiness, dry mouth, dizziness, blurred vision, stomach upset **and so on**.'
(https://epaper.ntuh.gov.tw/health/201012/project_1_1.html)

4.68 建議儘可能每天睡足 7 到 8 小時。睡眠是讓身體主要器官休息、修復的時間，休息的越充分，身體抵抗感染的能力就越強。

'It is recommended to get **as** much sleep **as possible**, up to 7 to 8 hours a day. Sleep is the time for the main organs of the body to rest and repair. The more rest there is, the stronger the body's ability to resist infection.'
(www.kmuh.org.tw/www/kmcj/data/10409/7.htm)

4.69 切除手術是唯一有可能治癒的方法，也是目前胰臟癌患者長期存活的最佳選擇[. . .]。

'Resection is the only **possible** cure, and it is also the best choice for long-term survival in pancreatic cancer patients [. . .].'
(https://epaper.ntuh.gov.tw/health/201305/special_1_2.html)

4.70 甲狀腺癌若很小，存在甲狀腺結節若不去手術也可能一輩子沒事。

'If the thyroid cancer tumour is **very** small, existing in thyroid nodules, it **may** be OK for a lifetime without surgery.'
(https://bit.ly/3x6ULWw)

4.71 在父母拼命希望孩子感冒快快好起來的同時, 可能也讓孩子吃下太多的感冒藥甚至抗生素, 久而久之孩子正常的免疫力也可能因此受到影響[...]。

'While parents desperately hope that their children's cold will get better quickly, they **may** also allow their children to take **too much** cold medicine or even antibiotics. If this continues for a long while, the child's normal immunity **may** also be affected [...].'
(www.femh.org.tw/epaperadmin/viewarticle.aspx?ID=4426)

4.72 胰臟癌的死亡率非常高，就算還能手術切除，存活時間也可能僅有一年左右[...]。

'The mortality rate for pancreatic cancer is **very** high, and even if the cancerous tissue can be surgically removed, the survival time **may** be **just about** one year [...].'
(www.cgb.com.tw/j2j0/cus/cus1/hel/hel2/20017.jsp)

Compared with *keneng*, the other epistemic stretchers play a minor role – that is, their frequency counts were less than 20. One or two examples illustrating some of them are cited below (see Excerpts 4.73–4.77). *Sihu* (似乎 'seem') also expresses uncertainty, but it makes a statement even less certain than *keneng*. If *sihu* in Excerpt 4.73 is replaced by *keneng*, syntactically it is acceptable, but pragmatically, the changed sentence would express a higher degree of certainty than the original version. However, it would be odd to replace *keneng* with *sihu* in some cases. For example, if *sihu* were used to describe side effects (see Excerpt 4.67), the sentence would suggest a rather unprofessional tone as if little were known about the medicine or insufficient research had been conducted. Furthermore, when advice is offered using *jin keneng* ('if possible') (see Excerpt 4.68), if it were replaced by *sihu*, it would not only be syntactically unacceptable but also pragmatically problematic because the advice would be far too uncertain to be convincing. *Buyiding*, which is placed before a verb phrase or an adjective, signifies a higher degree of uncertainty than *keneng* and *sihu* (see Excerpt 4.74).

Next, *xiangxin* (相信 '[I] believe/it is believed') can be an epistemic stretcher when the agent of the mental verb is the writer or a group of people including the writer, although the agent (*wo* 'I') is not always stated in the sentence, as zero-subject sentences are common in Chinese (Li and Thompson, 1979). Like the other epistemic stretchers, (*wo*) *xiangxin* allows the health professional to soften the medical information being conveyed but with a higher degree of certainty than uncertainty. We believe the use of *xiangxin* in the health context, whether or not the writer as the agent of the verb is present in the sentence, makes the health information appear more professional than mere speculation as it reinforces that the source of the opinion is the health expert. Presumably, whatever is given in the health information is based on reliable sources, and the given information is what the health professional believes to be true; therefore, the use of *I believe* or *it is believed* would not be essential. Nevertheless, when it is used, it expresses an awareness of possible exceptions (Excerpts 4.75–4.76). It is the seeming certainty with a hint of uncertainty that makes this expression elastic and, therefore, useful. For example, in Excerpt 4.76, the uncertainty expressed in the first half of the sentence is attenuated by the follow-up *xiangxin* in the second half, thus increasing the value of the given health information as the reader would feel frustrated if most of the given health information is highly uncertain. Numerous studies of epistemic stance based on English data have examined the pervasive use of *I think* in spoken interactions (Kärkkäinnen, 2003, 2006), yielding insights into subtly different meanings of *I think* in various contexts. Zhang and Sabet study how *I think* is used in L1 and L2 contexts, the latter of which involves speakers of Persian and of Chinese. Their study suggests that 'L1 speakers are speaker-oriented and assertive, the Persians are listener-centred and less authoritative, and the Chinese tend to take the middle-ground position' (2016: 334). The 'middle-ground position' reinforces the in-between position of the similar epistemic stretcher *xiangxin* in our health information data as it strengthens certainty without making it sound too assertive.

4.73 根據統計, 有過敏性疾病史的人, 包括氣喘病等似乎具有保護作用, 比較不易罹患胰臟癌。扁桃腺切除者, 患胰臟癌的機會也少。

'According to statistics, people with a history of allergies, including asthma **and so on**, **seem** to have a level of protection and have a smaller chance of developing pancreatic cancer. Those who have tonsillectomy have **less** chance of developing pancreatic cancer.'
(www.cgb.com.tw/j2j0/cus/cus1/hel/hel2/20017.jsp)

4.74 若曾經得過某一型的流感病毒, 不一定會對此型終身免疫, 因為病毒隨時可能有突變[. . .]。

'If you have ever had a certain type of influenza virus, you do **not necessarily** become immune to this type for life, because the virus **may** mutate at any time [. . .].'
(www.twhealth.org.tw/journalView.php?cat=2andsid=30andpage=1)

4.75 精神分裂症對於病人及家屬都是一個相當辛苦長期抗戰, 相信在接受完整的治療後, 都能有更快樂的人生。

'Schizophrenia is a **very** hard and long-term battle for patients and their families. **It is believed** that after receiving complete treatment, they can have an even happier life.'
(www1.cgmh.org.tw/intr/intr2/c3360/E_LYH(Schizo).htm)

4.76 直至現在，思覺失調症的真正成因仍未能確定，但相信是腦部的生化物質受到影響。

'Until now, the true cause of schizophrenia has not been determined, but **it is believed** that the condition is affected by the biochemical substances in the brain.'
(wwwv.tsgh.ndmctsgh.edu.tw/unit/10058/17019)

4.77 術前輔助性化學治療 (或合併化學放射治療) 可提高 R0 手術的機會，甚至有機會讓原本無法切除的局部晚期胰臟癌轉變為可切除的。

'Preoperative adjuvant chemotherapy (or its combination with chemoradiation therapy) can increase the chance of R0 surgery [i.e., complete resection], and it is even **likely** that a previously unresectable localised pancreatic cancer at an advanced stage will become resectable.'
(https://medinsight.ylhealth.org/article/58)

Youjihui (有機會 'likely') is similar to *keneng* in meaning; if the former were to be replaced by the latter in Excerpt 4.77, the information would be equally acceptable. However, the two stretchers are very different pragmatically. While *keneng* appears in sentences that state desirable or undesirable phenomena, *youjihui* is usually followed by something positive or expected. Should *youjihui* replace *keneng* or *youkeneng*, especially where the health situation is undesirable (e.g., Excerpts 4.66–4.67), the sentence would seem odd and inappropriate: it would create a sarcastic tone as it would go against the favourable situation implied by *youjihui*.

4.4 Correlations between the Four Categories and Six Diseases

This section examines whether correlations exist between the use of EL and the six health topics. If they do, then how can we explain them? We address these issues from two viewpoints. First, we explore possible correlations from a macro perspective (i.e., based on the overall distribution of EL in disease-specific sub-corpora). Then, we have a closer look by comparing the top 10 elastic terms in each of the six sub-corpora or in the three disease clusters. We identify specific elastic terms that were particularly salient in disease-specific sub-corpora.

Figure 4.7 presents the standardised frequency counts of EL in the six sub-corpora. Two distribution patterns, presented in decreasing order of the four categories, emerged. The pattern SC-AQ-GE-EP was found in four of the sub-corpora: cold, flu, thyroid cancer and pancreatic cancer. By contrast, another pattern SC-GE-AQ-EP was manifested in the two mental-condition sub-corpora. Specifically, while in both patterns scalar stretchers were the most common category and epistemic stretchers constituted the least frequent one, the order of the other two categories (i.e., AQ and GE) differed. The common-disease and cancer clusters used more approximate stretchers than general

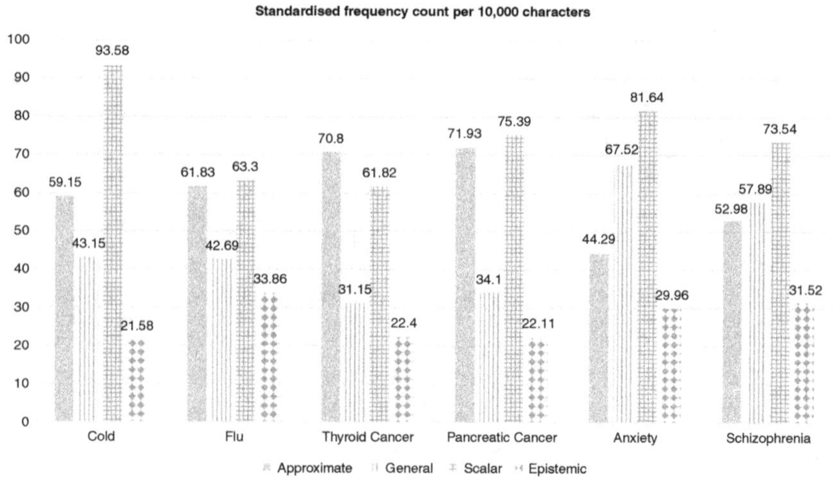

Figure 4.7 Overview of the distribution of the four categories of EL in six disease sub-corpora in the Chinese corpus

stretchers, but the mental-condition cluster used more general stretchers than approximate stretchers. This difference suggests that health information concerning mental conditions relies less on quantification than its non-mental-condition counterparts.

In terms of severity of disease, approximate stretchers appeared consistently more often in each of the more severe sub-corpora across the three clusters: flu > cold, pancreatic cancer > thyroid cancer, and schizophrenia > anxiety disorder. This may suggest that the more serious a health condition is, the more quantification is used, but this might be restricted only to a comparison of a specific type of health condition, as in each of the three clusters of diseases used in the current study.

The tendency to use more approximate stretchers in the sub-corpus of a more severe disease in a cluster is also applicable to the other three categories of EL, but this is the case only to a lesser extent. General stretchers appeared more frequently in two of the sub-corpora featuring the more severe disease: flu and schizophrenia. Epistemic stretchers were also more frequently used in flu and in pancreatic cancer – that is, the more severe diseases in the common-disease and cancer clusters. Scalar stretchers were found to appear more frequently in pancreatic cancer than in thyroid cancer, the tendency being found only in the cancer cluster. These tendencies suggest that the use of EL might or might not increase as the severity of the disease increases. Nevertheless, one or more specific categories of EL may be used more frequently in the more severe condition in a cluster than the less severe one in it.

To better understand possible correlations between the four categories of EL and information about different diseases, we need to look closely at what elastic terms tended to appear in each sub-corpus and why they appeared relatively frequently. Correlations might be more visible not in terms of the severity of the disease but in light of the nature of the disease.

Table 4.1 shows the top 10 elastic terms in the six health conditions. We focus on each cluster of diseases at a time. We first concentrate on the common-disease cluster: cold and flu. Although the order of their standardised frequency count differs, seven of the elastic terms on the two lists are identical. For example, among the top five, three of the elastic items occurred across the two sub-corpora and in the same order: *deng* (等 'and so on'), *keneng* (可能 'possibly/may') and *chang* (常 'often'), the three terms that were also the most frequently used general, epistemic and scalar stretchers in the whole corpus, respectively. The frequency counts of *keneng* and *deng* in flu were the highest among the six diseases. This might be due to the ever-changing nature of flu viruses, hence the need to soften the statement. On the other hand, the high frequency of *deng* indicates both the complexity of the disease and some assumptions about it (that need not be all spelt out as it is impossible to compile a complete list of the complex causes and interactions of the items mentioned).

Two other striking observations can be made about the cluster containing the two common health conditions. First, in the cold sub-corpus, two scalar terms figured prominently: *duo* as the second most frequent elastic item and *geng* as the fifth on the list. These were not, however, found on list for their flu counterpart. This suggests that, while some stretchers are relatively frequently used across the six sub-corpora irrespective of the disease being discussed, some other stretchers are more likely to be used in disease-specific health information. For example, the standardised frequency of *duo* as a scalar stretcher was over 25 per 10000 Chinese characters in the cold sub-corpus, the highest standardised frequency count of this elastic term in the whole corpus. This is due to the common advice given to speakers of Chinese when they have a cold: *duo he shui* (多喝水 'drink water frequently'), *duo xiuxi* (多休息 'rest frequently') and *duo chi shenluse shucai* (多吃深綠色蔬菜 'eat dark green vegetables frequently'). However, to cope with the flu, it is far from enough to simply advise people to act on their own; rather, it is important to educate the public about the risk of the flu (Excerpt 4.78) and about vaccination (4.79), as having a flu is more severe than catching a cold. Therefore, we can understand why *duo* as a scalar stretcher is strongly correlated with the cold dataset but not the flu one. *Geng* (更 'more'), also a scalar stretcher, was ranked fifth, and if we look at some examples where it is used, we can understand why it is commonly used. It intensifies aspects of health information involving comparisons and is often embedded within the delivery of advice (Excerpt 4.80) or warning (4.81), thus alerting the reader to whatever should be noted

Table 4.1 *Top 10 elastic terms in the six medical conditions (frequency per 10,000 characters)*

	ANX	#	SCHIZ	#	COLD	#	FLU	#	THYR	#	PANC	#
1	等 *deng*	33	可能 *keneng*	29	等 *deng*	31	等 *deng*	36	約 *yue*	24	約 *yue*	26
2	可能 *keneng*	25	等 *deng*	28	多(SC) *duo*	26	可能 *keneng*	31	可能 *keneng*	21	常 *chang*	20
3	常 *chang*	21	很 *hen*	15	可能 *keneng*	18	常 *chang*	17	常 *chang*	19	等 *deng*	20
4	很 *hen*	16	常 *chang*	15	常 *chang*	18	約 *yue*	10	等 *deng*	17	可能 *keneng*	18
5	過度 *guodu*	13	更 *geng*	11	更 *geng*	14	以上 *yishang*	10	很 *hen*	9	通常 *tong-chang*	10
6	多(AQ) *duo*	10	多(AQ) *duo*	9	很 *hen*	9	多(SC) *duo*	9	多(AQ) *duo*	8	很 *hen*	10
7	更 *geng*	9	一些 *yixie*	9	通常 *tong-chang*	9	通常 *tong-chang*	7	以上 *yishang*	7	大部分 *dabufen*	10
8	一些 *yixie*	7	通常 *tong-chang*	8	多(AQ) *duo*	8	以下 *yixia*	7	多SC *duo*	7	多(AQ) *duo*	9
9	許多 *xuduo*	7	許多 *xuduo*	8	太 *tai*	8	很 *hen*	6	通常 *tong-chang*	6	更 *geng*	9
10	常常 *chang-chang*	6	多(SC) *duo*; 約 *yue*	7	以上 *yishang*	7	多(AQ) *duo*; 極 *ji*	5	大部分 *dabufen*	6	少(SC) *shao*	6

when responding to having a cold, a common health condition that many can cope with on their own. In short, *duo* and *geng* in the cold sub-corpus have the highest frequency counts in the whole corpus, and this shapes and is shaped by the nature of a cold as a condition that can be improved by a patient following the suggested advice (e.g., to implement a healthy diet, drink more water and rest more).

4.78 流感併發重症多見於老年人、小孩, 以及患有心、肺、腎臟及代謝性疾病或免疫功能不全者。

'Severe cases of influenza are **more** common in the elderly, children, and those with heart, lung, kidney and metabolic diseases or immune deficiency.' (www.jungongphc.taichung.gov.tw/1037520/post)

4.79 為了防止得到流行性感冒可以事先接種感冒疫苗, 但病毒疫苗只針對特定病毒才有反應, 不同病毒則無效果[...]。

'In order to prevent influenza, you can get a flu vaccine in advance, but the vaccine responds to specific viruses **only**, and it has no effect on other viruses [...].'
(www.kingnet.com.tw/news/single?newId=19801)

4.80 如果服[感冒]藥後三天症狀並沒有獲得改善或是變得更加嚴重, 就應該就醫[...]。

'If the symptoms do not improve or become **more** serious three days after you take the [cold] medicine, you should seek medical attention [...].'
(www.cgmh.org.tw/cgmn/category.asp?id_seq=1601002#.YI4KWcDis2x)

4.81 [發燒時]睡冰枕不但不能降體溫, 還會讓小朋友感覺很冷, 促使身體需要製造更多熱量因應, 反而造成病體更虛弱。

'[In case of a fever], sleeping on an ice pillow not only fails to lower the body temperature but also makes the child feel **very** cold, prompting the body to use **even more** calories to respond, and thus making the sick body **even** weaker.'
(www.commonhealth.com.tw/article/62597?from=search)

Second, three stretchers are prominent in the flu sub-corpus but are not on the top-10 list for that of the cold. One of them is *yue* (約 'about'; e.g., Excerpts 4.82 and 4.83). This may be due to the relative complexity of influenza compared with colds. The complexity of influenza must have attracted much attention and research and makes it possible to state aspects of the health condition more in quantitative terms in the flu sub-corpus than in that of the cold. This observation is also reinforced by the two cancer sub-corpora, as *yue* tops the lists of elastic terms in the cluster (see Table 4.1). The other two terms that are on the flu list are *yishang* (以上 'over') and *yixia* (以下 'under'), their frequency counts in the flu sub-corpus being the highest in the whole Chinese corpus. Excerpts 4.84–4.87 show that the two stretchers were used to stretch age, time range and virus types. Many of their uses relate to the age range in which people can receive a free vaccine as it is covered by Taiwan's National Health Insurance. As such, their highest standardised frequency counts in the flu data are partly due to the disease, as the use of the terms often concerns the use of flu vaccines (see 4.84–4.86) and is partly related to the country's health policy.

4.82 [流感疫苗]保護效果亦約只能維持1年, 因此建議每年均須接種 1 次。

'The protective effect [of an influenza vaccine] can last for **just** **about** one year, so it is recommended that people be vaccinated once a year.' (https://bit.ly/3KkWV8P)

4.83 在高危險群之[流感]病患, 其嚴重之併發症亦可能導致死亡, 根據估計約每 5,000~10,000 名患者, 就會有1人死亡。

'In the high-risk group of [flu] patients, serious complications **may** also lead to death. According to estimates, **about** 1 person will die for every 5,000 to 10,000 patients.'
(https://prevention.hcshb.gov.tw/News_Content.aspx?n=471ands=84029)

4.84 除了醫護人員和六十五歲以上的老年人口, 以及延續去年為了防治禽流感而增加的禽畜業者外, 今年又納入了二歲以下的幼兒可接受免費提供的流感疫苗接種。

'In addition to medical staff, the elderly population **over** 65 and people who work in the poultry industry (a group added to the list in order to prevent bird flu last year), children **under** two years of age are also included this year among those who can receive free flu vaccination.'
(www.kmuh.org.tw/www/kmcj/data/9311/6.htmhttp)

4.85 八歲以下的兒童若為初次接種, 須間隔一個月以上施打兩劑[. . .]。

'Children **under** the age of eight must be given a second dose **more than** one month after the first vaccination [. . .].'
(www.kmuh.org.tw/www/kmcj/data/9311/6.htmhttp)

4.86 十二歲以下兒童只適合接種副作用比較小的裂解病毒疫苗[. . .]。

'Children **under** the age of twelve are suitable for **only** split-virus vaccines, which have relatively mild side effects [. . .].'
(http://w3.tpsh.tp.edu.tw/organization/osa/osa05oldnew/health/437.htm)

4.87 一般會引起感冒的病毒至少有百種以上[. . .]。

'Generally, there are **more than** 100 different viruses that cause the common cold [. . .].'
(www.tcmg.com.tw/paper/paper-981002.htm)

Let us turn to the cancer cluster, concerning which four striking points are made (see Table 4.1). First, in the two cancer sub-corpora, seven of the elastic terms are identical across the top-10 lists although their order is slightly different: *yue* (約 'about'), *keneng* (可能 'may/possibly'), *chang* (常 'often'), *deng* (等 ('and so on'), *hen* (很 'very'), *duo* (多 'many/much') and *tongchang* (通常 'usually'). These overlap with the six stretchers shared between the cold and flu top-10 lists except *yue* ('about'), which was on the flu and cancer lists but was not on the cold list. This seems to suggest the tendency of *yue* ('about') to occur in health information concerning relatively severe diseases. This is also reinforced in the schizophrenia data (see Table 4.1). Second, the top four elastic terms on the two cancer lists represent four categories of EL: approximate (*yue*), epistemic (*keneng*), scalar (*chang*) and general stretcher (*deng*). This phenomenon is not found in the other four sub-corpora, suggesting that a less fluctuating pattern of collaboration among the four categories is more likely to be found in the cancer cluster. If we associate this phenomenon with the overall distribution of the four categories of EL in the cancer cluster (see Figure 4.7), it can be confirmed that the counts of the approximate and scalar stretchers were closer in the cancer cluster than in the other two clusters, which used many more scalar than approximate stretchers. The approximate stretcher *dabufen* (大部分 'majority/a large part') contributed to increasing the overall counts of this category of EL in the cancer cluster (see Excerpt 4.88; see Table 4.1), as it was not found at all on the top-10 lists in the other two clusters.

Third, *yue* (e.g., Excerpt 4.89) is the most frequent elastic term in the two cancer sub-corpora, something not found in any of the other sub-corpora. In fact, a close look at the top 10 elastic expressions based on the cancer cluster (see Table 4.1) reveals that the category of approximate stretchers constituted the largest part in the thyroid cancer sub-corpus (*yue*, *duo*, *yishang*, *dabufen*) and that the category represented the second largest proportion in the pancreatic cancer sub-corpus (*yue*, *dabufen*, *duo*), only surpassed by the category of the scalar stretchers. The high frequent use of this category is not found on the top-10 lists of all the other four diseases. The significance of the approximate stretchers is confirmed by the high-frequency use of *yue*, the most frequently used stretcher of its type in the two cancer sub-corpora and in the whole corpus. In fact, the frequency counts of *yue* in the cancer cluster were the highest among the three clusters. This suggests that it is strongly correlated with cancer. Fourth, although the general stretcher *deng* (e.g., Excerpt 4.90) was ranked high on the two lists, its frequency counts in the cancer cluster were the lowest among the three clusters. This suggests that when writing about cancer, the health professional using Chinese as L1 is more cautious of using the term, possibly because cancer is regarded as relatively critical and many omissions of detailed health information concerning it are not appropriate.

4.88 大部分胰臟癌長在體部或尾部的病患，發現時大多很晚期，已無法進行手術切除。

'**Most** patients whose pancreatic cancer grows on the body or tail of the pancreas are **mostly** diagnosed at a **very** late stage, and the cancerous tissue cannot be surgically removed.'
(http://web.tccf.org.tw/lib/project/books/book02.php)

4.89 [胰臟癌中]胰臟頭部的發生率約 60%、體部約 15%、尾部約 5%、侵犯整個胰臟則約 20%。

'The incidence rate for pancreatic head [cancer] is **about** 60%, the rate for the pancreatic body is **about** 15%, the rate for the tail is **about** 5%, and the rate for the entire pancreas being affected is **about** 20%.'
(https://epaper.ntuh.gov.tw/health/201305/special_1_2.html)

4.90 胰臟癌不易早期發現, 常見的症狀包括: 腹痛、體重減輕以及黃疸等[. . .]。

'It is not easy to detect early-stage pancreatic cancer. The symptoms that **often** appear include abdominal pain, weight loss, jaundice **and so on** [. . .].'
(www.kmuh.org.tw/www/kmcj/data/9901/14.htm)

Next, we turn to the two top-10 lists concerning the mental-condition cluster (Table 4.1). Three salient patterns can be identified, supporting correlations between the use of EL and health information concerning the two mental conditions. First, in this cluster, the high-end stretcher *hen* (很 'very') had the highest standardised frequencies, at more than 15 per 10,000 characters, among the three clusters. In fact, the proportions of the scalar stretchers on the two lists are rather large, as they constitute five of the top 10 terms on each. Apart from the shared *chang* (常 'often'), *hen* (很 'very'), and *geng* (更 'more'), the additional two are *guodu* (過多 'too') and *changchang* (常常 'often') on the anxiety list and *tongchang* (通常 'usually) and *duo* (多 'frequently') on the schizophrenia list. This suggests that scalar terms, *hen* (很 'very') in particular, are used much more frequently than other categories of EL. Some examples are given in Excerpts 4.91–4.94. High-end stretchers intensify the statements being made; furthermore, they also serve second-order functions such as providing emotional support (4.35–4.37), gently advising (4.29–4.30), describing a tendency (4.91, 4.93) and correcting a health misconception (4.92), among others, particularly when they are combined with one or more elastic terms.

4.91 大部分的精神分裂症患者在表現出明顯的精神病態之前, 都會有一段不算短的前驅期(通常可達一年以上), 像是覺得注意力很難集中[. . .]。

'**Most** patients with schizophrenia have a not significant prodromal period (**usually** up to one year or even **more**) before there is an obvious psychosis; for example, they find it **very** difficult to concentrate [. . .].'
(https://health.ntuh.gov.tw/health/new/6023.htm)

4.92 一般人常把焦慮疾患歸因於「心理壓力」。這是錯誤的, 焦慮疾患與憂鬱症一樣, 是「生病」, 不是單純的心因性反應。壓力通常只是促發[焦慮疾], 或是加重因子而已。

'People **often** attribute anxiety disorders to "psychological stress". This is wrong. Anxiety disorders, like depression, are "sickness", not purely psychogenic reactions. Stress is usually **just** a triggering or aggravating factor [for anxiety disorders].'
(www1.cgmh.org.tw/intr/intr2/c3360/E_LCY(anxiety).htm)

4.93 如果確定罹患精神分裂症, 病人很可能需要一輩子服藥、需要親人照顧。

'If it is confirmed that the patient has schizophrenia, the patient will **most likely** need to take medicine for the rest of their life and be cared for by relatives.'
(https://bit.ly/3NVyXD0)

4.94 大多數的患者皆需長期服藥, 切勿自行停藥, 否則每次復發, 祇會讓病情更形惡化。

'**Most** patients need to take the medicine for a long time. Do not stop the medicine solely on your own initiative, otherwise each relapse could then make the condition **even** worse.'
(www.ysvh.gov.tw/ysvh/code_upload/HealthCate/file1_636_5425246.pdf)

Second, although the scalar category was also used most frequently in the cold and pancreatic cancer sub-corpora, the exact scalar terms used varied. For example, while *duo* was frequently deployed in the cold dataset, *guodu* (過度 'too much') was frequently used in the anxiety sub-corpus but not in any of the other datasets. This is attributed to the nature of anxiety disorder, which features a much higher degree of dangerous anxiety than harmless anxiety. *Guodu* lends itself to doing the job of making a distinction (Excerpt 4.95).

4.95 [焦慮症患者]會有過度擔心小事, 胡思亂想而無法控制的情況 [...]。

'[Patients of an anxiety disorder] worry **too much** about trivial matters, are lost in various fancies and conjectures and can't control them.'
(www1.cgmh.org.tw/intr/intr2/c3360/E_HsuSJ.htm)

4.96 每個人多多少少會有一些強迫意念、強迫行為, 這不見得是強迫症。
必須是「不合理」而且帶來重大痛苦, 或佔據許多時間[...]。

'Everyone **somehow** has **some** obsessive thoughts and compulsive behaviours, and this does not have to count as an obsessive-compulsive disorder. It must be "unreasonable" and cause great pain or take up **a lot of** time [...].'
(https://health99.hpa.gov.tw/material/3231)

4.97 有許多[精神分裂症]病人腦海裡仍浮現著許多奇怪的聲音或想法，但他們已經學會不要在意。

‘**Many** patients [of schizophrenia] still hear **many** strange sounds or have **many** strange thoughts in their minds, but they have learnt not to care.’ (https://health.businessweekly.com.tw/AArticle.aspx?id=ARTL000022323ht)

4.98 只要社會大眾有更多認識, 將之[思覺失調症]視為千百種慢性病之一, 患者亦願意接受正確治療，長期服用藥物控制病情，無形中也為社會減少許多隱憂。

‘As long as the general public has **much more** knowledge and regards it [schizophrenia] as one of thousands of chronic diseases, and patients are also willing to receive the correct treatment while taking medication on a long-term basis to control their condition, **many** hidden worries for society will be reduced.’ (www2.mohwpaper.tw/inside.php?type=historyandcid=203)

Third, compared with the cancer and flu sub-corpora, the two mental health sub-corpora use *yue* much less frequently; it is at the bottom of the top-10 list for schizophrenia and does not appear on the anxiety disorder list. This suggests that when dealing with mental-health information, health professionals writing in Chinese rely much less on statistics, and that is why the *yue*-plus-a-number construction was least used. Instead, as Excerpts 4.96–4.98 show, they resort to other approximate stretchers such as *duo* (多 ‘many/much’), *yixie* (一些 ‘some’), and *xuduo* (許多 ‘many/ much’), the last two of which are not found on the top-10 lists based on the other four sub-corpora. This suggests that when delivering information about mental health, health professionals who are L1 speakers of Taiwan Mandarin tend not to use numbers that are rounded up or down. This might be attributed to the relative difficulty in accessing data related to mental health or to the sensitive nature of mental health that makes it undesirable to quantify aspects of mental health information in statistical terms.

4.5 Concluding Remarks

This chapter presents the forms of EL in Chinese health information. Four categories of EL were found in the Chinese data. Approximate stretchers express vague quantity – for example, *yue* (約 ‘about’), *yishang* (以上 ‘over’), *yixia* (以下 ‘under/less than’), *xuduo* (許多 ‘many/much’), *duo* (多 ‘many/ much’), *yixie* (一些 ‘some’) and *ji* (幾 ‘several’). General stretchers consist of two types: general extenders (e.g., *deng* 等 ‘etc./and so on’, *dengdeng* 等等 ‘and so forth’, *gezhong* 各種 ‘all sorts of’) and general expressions (e.g., *shiqing* 事情 ‘matters/ stuff/thing[s]’, *mouren* 某人 ‘someone’, *mouxie* 某些 qualitative ‘some’, *youren* 有人 ‘someone’, *youshi* 有時 ‘sometimes’ and *youde* 有的 qualitative ‘some’). Scalar stretchers tone the scale up or down or show the strength or extent of a feature, phenomenon or behaviour. Chinese high-end scalar stretchers, which scale the degree upwards, include *ji* (極 'extremely'), *hen* (很 'very'), *chang* (常 'often'), *tongchang* (通常 'usually'), *duo* (多 'frequently') and *geng* (更 'more'). By contrast, low-end scalar stretchers, which scale the degree downwards, include *shao* (少 'rarely/little') and *qingwei* (輕微 'slightly'). Epistemic stretchers express the speaker's evaluation of and attitude towards the statement being made in terms of possibility. Chinese epistemic stretchers cover *keneng* (可能 'may/possibly'), *sihu* (似乎 'seem'), *(wo)xiangxin* ([我]相信 'I believe'), *(wo)juede* ([我]覺得 'I think'), *huoxu* (或許 'perhaps') and *haoxiang* (好像 'seem like'). The top 10 elastic expressions are as follows: *deng* (等 'etc.'), *keneng* (可能 'likely/may/possibly'), *chang* (常 'often'), *yue* (約 'about'), *hen* (很 'very'), *duo* (多 'frequently'), *geng* (更 'more'), *duo* (多 'many/much'), *tongchang* (通常 'usually') and *xuduo* (許多 'many/much').

The pragmatic functions of EL were also investigated. A total of eleven functions of EL in the health context were identified. Six of them are first-order, as these functions are fulfilled on the lexico-grammatical level and identified based on the propositional meanings of the elastic items used. The first-order functions are softening, intensifying, deintensifying, approximating, avoiding and shortening. A first-order function served by an elastic term may also have a second-order function, especially when the health context and the co-text are considered. Five second-order functions of EL were also identified: describing tendency, reporting medical research, correcting health misconceptions, advising gently and supporting (the target reader) emotionally.

The standardised frequency counts of EL were calculated and analysed. In the Chinese data, the most frequently used elastic items are scalar stretchers, followed by approximate and general stretchers, with epistemic stretchers coming in fourth place. Specifically, the pattern in decreasing order is SC-AQ-GE-EP. Scalar stretchers are most used possibly because they can perform a wide range of functions and assist in augmenting health information via intensification and in presenting details involving comparisons. Whether the pattern identified has any cultural significance is discussed in Chapter 6.

The standardised frequency distribution of the top 10 elastic items of each of the four categories of EL reveals two tendencies: a gradual versus a sharp decrease. While the top 10 approximate (Figure 4.3) and scalar (Figure 4.5) stretchers exhibit a gradual decrease in the use of such elastic items, their general and epistemic counterparts show a drastic decrease (Figures 4.4 and 4.6). More specifically, *deng* and *keneng* are used far more frequently than any other stretchers in their categories. In terms of approximate stretchers, *yue* (約 'about') followed by a number is the most-used approximate stretcher, but the majority of approximate stretchers are non-number based, such as *duo* ('many/

much'), *xuduo* (許多 'many/much'), *yixie* (一些 'some') and *henduo* (很多 'many/much'). In terms of scalar stretchers, nine out of the top 10 items in this category are high-end stretchers. *Chang* (常 'often/usually') is the most frequently used scalar expression and is also consistently the most common scalar term in each of the six disease-specific sub-corpora (see Section 4.4). This supports the observation that healthcare information for the public concentrates more on what is often the case with a condition rather than on exceptions. At the same time, its high frequency is motivated by the wide-ranging functions *chang* (常) may serve, including describing tendency, gently advising, supporting the target reader emotionally and correcting a health misconception. The second most frequently used scalar stretcher is *hen* (很 'very'), an intensifier, which amplifies the interpersonal force of an evaluative statement, thus engaging the reader. As to the all-time favourite general stretcher, *deng* (等 'etc.'), it allows the health professional to showcase the complexity of a health condition and/or a range of options in a concise, manageable way. *Keneng* (可能 'possibly/may') is the most favoured epistemic stretcher in the Chinese corpus due to its flexibility in interpretation.

Possible correlations between the four categories of EL and three clusters of health conditions are also explored. First, two overall patterns of frequency distribution in relation to the six diseases are identified. In decreasing order of frequency counts, they are SC-AQ-GE-EP and SC-GE-AQ-EP. The former, which is identical to the distribution pattern of the Chinese data in full, is found in the common-disease and cancer-related clusters. The latter is found in the mental-condition cluster, suggesting that quantification is less used in mental health information than in physical conditions. Second, there may be more uses of a specific category of EL as the severity of the disease increases, but this is not found across all the categories. The cases identified are as follows: more use of approximate stretchers in the more severe condition across the three clusters; more use of general stretchers in flu and schizophrenia, of scalar stretchers in pancreatic cancer, and of epistemic stretchers in flu and in pancreatic cancer. Third, a specific elastic term may be used most frequently in relation to a specific condition or a cluster of diseases. For example, *yue* (約 'about') has the highest average count in the cancer cluster but the lowest count in the mental-health cluster, suggesting that while number-based quantification tends to be used more frequently when the condition does not relate to mental health and relatively critical, it is less used when the information deals with mental conditions, which are personal and sensitive. While the common-disease cluster has the highest average count of *deng* (等 'etc.'), the cancer cluster has the lowest occurrences of this term. This may relate to the nature of the diseases. By contrast, when information concerning common diseases is delivered, some health information may be assumed, and the unstated assumption is acceptable. However, for critical conditions such as cancer, *deng* is least used. Key

Table 4.2 *Correlations between the four categories of EL and three clusters of health conditions*

	COLD and FLU	THYROID (THY) and PANCREATIC (PAN) CANCER	ANXIETY DISORDER (ANX) and SCHIZOPHRENIA (SCHIZ)
Approximate	• used more frequently in the more severe disease (FLU) • highest counts of *yishang* (以上 'over') and *yixia* (以下 'under/less than') in FLU	• used more frequently in the more severe disease (PAN CANCER) • highest average count of *yue* (約 'about') in the cluster • average count of this category of stretchers being closest to that of scalar stretchers • highest average count *of dabufen* (大部分 'majority') in the cluster	• used more frequently in the more severe disease (SCHIZ) • highest average counts of *yixie* (一些 'some') and *xuduo* (許多 'many') in the cluster • least use of *yue* (約 'about') in the cluster
General	• used more frequently in the more severe disease (FLU) • highest average count of *deng* (等 'etc.') in the cluster	• least use of *deng* in the cluster	• used more frequently in the more severe disease (SCHIZ)
Scalar	• highest counts of *duo* and *geng* (更 'more') in COLD	• used more frequently in the more severe disease • average count of this category of stretchers being closest to that of approximate stretchers	• highest average count of *hen* (很 'very') in the cluster • highest count of *guodu* (過度 'too much') in ANX
Epistemic	• used more frequently in the more severe disease (FLU) • highest count of *keneng* (可能 'may/ possibly') in FLU	• used more frequently in the more severe disease	• highest average count of *keneng* (可能 'may/ possibly') in the cluster

highlights concerning the correlations between EL and the six health conditions are summarised in Table 4.2.

In short, there appears to be a combination of contributing factors that affect and shape the use of EL in the Chinese data: the nature of the medical condition (e.g., disease severity, the sensitive nature of mental conditions), the applications and restrictions of medicine (e.g., the groups suitable or unsuitable for vaccines), the country's health policy (e.g., the groups eligible for free treatment), the written mode, the health professional's stance towards the health information, and the potentials and constraints of an elastic/vague term (e.g., *keneng* versus *sihu*; *hen* versus *guodu*). Social conventions in language use are also a significant factor, an issue that is addressed in Chapter 6.

5 Elastic Language Used in English

This section discusses the use of EL in online English medical data collected for this study. A total of 209 websites were used: professional websites (50.2%), private/public hospital websites (35.9%) and government websites (13.9%). The relative sizes of the corpus by disease are as follows: pancreatic cancer (14.8%), thyroid cancer (27.3%), cold (11.5%), influenza (13.4%), anxiety (25.8%) and schizophrenia (7.2%).

The English corpus consists of a total of 281,762 words. The word distribution among the six diseases is anxiety (100,565 words, 35.69%), thyroid cancer (48,544 words, 17.23%), pancreatic cancer (45,208 words, 16.04%), influenza (40,037 words, 14.21%), the common cold (27,737 words, 9.84%) and schizophrenia (19,671 words, 6.98%). Where appropriate, the quantitative data analysis was based on standardised word counts (per 10,000 words) to address the problem of different data sizes.

Based on the data, this chapter discusses the forms and functions of EL in the context of the six medical conditions. The forms are distributed across four categories, and there are 11 pragmatic functions that emerged in the data, as discussed in Section 5.2 below.

5.1 Pragmatic Forms of Elastic Language

The data collected for this study support a classification of four categories of EL forms: approximate stretchers, general stretchers, scalar stretchers and epistemic stretchers (Zhang, 2015). They are discussed here to establish the terms of reference for this study.

Approximate stretchers (AQ) denote an imprecise amount. The context in which approximate stretchers are used is usually when there is uncertainty in the mind of the language user, which prevents him or her from using precise numbers (Folkman et al., 1979).

General stretchers (GE) create a global meaning, through general nouns and general extenders. The general nouns are 'maximally generic' (Andersen, 2010: 36), serving the situations where 'the required expressions are not known, cannot be retrieved (e.g., due to memory lapses) or cannot be mentioned (e.g., taboo words)' (Parvaresh, 2018: 170). General extenders (Overstreet & Yule, 1997) imply meaning drawn on shared knowledge, experience and conceptual schemes.

Scalar stretchers (SC) scale up or down the force of an utterance (e.g., *very*, *a little*). They enable the speaker to adopt a more or less assertively confident voice (Bradac et al., 1995; Hyland, 2000; Zhang, 2011). For example, *very* can push up the tone of utterance (Zhang, 2011), thus maximising the language user's attitudinal visibility (Hyland, 2005). However, studies show that people tend to hedge their utterances rather than boost them (Hyland, 2000, 2005; Powell, 1985).

Epistemic stretchers (EP) express possibility (e.g., *maybe*, *sort of*, *I think*). The user indicates that what is said is his or her subjective opinion rather than fact, lacking 'the commitment of the speaker to that which she [...] asserts' (Rowland, 2007: 82). The highlighting uncertainty on the part of the speaker makes speech less authoritative and less assertive (Carter, 2003: 11).

The 10 most frequent words overall in the data are listed in Figure 5.1. In terms of total word count, EP is first (2,072), SC second (1,802), AQ third (1,607) and GE last (494). This means that, as far as the use of the EL collected for this study is concerned, the users tend to speak in probable tones the most, enhance the strength of their utterances second, convey medical quantitative information vaguely third and speak in general terms last.

As shown in Figure 5.1, the word *may*, which refers to possibility, occurs the most frequently in the data (2,072 times). The second highest occurring term, *some*, refers to a small and vague quantity. The third one, *usually*, links with a common practice, and the fourth one, *more*, highlights an upwards but

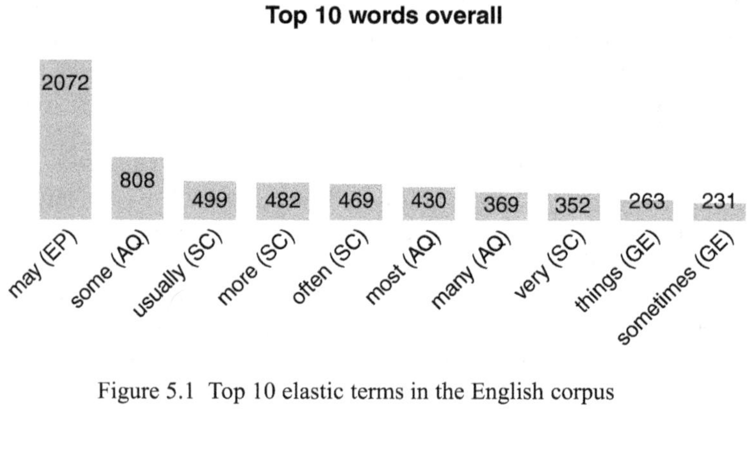

Figure 5.1 Top 10 elastic terms in the English corpus

unspecific comparison. The fifth, *often*, refers to a regular pattern, and the sixth, *most*, indicates a vaguely defined majority. The seventh, *many*, signifies a significantly higher number than is usually expected (Moxey and Sanford, 1993). The eighth, *very*, is a typical scalar word to accentuate the degree of something. The ninth, *things*, refers to unspecific items, and finally the tenth, *sometimes*, presents a non-regular and vague frequency.

5.2 Pragmatic Functions of Elastic Language

EL allows 'a speaker to take refuge in strategic imprecision' (Leech, 2000: 695) and 'to avoid an excess of precision' (Crystal and Davy, 1979: 112). EL is used regularly in everyday conversations, which can manage conversational implicature and serve social functions such as engendering camaraderie and softening implicit criticisms (Jucker et al., 2003: 1737). The data collected for this study tests and strengthens the existing research findings based on written monologue data drawn from online medical websites.

Two main categories of EL function emerged in the data: first-order (manifested through individual types of EL form) and second-order (manifested through multiple EL forms) pragmatic functions. As previously discussed in Chapter 4, the first order includes six sub-categories: softening, avoiding, intensifying, deintensifying, approximating and shortening. The second order includes five sub-categories: describing tendency, reporting, correcting, advising gently and supporting the reader emotionally .

The first six first-order functions are common functions (Hyland, 1998a, 1998b; Zhang, 2015), but the latter five second-order functions are less well-known and reveal more specifically the use of EL in the context of online healthcare data.

Functions are context-dependent, making it meaningless to generalise without considering variables such as social class, age and gender (Cheshire, 2007). As Overstreet (2011: 308) notes, 'the particular function of a vague expression has to be interpreted locally in context'. This study adopts a data-driven approach. The corpus excerpts extracted from the data provide authentic information on both the actual linguistic realisations and the contexts in which they are used. In this way, the evidence for the pragmatic function of EL is expected to be explicit and convincing. For this reason, the analysis presented in the following section is based on contextualised excerpts selected from this study's data.

5.2.1 Softening

The data show that EL is used to qualify the certainty of health information, serving purposes such as self-protection and politeness. This supports Adolphs et al.'s (2007) findings, when they observed that health professionals in hospital consultations use vague modifiers and general extenders to mitigate directives and soften distressing subjects for patients. EL 'nearly always enables polite and non-threatening interaction' (Carter, 2003: 92). Carter and McCarthy (2006: 202) suggest that VL 'softens expressions so that they do not appear too direct, or unduly authoritative or assertive'. Locher (2010) also found that medical professionals mitigated their expressions of advice-giving by using indirectness and hedging. Pounds (2018) investigated the discourse features used by medical experts on a UK healthcare site to achieve a patient-centred communication style, which is characterised by empathetic expressions and mitigated advice-giving.

5.1 The most common form of treatment is surgery, whereby a section or the whole thyroid gland is removed (partial or total thyroidectomy). As a preventative measure, the surgeon **may** also remove nearby lymph nodes (called a neck dissection).
(www.cancer.org.au/about-cancer/types-of-cancer/thyroid-cancer.html)

Excerpt 5.1 explains that the most common treatment for thyroid cancer is to remove the thyroid. In addition, a neck dissection is also a possibility. Here, the use of the epistemic stretcher *may* indicates that the choice of a neck dissection is not for certain but, rather, a possibility.

5.2 Professor Cyndi Shannon Weickert, the Macquarie Group Chair of Schizophrenia Research, has discovered that people with schizophrenia are **more likely** to inherit a gene that codes for a faulty oestrogen receptor in the brain. Together with the Schofield Group, they are also investigating another gene that plays an important role in the development of neural connections in the brain during early development.
(www.neura.edu.au/health/schizophrenia/extra-information/)

Scientists are unable to talk categorically about many medical phenomena, including schizophrenia. In Excerpt 5.2, Professor Weickert believes there is a possible link between a faulty gene and schizophrenia but is not sure about it. The use of the epistemic stretcher *more likely* can to some extent protect Professor Weichert from the risk of being wrong (Brown and Levinson, 1987; Zhang, 2015).

5.2.2 Avoiding

The data show that general stretchers tend to perform avoiding functions. General words such as *things*, *someone* were used to avoid presenting specific health information. The circumstances under which these items were used include situations where there was (1) a lack of precise information, (2) no need to be specific, (3) the delivery of sensitive or undesirable information (Cutting, 2015) and (4) information that is too complex to be specific.

5.3 Medullary carcinoma is an intermediate type of thyroid cancer, **somewhere** between differentiated and undifferentiated and anaplastic thyroid cancers, which thankfully is very rare, has a very poor prognosis.
(https://havasentclinics.com/head-neck-cancer/thyroid-cancer/)

The general stretcher *somewhere* is used to compare medullary carcinoma with other types. There are two main types of thyroid cancer: differentiated and undifferentiated. It is a complex issue to locate precisely where the medullary carcinoma sits between the two main types. Therefore, *somewhere* serves the function of providing a roughly defined position.

5.4 An exam of the body to check general signs of health, including checking for signs of disease, such as lumps or swelling in the neck, voice box, and lymph nodes, and **anything else** that seems unusual. A history of the patient's health habits and past illnesses and treatments will also be taken.
(www.rarecancers.org.au/directory/4/thyroid-cancer)

There are many things that can be included on a checklist for a diagnosis of a given thyroid cancer, so presenting an exhaustive list seems impossible. Even if it is possible, it may not be necessary. In Excerpt 5.4, the general stretcher *anything else* is used to indicate that a full list is not important or is unnecessary.

5.5 The limitation of these approaches is that they do not gain an understanding of why **someone** gets anxious in the first place, what causes anxiety. This is where psychotherapy can be effective and also help to prevent anxiety returning down the track.

Anxiety often happens because there is **something** we cannot bear to think about or to feel, perhaps to suffer. Anxiety acts like a blanket covering over our experience so that we cannot focus on what makes us uncomfortable. It is a psychological avoidance device.
(https://healthengine.com.au/info/psychotherapy-for-anxiety)

There are approaches that can be utilised to help manage anxiety, however psychotherapy addresses the underlying reasons for anxiety. The general stretcher *someone* is used here because it is impossible to name a real anxiety sufferer due to issues such as sensitivity and confidentiality. When discussing the reasons for anxiety, *something* is used, perhaps due to a lack of adequate knowledge of the specific things that cause an individual's anxiety.

The function of 'caution' tends to occur in the case of inconclusive data and incomplete work, as EL indicates tentativeness and carefulness (Salager-Meyer, 1994: 151). EL shows honesty in conveying scientific scepticism and doubt (Myers, 1996), and 'cautionary language may be advantageous, or even requisite' (Cutting, 2012: 286).

5.2.3 *Intensifying*

This function enhances the degree of a medical phenomenon, highlights an aspect of health information or increases the strength of a medical claim.

5.6 Thyroid problems are incredibly common and strike women **far more often than** men. An underactive thyroid is the most common disorder, but the thyroid gland can also become overactive, enlarged (goitre), become cancerous or develop nodules.
(https://sandracabot.com/thyroid-awareness-week/)

In Excerpt 5.6, the scalar stretcher *far more* is used to present the increase in frequency that women get thyroid cancer than men. The degree of extremity of *far more often* is much higher than of *often* alone because *far more* pushes the frequency upwards.

5.7 If your loved one is hesitant about entering hospital, trusting a psychiatrist or taking medication, it is important to let them know that hospitalisation may be **very** brief and may give them a safe space to deal with that they are going through. You can also let them know that psychiatrists are there to help. Finally, let them know that medication can **very** often be **very** helpful in reducing disturbing phenomena that they are experiencing.
(www.onedoor.org.au/advocacy/about-mental-illness/schizophrenia)

In Excerpt 5.7, three scalar stretchers (i.e., *very*) are used to highlight the possible short length of hospitalisation and the higher probability of the excellent effectiveness of medication. The use of *very* three times aims to emphasise the necessity of getting help from doctors.

5.2.4 *Deintensifying*

In contrast to the intensifying function discussed previously, the deintensifying function serves to lessen the degree or extent of a medical phenomenon such as a symptom or severity.

5.8 It is estimated that there will be 3,123 new cases of pancreatic cancer in 2016, ranking the disease as the 10th most commonly diagnosed cancer type in Australia. The risk of pancreatic cancer increases with age, with the average age at diagnosis 70 years and men at a **slightly** higher risk than women. The lifetime risk of developing pancreatic cancer is approximately 1.5%.
(https://www.cancercouncil.com.au/pancreatic-cancer/diagnosis/)

In Excerpt 5.8, the writer mixes precise and elastic information to meet the demands of the situation. The paragraph starts with precise statistics in the first half but turns to EL in the second half, with the help of *slightly*. When describing the gender difference in pancreatic cancer cases, the scalar stretcher *slightly* is used for the risk rate of men compared to women. The writer in this case may not have precise statistics to hand, or a non-precise utterance may be deemed good enough for the public.

5.9 Schizophrenia can appear to be **somewhat** different in different people. Some people experience more hallucinations and delusions, while others primarily experience disordered thoughts and speech. Some people also experience depression and mania (symptoms seen in people with bipolar disorder) which is characteristic of schizoaffective disorder.
(www.neura.edu.au/health/schizophrenia/extra-information/)

Excerpt 5.9 states that schizophrenia may affect people in different ways. The scalar stretcher *somewhat* indicates that the degree of difference is not huge. The function here is to deintensify the degree, rather than intensify it.

5.10 Often our breathing is shallow and fast when we're anxious, due to the mistaken idea (thought) that we can't breathe and need oxygen. In fact, this process gives us too much of the stuff and this affects our breathing! This can be remedied simply by holding one's breath **a bit** longer.
(www.360.org.au/News/How-can-we-better-manage-anxiety)

The scalar stretcher *a bit* scales down the length of time one needs to hold one's breath for, meaning we should not hold it for too much longer, just a short while. Similar to Excerpt 5.9, the function of *a bit* here is to reduce rather than increase the strength of a medical statement.

5.2.5 Approximating

This function makes the quantitative health information, with or without a specific number, flexible. In this category, the job of an elastic expression is to make a precise number elastic to form an approximation, to present elastic quantity or to make an approximation even more elastic. Approximation is used for cognitive economy, namely 'underspecification is achieved by selecting only the really relevant information and thereby avoiding redundancy' (Schwarz-Friesel and Consten, 2011: 351; Cheng and O'Keeffe, 2015: 374).

5.11 There are **several** different types of thyroid cancer, the most common is papillary thyroid cancer, which usually grows in one lobe of the thyroid gland (**about** 70–80% of all cases). Follicular thyroid cancer accounts for **about** 20% of thyroid cancers.
(https://healthand.com/tw/topic/general-report/thyroid-cancer)

In Excerpt 5.11, the elastic quantifier *several* is used to present the types of thyroid cancer in a non-precise fashion. The approximate stretcher *about* functions on both an elastic number (70–80%) and a non-elastic number (20%) to make the items it modifies either more elastic (70–80%) or become elastic (20%). Possible reasons for making approximation here are that the writer may not know the exact number or thinks the exact number is not important in this case.

5.12 Luckily, the odds of beating thyroid cancer tend to be very good: The 5-year survival rate for stage I and stage II papillary or follicular thyroid is **nearly** 100%. (https://www.womenshealth.com.au/4-signs-of-thyroid-cancer-you-should-watch-out-for)

The prognosis for surviving thyroid cancer is *nearly* 100%, which is an approximation. The writer probably does not have an exact figure at hand here and expects that an elastic number should do the job. *Nearly* 100% is a partial elastic number (Channell, 1994): 100% is the upper limit of *nearly* 100%, but the lower limit is unspecified. A partial elastic number differs from a whole elastic number, such as *about* 20, in that the latter's upper and lower limits are both elastic. As opposed to *nearly* n, the other type of partial elastic number, such as *more than* n, has a precise lower limit (n) but a vague upper limit.

5.13 Antigenic shift can also occur if an influenza virus that normally infects an animal species 'makes the jump' to humans. Antigenic shift is a rare event, occurring just once every 10 years **or so**, somewhere in the world. The new strain is very different to existing strains and so catches our immune systems by surprise. The result can be the flu outbreak or epidemic. (https://healthand.com/tw/topic/general-report/the-flu-influenza)

The time span in this excerpt is described as '10 years *or so*' (*or so* makes an elastic number), probably because the writer is not able to provide a precise number. An elastic number seems to be necessary in situations like Excerpt 5.13.

5.2.6 Shortening

This function highlights exemplary items from a long list, as a full exhaustive list is either unavailable or unnecessary (Ruzaitė, 2004, 2007). The data show that a shortened utterance with the help of EL is more effective than a full list.

5.14 Surgery is particularly advantageous in younger patients, those with eye disease, those with suspicion for cancer, those with large glands with pressure symptoms (difficulty in breathing, swallowing, **etc**.), or in whom medical management is difficult or not tolerated. (www.drsenarathedirimanne.com.au/thyroid-surgery/)

The writer states that surgery is advantageous for a number of groups of patients, including those with large glands and pressure symptoms. In brackets, examples of such symptoms are provided instead of giving a long list, and only two exemplary items are given. The general stretcher *etc.* serves to shorten the long list, which is deemed to be unnecessary here in the view of the writer, otherwise more items would have been provided.

5.15 Strategies can be used to decrease your arousal level, if it is too high. This will hopefully increase your sense of control and safety, and help you to face difficult memories and triggers associated with the trauma. A few important tips:
Exercise regularly, and eat a well-balanced diet with regular meals.
Do something relaxing each day.
Find a quiet and relaxing place.
Clear your mind.
Practice the slow breathing method for one minute.
Relax your muscles.
Enjoy the feeling of relaxation.
Practice once or twice every day for at least 8 weeks.
Reducing use of stimulants, such as coffee and cigarettes.
Don't use alcohol or other drugs to help cope. They make it worse.
Plan to do nice things each day.
Get back to a normal routine – regular sleep, meals, **and so on**.
To reduce symptoms of anxiety, learn to slow your breathing by following these directions.
(https://thiswayup.org.au/how-do-you-feel/)

Excerpt 5.15 discusses the strategies for managing anxiety. The writer provides a list of things that may work. When talking about the 'get back to a normal routine' strategy, two exemplary items are mentioned: regular sleep and regular meals. After that, the general extender *and so on* is used, indicating that the writer expects the reader to get the idea from the two items mentioned. All other items that fall into the 'normal routine' category would be understood by the reader, as the writer expects.

5.2.7 Describing Tendency

This function is to describe a common clinical scenario or a medical tendency using EL, without involving any specific numbers. This type of EL presents factual information, with no added tones such as a defensive tone.

5.16 Treatment for thyroid cancer **usually** includes surgery, thyroid hormone replacement therapy and radioactive iodine treatment. **Some** people also need external radiotherapy or chemotherapy.
Most people receive a combination of treatments. The type of treatments your doctor recommends will depend on the type and stage of thyroid cancer that you have. Discuss any preferences or concerns about treatment with your medical team.
(www.riverinacancercare.com.au/patients/cancer-information/types/head-and-neck-cancers/thyroid)

In Excerpt 5.16, a common scenario of thyroid cancer treatment is presented. First, the scalar stretcher *usually* is used to highlight common practices in its treatment: surgery, hormone replacement therapy and radioactive iodine treatment. In addition to this, external radiotherapy or chemotherapy could also be necessary for *some* people. The writer also points out that a combination of the above treatments can be the pattern for *most* people.

5.17 Influenza, or 'the flu' for short, is an infectious viral disease. The flu has plagued humanity for **thousands of** years, with epidemics reported as far back as ancient Greece and Rome. Today, despite the availability of vaccines, the flu is still **very** common throughout the world, **usually** emerging at wintertime.
(https://healthand.com/tw/topic/general-report/the-flu-influenza)

The three elastic expressions in Excerpt 5.17 depict a general picture of flu: it has been going on for *thousands of* years, is still *very* prevalent in the modern world and *usually* occurs in winter. How flu tends to behave is conveyed through the use of these three elastic expressions.

5.18 There is no cure for a cold, but getting **lots of** rest and drinking **plenty of** fluids may help your recovery. There are also **some** over-the-counter medications that can help to relieve some of the symptoms.
(https://healthand.com/tw/topic/general-report/the-common-cold)

Similarly, Excerpt 5.18 describes tendency and gives common advice on how colds can be dealt with. There are three things to be done: get *lots of* rest, drink *plenty of* fluids and take *some* medication. The elasticity in the language used here creates no issues for the reader, otherwise the writer would have swapped it for precise language.

5.2.8 Reporting (Medical Research)

This function features as reporting others' evidence-based medical research findings. It differs from other functions in that the writer talks about other people's opinions rather than his or her own.

5.19 **Some** studies have suggested that people with schizophrenia develop enlarged ventricles, natural connected spaces in between the folds of the brain that carry cerebral spinal fluid, but this finding is not present in all people with schizophrenia.
(https://www.neura.edu.au/health/schizophrenia/extra-information/)

The elastic expression *some* is used here to report studies on schizophrenia research. The writer here cites findings that schizophrenia patients – though not all of them – may develop enlarged ventricles. *Some* indicates a small number, and its elasticity also enables the writer to give no information regarding who these authors are, which may suit the writer's preference.

5.20 There is **some** evidence that the first 5–10 years of schizophrenia are really critical. In this timeframe, the more times a patient has what we call an acute relapse, where the symptoms get worse, the worse the illness becomes over the long term.
(https://healthengine.com.au/info/schizophrenia-1-about-schizophrenia)

Excerpt 5.20 is similar to Excerpt 5.19, where *some* evidence brings out the finding that the critical period of schizophrenia treatment is the first 5–10 years. However, there is a difference between the two excerpts: 5.19 uses the plural but 5.20 uses the singular. This suggests that the former focuses on the quantitative perspective, whereas the latter case has a qualitative focus. This supports the findings in Le and Zhang's (2018) study, where *some* can convey quantitative or qualitative information depending on the context.

5.2.9 Correcting

This function assists in introducing a common medical misconception that is to be dismissed.

5.21 Myth 5: Vaccination will make me ill.
Probably not . . .
Serious adverse reactions to the flu vaccine are rare. The most common reactions are redness and swelling at the injection site.
Allergic reactions are rare but may occur in people with a severe egg allergy – such people should not receive the influenza vaccine.
(https://www.immunisationcoalition.org.au/diseases/influenza)

In Excerpt 5.21, the writer introduces in the misconception ('myth') that vaccination will make people ill, then corrects it using the epistemic stretcher *probably not*. While the writer is not absolutely sure, it is highly likely that vaccination will not make people ill.

5.22 The common cold is an acute infection of the throat and nasal passages. It **may** be caused by several different viruses, the most common of which are rhinoviruses. The term 'common cold' refers to a set of symptoms, rather than a specific disease. Mild influenza **may** have similar symptoms to the common cold. Mild 'strep throat', which is caused by bacteria, **may** be incorrectly classified as a common cold, though usually it is easy for a doctor to distinguish between the two.
(https://healthengine.com.au/info/common-cold)

The writer points out there *may* be confusion between mild influenza and the common cold. The reasons why *may* is used may come down to politeness (Aijmer, 2013), a lack of certainty or self-protection (avoiding being challenged) (Cutting, 2012). For 'self-defence' purposes, the writer here avoids certainty to minimise the threat to him or her if it turns out they have their facts wrong (Trappes-Lomax, 2007).

5.23 **Many** people think that people with schizophrenia have 'dual', 'multiple' or 'split' personalities. This is not correct. People with schizophrenia have one personality, just like everyone else.
(http://www.mydr.com.au/mental-health/schizophrenia-medicines)

In Excerpt 5.23, the writer uses *many* to highlight the fact that the mistaken opinion– that is, schizophrenia sufferers have multiple personalities – is widely spread. This justifies the need to correct it: schizophrenia sufferers have just one personality and, therefore, do not differ from other people in this respect.

5.2.10 Advising Gently

This function is to make the delivery of health advice less strict.

5.24 You **might** feel overwhelmed, scared, anxious or upset if you have been diagnosed with cancer – these are all normal feelings. It's **very** important to have support from family, friends, health professionals or other services to help you cope with cancer.
(www.cancercouncil.com.au/pancreatic-cancer/diagnosis/)

In Excerpt 5.24, medical advice is given in an elastic fashion, with the help of *might* and *very*. The use of *might* gives an impression of a non-forceful statement, rather than saying that a cancer diagnosis will definitely make the patient feel bad. The use of *very* enhances the degree of importance of having support, but the degree to which it is enhanced cannot be precisely measured.

5.25 Drink plenty of fluids: Extra fluids are needed to replace those lost through sweating due to fever. If your urine is dark, you need to drink more. Try to drink a glass of water or juice or an equal amount of **some other** fluid every hour while you are awake.
(www1.health.gov.au/internet/main/publishing.nsf/Content/panflu-individuals-households-lp-1)

The advice given in Excerpt 5.25 is to drink fluids when one has a fever. The three elastic expressions in the excerpt make the advice less strict, as it is either problematic or unnecessary to specify a precise amount in the case of how much to drink or give precise types of *some other* fluid.

5.26 **Frequently** wash your hands, especially before eating.
Keep your fingers away from your eyes, nose and mouth.
Avoid sharing cups, glasses and cutlery.
Avoid close contact with cold sufferers.
Make sure you get immunised against influenza just before winter every year to avoid getting the flu.
(www.mydr.com.au/respiratory-health/colds-commonsense-not-antibiotics)

In Excerpt 5.26, advice is given on washing hands. The elastic expression *frequently* is used here, because it is impossible to advise on a precise number of hand washes. The elastic advice indicates the idea that one should wash one's hands more than the average number of times to keep colds and the flu at bay.

5.2.11 Supporting Emotionally

This function is to provide emotional support to patients by using EL.

5.27 If thyroid cancer is suspected, your doctor **may** order a number of tests. The tests you **may** have depend on your specific situation. Waiting for the test results can be a stressful time. It **may** help to talk to a friend, family member or health professional.
(www.cancercouncil.com.au/thyroid-cancer)

The writer shows empathy towards cancer sufferers and provides emotional support here by encouraging them to talk to people. The epistemic stretcher *may* functions here as a shield to mitigate the tone of the suggestion, to make it more acceptable to the addressee.

5.28 Psychosis can be incredibly stressful for both the person experiencing it and those around them. Becoming distressed yourself can cause the situation to escalate more quickly, so try your best to stay calm. SHOW COMPASSION remember that the person is **likely** to be feeling scared and confused. Where you can, keep them company and reassure them that they're not alone. Showing that you care and not judging them can mean more than you imagine.
(https://healthengine.com.au/info/schizophrenia-1-about-schizophrenia)

The writer encourages the schizophrenia patient's family and friends to show compassion to the patient, as he or she is *likely* not feeling at their best. Note that the elastic expression here functions to make the writer less imposing and more softly-spoken. The point the writer is making here is that emotional support is important in the treatment of schizophrenia patients.

5.29 Self-care treatments are simple strategies that can be done from home that **may** help to manage generalised anxiety disorder and help prevent it from becoming worse. Self-care treatments **may** include allocating time to relax, exercising regularly and avoiding stimulants, such as alcohol and caffeine. Self-care **may** also involve recognising triggers that cause you anxiety and learning to deal with these situations.

As with **many** mental health issues, support from family members and close friends can play an important role in recovery.
(https://healthand.com/au/topic/general-report/generalised-anxiety-disorder)

The writer discusses self-care in the sense of being mentally relaxed, physically strong and so on. The epistemic stretcher *may* is used three times in the first paragraph with an aim to make the suggestions and emotional support less authoritarian and more persuasive, as EL can be used to avoid appearing overly confident (Ruzaitė, 2007: 168). EL can also persuade and exert 'power' on the reader (Cutting, 2012: 286) – namely, vagueness is more persuasive (Lombardi Vallauri, 2016). The writer encourages the reader to seek help from their loved ones because it is important in their recovery – this also applies to *many* other mental issues. The approximate stretcher *many* is used here to highlight the significance of seeking help in managing mental health conditions.

5.3 Correlation between Frequency of Elastic Language and the Six Medical Conditions

This section discusses the pragmatic forms of EL (i.e., four categories) and its distributional difference in the six diseases/conditions.

5.3.1 Frequency of the Four Categories of Elastic Expressions and Top 10 Lexical Items

The four categories of elastic expressions, together with their overall distribution, are shown in Figure 5.2.

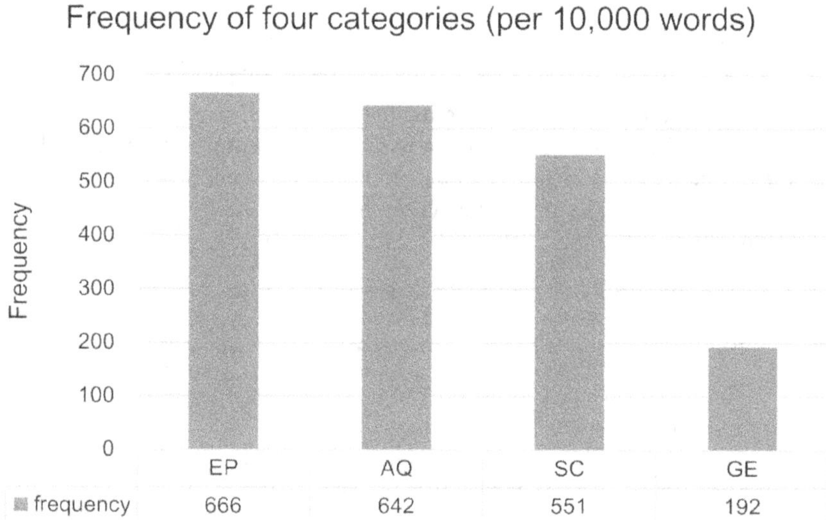

Figure 5.2 Overall distribution of the four categories of EL in English
Note: EP = epistemic stretcher, AQ = approximate stretcher, SC = scalar stretcher and GE= general stretcher.

Figure 5.2 shows that, in the online healthcare information collected for this study, EP is used the most, about three times more than GE. This suggests that the writers tend to communicate medical information by using epistemic expressions, due to factors such as the uncertainty of medical information (Adolphs et al., 2007; Bryant and Norman, 1979; Sarangi and Clarke, 2002) and the need for self-protection in the dissemination of medical information.

Figure 5.3 shows that for the category of approximate stretchers overall, *some* is used most often and *at least* is used the least – about 10 times less often. Quantifiers (without a specific number) are used twice as much as approximators (with a specific number): 1,734 (*some, most, many, a few*) versus 802 (*about, over, more than, up to, or more, at least*). The top three on the list are all quantifiers, suggesting that, when describing amounts, non-numerical expressions are preferred in the data.

In Figure 5.4, *things* referring to general entities is used the most, with the next most frequent expression, *sometimes*, referring to unspecified time. In this category, *some*, unlike *some* in the category of approximate stretchers, does not refer to quantity but to quality. For example, *some* in 'I read *some* book, but cannot remember the name', refers to the level of quality rather than quantity.

There are very few general extenders (Holmes, 1995) in the data, such as *things like that, and all that*, probably due to the nature of written discourse. General extenders tend to occur in conversations rather than in written communications (Terraschke and Holmes, 2007).

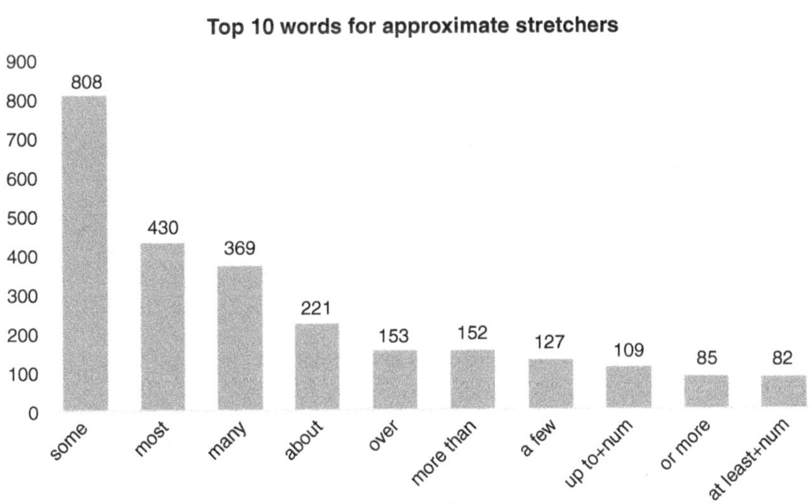

Figure 5.3 Top 10 approximate stretchers in the English corpus

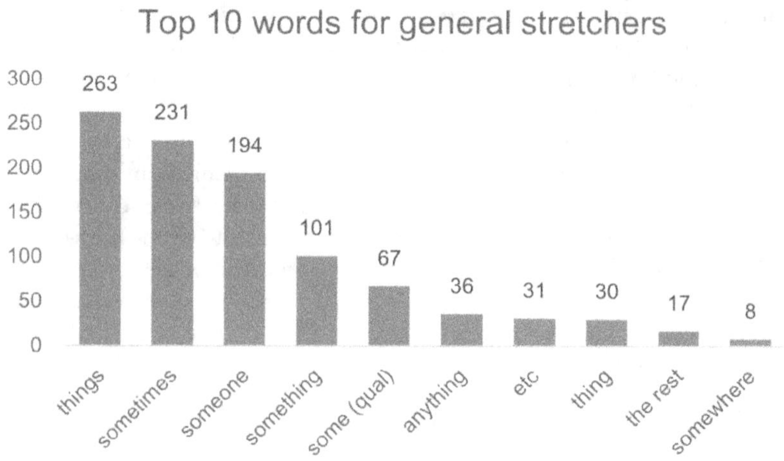

Figure 5.4 Top 10 general stretchers in the English corpus

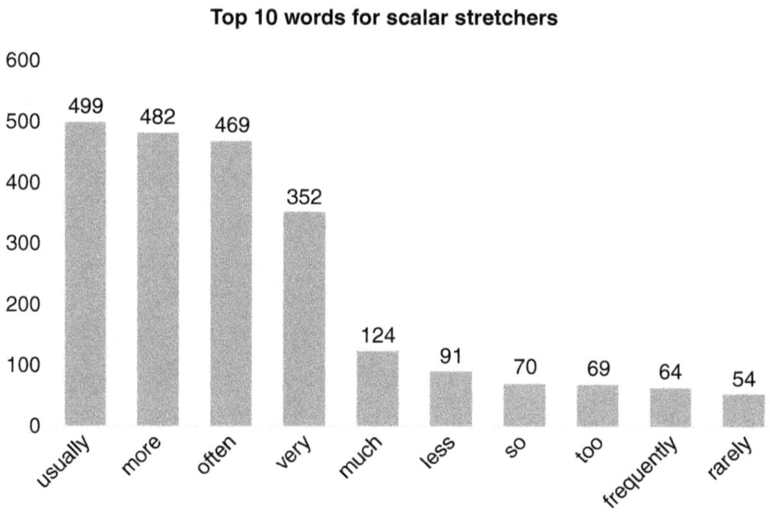

Figure 5.5 Top 10 scalar stretchers in the English corpus

According to Figure 5.5, *usually* is used the most frequently and tends to present a tendency or a common phenomenon in medical information. The next two are *more* and *often*, where they function in a similar way to *usually*. These three frequently used expressions indicate that in online healthcare

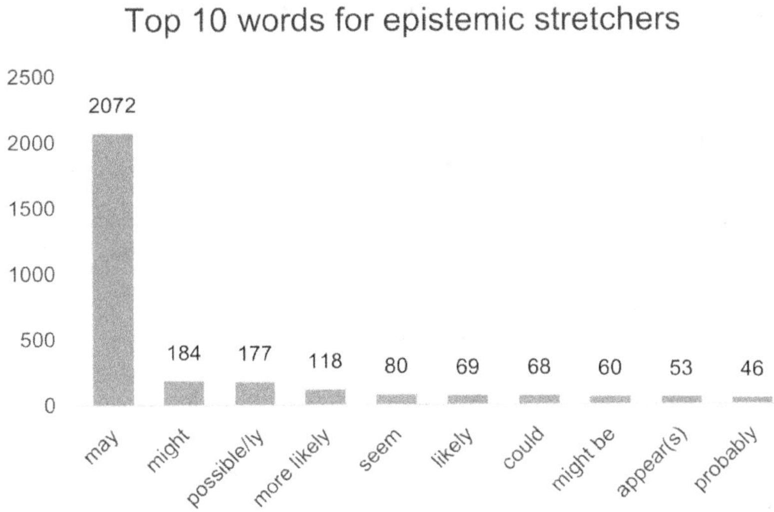

Figure 5.6 Top 10 epistemic stretchers in the English corpus

information, the writers tend to mention common patterns of medical phenomena or people's behaviours using heightened scalar stretchers. The fourth one on the list is *very*, with which the writer can emphasise and enhance a claim. The least used is *rarely*, for which the infrequency may be due to a lack of mentions of rare phenomena in online medical information dissemination or the possible negative tone of *rarely*.

Figure 5.6 shows that for epistemic stretchers *may* is clearly favoured far more than any other items in the group. It appears 20 times more than every other item on the list. Meaning-wise, there is a continuum among the ten items: some items (e.g., *seem*,[1] *appear(s)* and *might*) are at one end (weaker probability), with others at the stronger end (e.g., *more likely* and *probably*). *May* sits somewhere in the middle, which is likely the reason *may* is the most common. *May* expresses a possibility (not too much, not too little), so it is likely to suit more situations than most other items on the list.

5.3.2 Elastic Language Distribution in Six Medical Conditions

Table 5.1 shows that the average rate of EL in the corpus is 3.39%. EL is used most in schizophrenia information and the least in flu information. Except in

[1] *Seem* also includes *seems, seeming, seemingly* here.

Table 5.1 *Distribution of elastic expressions across the six medical conditions*

Condition	SCHIZ	COLD	ANX	THYR	PANC	FLU	Total
EL	801	1,041	3,631	1,606	1,343	1,119	9,541
Total word	19,671	27,737	100,565	48,544	45,208	40,037	281,762
% EL	4.07%	3.75%	3.61%	3.31%	2.97%	2.79%	3.39%
Ranking	1	2	3	4	5	6	

Note: Schizophrenia (SCHIZ), anxiety (ANX), thyroid cancer (THYR), pancreatic cancer (PANC) and influenza (FLU).

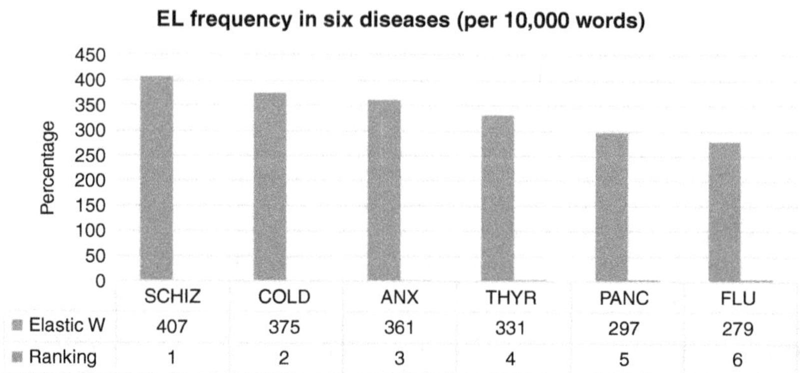

Figure 5.7 Standardised EL frequency across the six diseases

cold information, there is a correlation between the frequency of EL and the sensitivity or severity of the disease information. Both schizophrenia and anxiety are at the top of the list, perhaps because both are mental conditions and more sensitive. This result is in line with the findings of Zhang (2013), where EL was used more in sensitive conversation topics. After the two mental conditions, the two cancer cases (pancreatic and thyroid cancer) use more EL, suggesting that EL is used more for severe diseases. The correlation between EL use and the severity of the case is also found in Zhang (2015). The flu information is found to use the least EL, which is less sensitive and severe compared with the abovementioned mental conditions and cancer cases.

The ranking in Table 5.1 indicates that the writers are less sure about schizophrenia, colds and anxiety than about thyroid cancer, pancreatic cancer and the flu. Given the amount of EL used in the data, the writers may be most sure or less pragmatic about the flu, but much less sure and more pragmatic about schizophrenia.

Figure 5.7 elaborates further on the information presented in Table 5.1 by providing the frequency per 10,000 words. We can see that for every 10,000 words in the corpus, there are 407 elastic expressions for schizophrenia, 32 fewer elastic expressions in the information on colds and 128 fewer elastic words in the information on flu. This shows that information on the Internet about psychological conditions is more elastically phrased than it is for most of the other diseases.

5.4 Correlations between Pragmatic Forms, Pragmatic Functions and Six Types of Diseases

This section looks at the relationships between (1) pragmatic forms and their functions, and (2) pragmatic forms and six diseases. These analyses show the interconnection between form, function and medical condition, revealing further tendencies.

5.4.1 Pragmatic Forms and Their Functions

There is a correlational difference between first-order (individual-utterance-focused) and second-order (holistic-discourse-focused) pragmatic functions. For those that are first order, there are correlations between pragmatic forms and functions; for those that are second order, there is no such neat correspondence, as the second-order functions tend to employ a wider range of pragmatic forms with a limited one-to-one match.

Based on the data analysis presented in Section 5.2, for the first-order pragmatic functions, the following correspondences may hold.

1. The softening function tends to be performed by the epistemic stretcher.
2. The avoiding function tends to be performed by the general stretcher.
3. The intensifying function tends to be performed by the scalar stretcher.
4. The deintensifying function tends to be performed by the scalar stretcher.
5. The approximating function tends to be performed by the approximate stretcher.
6. The shortening function tends to be performed by the general stretcher/ general extender.

For the second-order functions, including tendency describing, reporting, correcting, advising gently and supporting emotionally, there is no tendency to focus on a specific form. Instead, they use more than one form, often a range of forms. This is because the nature of the second-order functions is such that they perform a general function carried out by multiple elastic forms.

5.4.2 *Pragmatic Forms and the Six Diseases*

In Section 5.3.2, a trend emerged in the data showing that the more severe or sensitive a medical condition is, the higher the frequency of EL used. Anxiety and schizophrenia information advises on potentially stigmatising chronic illnesses, and it used more EL than information such as that on the flu in this study. This is because people tend to use indirect language to describe diseases and their symptoms, especially talking about serious cases – for example, pre-symptoms of cervical cancer can be referred to as 'dysplasia' (literally 'wrong formation'), and a case of gross negligence on the part of the hospital was described as a 'medical mistake' (Mey, 2016b: 129).

As Figure 5.8 shows, within each of the six diseases, AQ is used most frequently within thyroid cancer information and again in flu information. It seems that imprecise quantities are preferred when professionals disseminate online information on these two diseases. On the other hand, EP tops the remaining four medical conditions: anxiety, schizophrenia, pancreatic cancer and colds. EP tends to be used to mitigate the certainty and authority of a claim made. Three out of the four cases are more sensitive (anxiety and schizophrenia, two mental conditions) and severe (pancreatic cancer). The findings presented in Figure 5.8 further strengthen the claim made previously that there is a correlation between sensitivity/severity and the use of EL.

For the other two types, scalar and general stretchers, neither occupy the top rank for any of the six medical conditions. However, scalar stretchers are used fairly frequently in describing colds and in schizophrenia information, suggesting that in these two cases, the writers need to either increase or decrease the

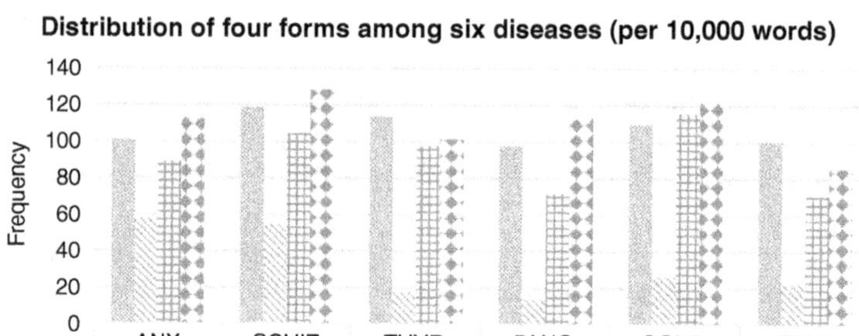

	ANX	SCHIZ	THYR	PANC	COLD	FLU
AQ	101	119	114	98	110	101
GE	58	55	17	14	26	22
SC	89	105	98	72	116	71
EP	113	129	102	113	123	86

Figure 5.8 EL frequency for the six diseases

Table 5.2 *Top 10 elastic terms in the six medical conditions (frequency per 10,000 words)*

	ANX	#	SCHIZ	#	COLD	#	FLU	#	THYR	#	PANC	#
1	may	73	may	76	may	70	may	51	may	77	may	92
2	some AQ	35	some AQ	39	more SC	30	some AQ	20	usually	27	some AQ	24
3	more SC	21	many	27	some AQ	28	usually	19	most AQ	24	usually	19
4	things	20	very	24	usually	27	most AQ	17	some AQ	23	often	18
5	often	19	often	23	often	16	very	11	very	19	most AQ	12
6	many	17	things	19	very	14	more SC	11	about	17	about	12
7	most AQ	12	someone	18	most AQ	13	up to	10	more SC	17	over	9
8	might	11	most AQ	17	many	12	over	10	often	14	many	8
9	someone	10	more SC	17	more likely	10	possible(y)	9	many	9	possible(y)	8
10	very	10	usually	16	more than	9	someone	8	(a) few	8	sometimes	8

strength of their claims. General stretchers, lacking specific information, seem to be less preferred in providing online medical information to the public.

As Table 5.2 shows, among the top 10 words used across the six diseases, *may* sits at the top for all six. As stated previously, *may* can express possibility as well as uncertainty, which suits both particular and universal scenarios when communicating medical information. The elastic quantifier *some* is ranked second from the top for four diseases out of six, and *some* also appears in third or fourth place for the remaining two diseases. This suggests that an imprecise quantity, such as *some*, also suits the dissemination of medical information. In Table 5.2, while *usually* is used frequently for the other four diseases, this is not the case for the two mental conditions. It seems that for the two mental conditions, *often* is preferred over *usually* when describing a tendency.

5.5 Concluding Remarks

The English data in this chapter show that the most prevalent elastic expression is *may*, which occurs 10 times more often than the least frequent, *sometimes*. The second most common expression, *some*, occurs four times more often than *sometimes*. This indicates that *may* is a much more popular choice of word than the remaining nine words on the top-10 list, explained by the fact that medical information is a matter of probability rather than being categorical.

6 Comparison between Chinese and English Regarding Elastic Language Use

This chapter compares the findings as presented in Chapters 4 and 5. While describing the similarities and differences in the results based on the Chinese and English data, we seek to explain the comparison from a cross-cultural perspective that considers multiple dimensions such as different diseases, health communication style, language-specific features, rhetorical convention and culture.

6.1 Pragmatic Forms of Elastic Language: Top 10 Elastic Expressions in Chinese and English

By comparing the lists of the top 10 elastic terms in the Chinese and English corpora, respectively (see Figure 6.1), we identify a few differences as well as similarities. Some of the top elastic terms in Chinese have English counterparts – not necessarily equivalents but words expressing similar or near-similar meanings – also found on the English top 10 list. They are *keneng* (可能) and *may*, *chang* (常)/*tongchang* (通常) and *usually/often*, *hen* (很) and *very*, *geng* (更) and *more*, and *duo* (多)/*xuduo* (許多) and *many/most*. These cover epistemic, scalar and approximate stretchers.

By contrast, there are also four striking differences, which shed light on significant cross-linguistic and cross-cultural differences. First, the number-one elastic term in the English corpus – the epistemic stretcher *may* – occurred more than twice as frequently as the second-ranked elastic term *some*. But the most-used stretcher in the Chinese data is the general extender *deng* (等 'etc.'), and the gap in frequency count between *deng* and the second-place word (*keneng* 可能 'may/possibly') is not as considerable as in the English data. This suggests that the epistemic stretcher *may* is used in English health communication to a much larger extent than any other stretcher in the English data. The significance of this finding is reinforced when the total frequency counts of the four categories of EL in the Chinese corpus and those in the English corpus are compared (see Sections 6.3–6.4), as epistemic stretchers are dominant in the English data. Second, while the most frequently used stretcher in the Chinese

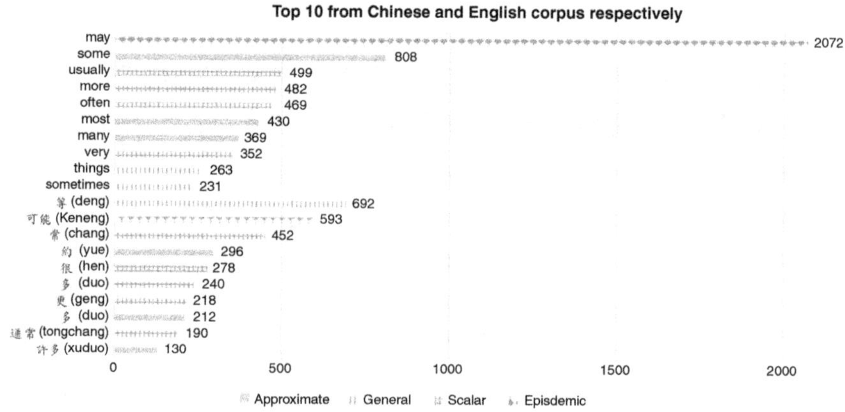

Figure 6.1 Top 10 elastic terms in Chinese and English

corpus is the general stretcher *deng*, the only stretcher of its kind on the Chinese top-10 list, the most-used general stretcher on the English top-10 list is *things* (see Section 6.3 below for further discussion). This difference might be due to a disparity in deep-rooted cultural assumptions between *deng* and *etc./and so on/and so forth*. In English, general extenders such as *etc.* are not considered very compatible with scientific writing. For example, an Australian university's site that helps with academic writing states: 'Avoid using run-on expressions' such as *and so on* and *etc.*[1] Health communication is usually expected to be based on scientific research and, therefore, general extenders tend to be avoided as well. Nevertheless, the same cultural assumption regarding general extenders in English is not held in Chinese. Instead, providing a short list that ends with *deng* allows for some details to be given while making the information concise for the reader. Furthermore, *deng* is not restricted to informal genres or occasions but is widely used across formal and informal discourse types as long as the unstated information is assumed to be shared or traceable. In other words, the established convention regarding a specific general extender affects whether and where it tends to be used.

Third, both *some*, when used to express quantity, and *sometimes* are found on the top-10 English list. By contrast, the Chinese elastic terms expressing similar meanings – for example, *yixie* (一些)/*youxie* (有些 'some') and *youshi* (有時 'sometimes') – are not on the top-10 Chinese list (Figure 6.1). This suggests information applicable to the medium-range quantity (i.e., between *few/little* and *many/much*) or to a moderate time frequency (between *rarely* and

[1] This quotation was retrieved on 8 April 2022 from https://bit.ly/3KmPFJD.

frequently) is significant to the writing of health communication in English, but less so in Chinese. Fourth, *yue* (約 'about') is on the Chinese list but not on its English counterpart. This suggests that quantitative information in health communication in Chinese relies on *yue* to a larger extent than *about* when it is used to deliver health communication in English. In other words, in terms of approximate stretchers, the English health information collected relies more on non-number stretchers (e.g., *some*, *most* and *many*) than on the number-based *about*.

Zhang (2015: 79) presented a list of the top 20 elastic terms based on a TV documentary series featuring authentic spoken conversations that took place at international airports and international mail centres in Australia. The top 10 terms on Zhang's (2015) list and our top-10 list of elastic terms in the English health data share only three words, *very*, *some* and *things*, suggesting that the overall use of EL is affected by topic and context. Chen (2007) identified the top 10 vague items based on the Hong Kong Corpus of Spoken English (HKCSE), which covers different spoken genres and contexts – for example, academic talks, business discourse, conversation and public discourse. The top-10 list in HKCSE and our top-10 list based on the English data share six items: *very*, *some*, *more*, *many*, *things* and *most*. This suggests that these vague/elastic terms are not restricted to spoken data but are also used in online written health discourse. There are four items that are on our top-10 list but not present on its HKCSE-based counterpart: *may*, *usually*, *often* and *sometimes*. The epistemic stretcher *may* is not on Chen's (2007: 165) list. This is not necessarily because it was used infrequently but because her study of VL did not cover epistemic items. The relatively high frequencies of the four elastic items found only on our list suggest EL use is to some extent genre-specific, an observation that reinforces Chen's (2007) finding. Three Chinese elastic expressions corresponding to three out of the four elastic terms in English – *keneng* (可能 'possibly/may'), *chang* (常 'often') and *tongchang* (通常 'usually') – are also found on the top-10 list based on the Chinese health data, thus further supporting the notion that EL use to some extent is genre-specific. Another way to further justify this observation is to examine the functions of EL because the same elastic term, when used in different discourse types, may have different functions. We next turn to the functions of EL in the health context.

6.2 Pragmatic Functions of Elastic Language

According to our accounts of the pragmatic functions of EL in Chinese and English, the eleven functions, either first- or second-order, are found in both corpora. This probably comes as no surprise since there are many elastic expressions in both languages, and the corpora consist of similar genres, which serve similar social functions. Based on the examples outlined in

Chapters 4 and 5, Table 6.1 shows the type(s) of elastic expressions usually associated with each of the eleven pragmatic functions. Elastic terms that can perform second-order functions are diverse and wide-ranging. Therefore, there is no direct connection between an elastic term and a specific second-order function. The identification of a second-order function is highly reliant on the context. Where appropriate, we highlight cues (cf. Gumperz 1982: 131–132) – that is, expressions signalling how a pragmatic function of one or more elastic terms is to be interpreted in the sentence where the elastic term or set of such terms occurs. The lexical cue is usually in the sentence, the preceding sentence or in the sentence that follows.

Table 6.1 *Pragmatic functions and their associated elastic terms*

First-order Function	EL in Chinese	EL in English
Softening	Epistemic stretchers – for example, *keneng* (可能 'may/possibly'), *sihu* (似乎 'seem'), *buyiding* (不一定 'not necessarily')	Epistemic stretchers – for example, *may, could, might, possible, possibly, likely, seem*
Avoiding	General stretchers: *mouxie* (某些 'some'), *mouzhong* (某種 'some sort'), *youren* (有人 'someone'), *shiqing* (事情 'stuff/thing')	General stretchers: *someone, something, somewhere, anything else, things*
Intensifying	High-end scalar stretchers: *hen* (很 'very'), *ji* (極 'extremely'), *xiangdang* (相當 'quite'), *yuan* (遠 'far'), *guo* (過 'over-/too'), *guodu* (過度 'too much'), *tai* (太 'too') and *geng* (更 'more')	High-end scalar stretchers: *more, far more, very, quite, most* (plus a modifier), *really*
Deintensifying	Low-end scalar stretchers: *jin* (僅 'just'), *shaowei* (稍微 'slightly'), *qingwei* (輕微 'a bit'), *youdian* (有點 'a little bit') and *xiexu* (些許 'a little')	Low-end scalar stretchers: *less, slightly, a bit, a little, somewhat*
Approximating	Approximate stretchers (with a number): *yue* (約 'about'), *dayue* (大 約 'about'), *yishang* (以上 'over'), *yixia* (以下 'under/less than'), *zhuoyou* (左右 'or so'); (without a number): *henduo* (很多 'many'); *bufen* (部份 'part of'), *youxie* (有些 'some')	Approximate stretchers (with a number): *about, approximately, more than, before,* after, *under*; (without a number): *many, some, a few*
Shortening	General stretchers – for example, *deng* (等 'etc.'), *dengdeng* (等等 'and so forth')	General stretchers: *etc., and so on, and so forth*

Table 6.1 (*cont.*)

First-order Function	EL in Chinese	EL in English
Second-order Function	EL in Chinese and cues that facilitate the identification of the function	EL in English and cues that facilitate the identification of the function
Describing tendency	Typically co-use of more than one stretcher of the same or different categories	Refer to the content in the first column
Reporting research	Cues: an approximate stretcher (e.g., *xuduo* 許多 'many/much', *youxie* 有些 'some') followed by a research-related noun (e.g., *yanjiou* 研究 'research/ studies', *faxian* 發現 'findings', *xuezhe* 學者 'scholar')	Cues: an approximate stretcher (e.g., *some*, *many*) followed by a noun signifying research (e.g., *studies*, *evidence*, *findings*)
Correcting	Cues: *cuo* (錯 'wrong'), *cuowu* (錯誤 'mistake'), *wuyiwei* (誤以為 'mistakenly believe'), *budui* (不對 'incorrect[ly]'), *misi* (迷思 'misconception') or a negative evaluative expression (e.g., *shideqifan* (適得其反 'counter-productive'), *tulaowugong* (徒勞無功 'futile')	Cues: *myth*, *incorrect(ly)*
Advising gently	Cues: imperatives, *duo* followed by a verb phrase (e.g., *duo xiuxi* 多休息 'rest frequently'), *qianyi* (建議 'you are advised to') and *bimian* (避免 'avoid . . . ')	Cues: imperatives (e.g., *we suggest that you . . . , it's very important to . . . , you need to . . .*)
Supporting emotionally	Cues: expressions indicating negative emotions (e.g., *jinhuangshicuo* 驚慌失措 'be seized with panic', *guodu dianxin* 過度擔心 'worry too much', *wufa kongzhi de qingxu* 無法控制的情緒 'uncontrollable emotions')	Cues: second-person pronoun (*you*), and words expressing negative emotions (e.g., *stressful*, *scared*, *confused*, *distressed*)

The expansion from the first- to the second-order functions echoes 'a path of development from a *more referential to a more interpersonal* function' (Overstreet, 2011: 309, emphasis added), as the first-order functions attend more to the propositional content of EL and the second-order functions deal more with the writer's interaction with the reader, whether it involves telling the reader about a health tendency, reporting health research, or advising or correcting him/her. Indeed, some interesting similarities and subtle, language-specific differences emerge when we juxtapose contrastive examples from the Chinese and English corpora collected for this study and relate them to their respective frequency distribution of EL (e.g., Figure 6.1). We highlight four points related to four functions, softening, shortening, correcting and advising gently, as they seem to serve as good examples for a cross-cultural comparison in terms of similarities and/or differences. As language is inseparable from culture (Hymes, 1962; Silverstein, 1976), our account of the similarities and differences is both cross-linguistic and cross-cultural.

First, *keneng* (可能 'likely/possibly') and *may* are the most used epistemic stretchers in the Chinese and English corpora, respectively. They each have a much higher frequency count than the next stretcher from the same category (cf. Figures 4.6 and 5.6). *Keneng* was used almost 40 times as frequently as *sihu* (似乎 'seem'), and *may* occurred almost 25 times as frequently as *might*. Despite their difference in grammatical status (i.e., *keneng* as an adjectival verb and *may* as a modal verb), they serve the same function of softening statements, and their being by far the most frequently used epistemic stretchers in the two corpora is not a coincidence but motivated by two factors. One is their potential for a combination with other stretchers in performing second-order functions – for example, describing tendency, advising gently and supporting emotionally. The other factor is their compatibility with the very nature of medicine, which is scientific but not always categorical. In English, *may* indicates a stronger possibility than *could* and *might*. Its relatively strong possibility allows the health professional to articulate medical facts that can have exceptions. *Keneng* in Chinese is more certain than other Chinese epistemic stretchers such as *sihu* ('seem') and, at the same time, its interpretations could cover a wide range of degrees of possibility as expressed by *may*, *could* and *might*, especially when it is modified by an adverb of degree (e.g., *youdian* 有點 'a bit' or *hen* 很 'very'. Even though a degree modifier is not present where *keneng* is used, the epistemic term can still be flexibly interpreted. As was pointed out in Chapter 4, this wide spectrum of probability degrees that can be accorded to *keneng* makes it possible to replace *sihu* with *keneng* but not vice versa (see Section 4.3.4). Despite the syntactic and semantic differences between *keneng* and *may*, they are the most appropriate epistemic stretchers in the Chinese and English health data because of their respective advantages over other epistemic terms in Chinese and English.

Second, the function of shortening a list is served by general extenders – for example, *deng* in Chinese and *etc.* in English. *Deng* is the most frequently used stretcher, at 692 counts (see Figure 6.1) in the Chinese corpus. Although *etc.* is used in the English data, at 31 counts in total (see Figure 5.4), neither *etc.* nor its equivalents (e.g., *and so on*, *and so forth*) are on the top-10 list of elastic terms in English. This difference in distribution suggests that the function of shortening a list is activated much more frequently when online health information is delivered in Chinese than in English. As has been pointed out in Section 6.1, the difference may be due to different cultural attitudes towards the use of the two general extenders: *deng* in Chinese and *etc.* in English. While *deng* (等) is a common, acceptable general extender in formal Chinese writing, *et cetera*, or its shortened form *etc.*, though having a formal connotation due to its Latin origin, is usually discouraged in scientific writing in English. The difference is underpinned by a set of sociocultural assumptions regarding a particular general extender – specifically, under what situation it is normally used, what it is conventionally used for and when it is to be avoided. Some previous studies based on conversational data have pointed out that general extenders such as *and so on*, *and things like that* and *and stuff like that* have a referential meaning (Dines, 1980; Jefferson 1990) and also serve an interpersonal function (e.g., to be polite or maintain solidarity; Overstreet, 1999, 2005). However, in contrast to the general extenders widely used in conversations, *etc.* is the one used in formal written health information and its use is quite limited. Instead, it is the general noun *things* that takes the lead in the category of general stretchers. *Things* does not necessarily replace the function of shortening, but *things* is admissible in the context of formal English writing due to its capacity for the creation of textual cohesion as it conveniently links with items mentioned in the text (Halliday and Hasan, 1976: 274–282).

Third, the way advice is delivered in Chinese and English is not always the same, and this affects and is also reflected in the overall frequency counts of EL. For example, in Chinese, when used as an adverb, *duo* is often placed before a verb to deliver gentle advice (see Chapter 4). Partly because it can modify a range of verbs and adjectives and partly because its being placed before a verb has become a formulaic way of offering advice in Chinese, *duo* as a scalar stretcher is on the top-10 list of Chinese elastic terms. The use of *duo* as an adverb is a case of grammaticalisation, as *duo* as a quantifier has changed to an adverb modifying verbs (Chen, 2008). The grammaticalisation does not completely remove the meaning of quantity from *duo* as an adverb because it can be understood to mean 'more', including more times or higher frequency. For example, *duo he shui* (多喝水) can be understood to mean 'drink water frequently' and/or 'drink more water', although *duo* as part of a construction should be an adverb.

By contrast, in English, *frequently* and *more* are two separate words. In our English corpus, we only occasionally find that English examples of advice formed using an imperative containing *frequently* – for example, *Wash your hands <u>frequently</u>, especially before eating* or *Eat small meals <u>frequently</u>, e.g. every 2–3 hours*. The elastic term *frequently* is not on the top-10 list of English elastic terms. In English, sometimes not specifying how frequently an action (e.g., *eating*) should be conducted could sound odd. For example, when someone has the flu, offering advice in English such as *Eat nutritional food frequently* might sound a bit odd as *frequently* can mean from every five minutes to every week. Instead, saying *Eat nutritional food regularly* would be more natural. However, in a similar context it is acceptable to say in Chinese *duo chi you yingyang de shiwu* (多吃有營養的食物 'Eat nutritional food frequently'). There appear to be different cultural constraints on how advice is delivered in different languages and cultures. In the similar health context, in Chinese *duo* followed by a verb phrase has become a common way of suggesting what is to be encouraged, and it is so widely used that *duo* plus a verb phrase has become a formulaic way of giving the addressee gentle advice to take a suggested action; in English, however, *frequently* does not have the same status.[2]

Fourth, the function of correcting is found in the Chinese and English corpora, but there appears to be one subtle difference. When misconceived health information is referred to, apart from using blatantly problematic terms such as *incorrect(ly)*, the term *myth* is often used in the English corpus, for example, *MYTH 1: Influenza is not serious. Influenza (the flu) is a highly contagious and for some people it's a potentially life-threatening disease*. *Myth*, which originally alluded to a literary genre (i.e., ancient stories), is a lexical term available in English to refer to a false idea or belief. Although the term *shenhua* (神話 'myth') is available in Chinese, according to our data, it is not used to refer to a misconception in the health context. In Chinese, some health professionals resort to *chengyu* (成語), a type of traditional Chinese idiomatic expression consisting of four characters or syllables, especially those idioms indicating a negative evaluation – for example, *shideqifan* (適得其反 'counter-productive'; see Excerpt 4.27), or *tulaowugong* (徒勞無功 'futile'; see 4.28). Such expressions are derived from classical Chinese and are often associated with old wisdom. We believe the use of these Chinese expressions to refer to a health misconception may have an effect similar to that of using *myth* when referring to incorrectly conceived health information delivered in English, because both seem to appeal to the connotative meaning of something centuries-old and classical (i.e., *chengyu* in Chinese and *myth* in English).

6.3 Frequency Distribution among the Four Categories

As has been pointed out, the overall pattern of the four categories of EL in Chinese in order of the most to the least used is SC-AQ-GE-EP (see Chapter 4) while its English counterpart is EP-AQ-SC-GE (Chapter 5). The difference is

[2] In the context of the COVID-19 pandemic, the advice *Wash hands frequently* has been constantly used. The use of *frequently* in the context seems to encourage a sense of urgency as washing hands as frequently as possible helps stop the spread. But *duo* in Chinese does not have a similar connotation.

striking, as the sequences of the two patterns are totally different except for the second-place category in both (i.e., AQ, approximate stretchers). The most frequently used category in the English corpus – epistemic stretchers – is the least used in the Chinese corpus. Furthermore, the most frequently used category of EL in the Chinese data is scalar stretchers, but it is ranked third in the English data.

The overall differences, together with the one similarity, suggest that, although approximate quantification is significant in both the Chinese and English data, the Chinese health information attends most to details that involve comparisons (*geng*), intensification (*hen*) and commonality (*chang*, *duo*), while the English counterpart acts mostly to make health statements less absolute (*may*, *might*, *possibly*) and to open a door for exceptions and counter-examples. On the one hand, the difference reflects variation in ways of delivering health information, even if it concerns the same health condition. The variation in the use of EL may be due to the complexity of medicine. The heavy use of epistemic stretchers in the English data indexes the health professionals' high awareness that medicine is not always categorical, and the information being delivered should reflect this aspect of medicine lest the information be misleading. By contrast, the heavier use of scalar stretchers than epistemic stretchers in the Chinese data evinces a different collective mindset that prioritises intensification and commonality. This emphasis pertains to a different dimension of medicine, as comparisons of symptoms, conditions and treatments are helpful to the reader, as is the description of health tendencies using *often* or *usually*. General stretchers are the third-place category of EL in the Chinese data, constituting over 60% of the standardised frequency count of the first-place scalar stretchers (see Figure 4.2). In the English data, general stretchers are the least used category of EL and represent approximately 30% of the most used category (see Figure 5.2), suggesting that the category is used to a lesser extent than its Chinese counterpart.

The brief comparison in the overall distribution of the four categories suggests that the ways the four categories are concocted in health communication vary in different cultures. We now take a closer look at each category and compare the most-used elastic terms of each category in the Chinese and English data. In terms of approximate stretchers, a very interesting contrast between the Chinese and English corpora emerges. In the English data (see Figure 5.3), the top three approximate stretchers are non-number ones – that is, *some*, *most* and *many*, followed by *about* and *over*, both of which occur with a round number. By contrast, in the Chinese data (see Figure 4.3), the first and third approximate stretchers – *yue* ('about') and *yishang* ('more than') – are followed or preceded by a number, and the second one *duo* may occur with a number when it appears in the linguistic environment with a verb such as *chaoguo* (超過 'exceed') or *gaoda* (高達 'be as high as'). In other words, as far as the top five approximate stretchers are concerned, online health information in English relies much more on non-number stretchers than number-based stretchers, while its Chinese counterpart does not have a huge gap between number and non-number-based stretchers. Furthermore, while *yixie* ('some') is ranked fifth in the Chinese data, about one-third of the count of the top stretcher *yue* ('about'), in the English data, *some* appears five times as frequently as the fifth-ranked stretcher, *over*. The enormously high frequency count of *some* approximately constitutes the adding up of the counts of *most* and *many*, ranked second and third, respectively. When delivering the quantitative aspect of health information in English, health professionals prefer *some* to *many*, *most* or *about*, suggesting the significance of details concerning 'next-to-most' phenomena in online health information. This may be due to the appropriateness of using the term for any quantity where a number is unavailable or unnecessary, as it fits such situations better than *many* or *most*. On the other hand, the common use of *some* also echoes the use of *may*, the most frequently used stretcher in the English data, in that both *some* and *may* contribute to qualifying statements, making them less absolute and more open to variation.

Regarding general stretchers, there is one striking similarity and one difference between the Chinese and English corpora. The similarity is that on their respective top-five lists (see Figures 4.4 and 5.4), three of the top five elastic terms are similar in meaning – specifically, *youshi* (有時) corresponding to *sometimes*, *mouxie* (某些) to qualitative *some* and *youren* (有人) to *someone*. The obvious difference is the number-one term: *deng* ('*etc*.') in Chinese versus *things* in English. In English, the general extender *things like that* tends to be used in conversations (Terraschke and Holmes, 2007). Nevertheless, based on our English corpus, the general noun *things* is the most frequent general stretcher, suggesting that it is not regarded as too colloquial to be used in written health information. We believe there are two reasons. One is that its advantage of being flexible in covering all manner of items and behaviours outweighs its association with more colloquial expressions. The other reason is that in writing, a general noun like *things* contributes to creating cohesion (Halliday and Hasan, 1976: 274–282) as *things* can cohere with many nouns mentioned in the text (e.g., *hallucinations* and *delusions*). By contrast, in the Chinese corpus, *deng* ('etc.') is the top general stretcher because, in Chinese writing, using *deng* has become a convention, and this may be attributed to the conciseness facilitated by *deng* as it both introduces a certain amount of information and helps prevent offering too much information. The difference in the most-used general stretcher in the Chinese and English data may be motivated by a respective rhetoric deeply rooted in the writing of health communication in Chinese and English. While Chinese health information relies mostly on the general extender *deng* for the expanding coverage of health information, English resorts most often to the general noun *things* for a wider application of the health aspect being described. Albeit in different ways, the two terms confirm the Maxim of Quantity being observed (Grice, 1975) and reveal how it is differently realised in health communication delivered in the two languages. There are sociocultural conventions and constraints that shape the use of EL (cf. Chapter 9).

Concerning the category of scalar stretchers, there appear to be striking similarities between the Chinese and English corpora. On their respective top five list of scalar terms (see Figures 4.5 and 5.5), although their order is not exactly identical, four of them are similar across the lists: *hen*, *chang*, *tongchang* and *geng* in Chinese correspond in meaning to *very*, *often*, *usually* and *more* in English, respectively.[3] Furthermore, all of the terms on the top-five lists of their kind are high-end stretchers. Indeed, only *shao* (少 'rarely/infrequently/less') appears on the top-10 list of Chinese scalar terms, and only *less* and *rarely*, both of which correspond to *shao*, occur on the English list. Compared with the English data (see Figure 5.2), the Chinese data utilise more scalar stretchers than any other category (see Figure 4.2). Nevertheless, the similarities between the Chinese and English data in the use of these high-end scalar stretchers imply their constant references to common health scenarios and intensifications. *Duo* in Chinese, when used as a scalar stretcher, has the meanings of *more* and *frequently*.[4] In the latter case, *duo* is often used to perform the function of advising. Although in English *frequently* could be used with imperatives to form advice, in our English data it does not occur as consistently as *duo* in Chinese. This may be due to the use of the construction '*duo*+verb' having become an expression in Chinese functioning as advice, but according to our data, its English counterpart has not gained the same status.

The comparison of the top five epistemic stretchers on the Chinese and English lists reveals an interesting similarity: there is an enormous gap in frequency count between the most frequently used stretcher and the next. *Keneng* (可能 'possibly/may') in Chinese occurred almost 40 times as frequently as *sihu* (似乎 'seem'; see Figure 4.6). On the English list, *may* appeared more than ten times as frequently as *might*, ranked second (see Figure 5.6). This similarity suggests that there is an overall favourite epistemic stretcher in online health information in Chinese and English. Compared with the second-place epistemic term on the list in Chinese and English, the favourite shows a relatively stronger possibility, suggesting that, when uncertainty arises, online health information prefers a relatively-strong-possibility epistemic stretcher than one that carries higher uncertainty.

[3] *Duo* and *much*, when used as a scalar stretcher, are not the same in meaning, as *duo* has the meaning of *frequently*, but *much* does not necessarily refer to time frequency.

[4] For example, *duo* in the expression *duo jia yidiandian qiaosi* (多加一點點巧思 'Add a bit more creative thought') is an adverb modifying the verb *jia* ('add') and carries a meaning similar to *more*, though in the English translation *more* is an adjective.

6.4 Correlations between the Four Categories and Six Types of Diseases

In terms of the distribution of the four categories of EL in relation to the six health conditions, the Chinese and English corpora each have their own distinctive patterns from the most-used to the least-used category of EL (see Figures 4.7 and 5.8). In the Chinese data, two patterns emerge: SC-AQ-GE-EP in information specific to four diseases (i.e., the common-disease and cancer clusters) and SC-GE-AQ-EP in the two mental-condition sub-corpora. By contrast, in the English data, two different patterns can be identified: EP-AQ-SC-GE, applicable to four health conditions (cold, pancreatic cancer, anxiety disorder and schizophrenia) and AQ-EP-SC-GE identified in the other two diseases (flu and thyroid cancer). Specifically, in the Chinese data, scalar stretchers occur most frequently, and epistemic stretchers appear least frequently across the six disease-specific sub-corpora. Nevertheless, in the English corpus, epistemic stretchers take the lead in four diseases, and approximate stretchers are the most-used category in the other two diseases while scalar and general stretchers consistently occupy third and fourth place, respectively.

In the Chinese data, the two patterns happen to correspond to non-mental and mental health conditions. One explanation is that the relatively sensitive nature of mental health could make quantification less desirable, and for this reason, approximate stretchers are less used (i.e., in third place). However, whether the health condition is mental or not does not help differentiate the two patterns derived from the English data, as the EP-AQ-SC-GE pattern is applicable to four of the conditions, including the two mental conditions. By contrast, information relating to thyroid cancer and flu utilises more cases of approximate stretchers than epistemic ones. One possible explanation is that the two diseases are among those suitable for quantification due to the complexity of flu virus types, vaccines and/or the availability of abundant clinical research on the diseases. The counts of approximate stretchers in the Chinese data are also relatively high (i.e., ranked second). Nevertheless, epistemic stretchers, the least used category of EL in the Chinese data, are used most in the English data. This finding suggests that other dimensions such as language and culture may affect the use of EL more than disease types (see Chapter 10 for further discussion).

As regards whether an increased use of a specific category of EL corresponds to the more severe disease in each disease cluster, the Chinese corpus demonstrates more correlations of this type than the English corpus. There are eight cases of such correlations in the Chinese data. For example, more uses of approximate stretchers correlated with the more severe disease in the common-disease cluster, the cancer cluster and the mental-condition cluster (see Figure 4.7). In the English data, only four cases emerge: more uses of approximate, scalar and epistemic stretchers correlated with the more severe disease in the mental-health cluster, and more counts of epistemic stretchers correlated with the more severe disease in the cancer cluster (see Figure 5.8). In other words, in the English data, the mental-health cluster exhibits three of the four cases, suggesting that sensitivity of mental-health conditions may facilitate such correlations in the English data. Even where possible correlations might not exist between the four categories of EL and the severity of the disease, it is also important to identify specific elastic terms in each category that play a salient role in relation to a specific disease or disease cluster.

Let us next compare how specific elastic terms in Chinese and English may relate to specific health conditions (see Tables 4.2 and 5.2). Some striking similarities are identified in the Chinese and English corpora. For example, three approximate stretchers in Chinese and their corresponding terms in English behave similarly: *hen* (很), *yixie* (一些) and *xuduo* (許多) and their corresponding English expressions – *very*, *some* and *many*, respectively – have their highest standardised frequency counts in the mental-condition cluster. Furthermore, *yue* is least used in the mental-condition cluster among the six diseases, and so is *about* in schizophrenia. These similarities suggest that the tendency patterns of the stretchers are highly correlated with the mental-condition cluster or a specific condition in the cluster. Next, the highest counts of *yue* and its English equivalent *about* fall in the cancer cluster in the Chinese and English data. This possibly suggests a shared health culture – that is, utilising numbers is common to information concerning cancer possibly because the condition is perceived as relatively severe and adopting approximate numbers helps to deliver more clearly key information concerning the disease than merely relying on the use of *many* or *a few*. Interestingly, the Chinese scalar stretcher *geng* (更) and its English equivalent, *more*, have the highest counts in the data about the cold probably because it is a very common, well-known condition, and, therefore, comparisons involving aspects of it can be more easily made. In addition, *dabufen* (大部分) and its near-equivalent term in English, *most*, have the highest counts in the data concerning thyroid cancer. This may suggest that *much* is known about the disease and, therefore, health professionals can write about the situation that applies to most people, whether it concerns the diagnosis, development or prognosis of the health condition.

There are also differences. For example, in the Chinese data, *deng* ('etc./and so on') is the most-used general stretcher in the common-disease cluster. By contrast, the most-used general term in the English data is *things*, especially in the mental-condition cluster. Another difference is that the Chinese epistemic stretcher *keneng* and the English term *may* have their highest counts in different health conditions: the mental-condition cluster and cancer cluster, respectively. All the differences suggest the identified tendencies of the stretchers are

Table 6.2 *Correlations between the four categories of EL and three clusters of health conditions*

	Approximate	General	Scalar	Epistemic
COLD and FLU	• ☑ C • *yishang* 以上 'over' and *yixia* 以下 'under/less than' (FLU)	• ☑ C • *deng* 等 'etc.'	• *duo* 多 'frequently/ much' and *geng* 更 'more' (COLD) • *more* (COLD) • *usually* (COLD)	• ☑ C • *keneng* 可能 'likely/ may/ possibly' (FLU)
Thyroid (THY) and Pancreatic (PANC) cancer	• ☑ C • *yue* 約 'about' • *dabufen* 大部分 'majority/most' • *most* (THY)	• least use of *deng* in the cluster	• ☑ C • *usually* (THY)	• ☑ C ☑ E • *may*
Anxiety disorder (ANX) and Schizophrenia (SCHIZ)	• ☑ C ☑ E • *yixie* 一些 'some' and *xuduo* 許多 'many' • least use of *yue* 約 'about' in the cluster • *many* and *some* • least use of *about* in SCHIZ	• ☑ C • *things*	• ☑ E • *hen* 很 'very' • *guodu* 過度 'too much' (ANX) • *very* and *often*	• ☑ E • *keneng* 可能 'likely/ may/ possibly'

Note: ☑C: the category of Chinese EL used more frequently in the more severe condition in the cluster; ☑E: the category of English EL used more frequently in the more severe condition in the cluster;
___ (): an elastic term with the highest standardised frequency count in (the specified condition);
___: an elastic term with the highest average frequency count in the cluster.

attributed to a combination of factors, including the health condition, rhetorical convention, language and culture. The comparative discussion in this section is summarised in Table 6.2.

6.5 Concluding Remarks

Quite a few elastic terms on the Chinese top-10 list are similar to their English counterparts or near-counterparts: *keneng* (可能) and *may*, *chang* (常)/*tong-chang* (通常) and *usually*/*often*, *hen* (很) and *very*, *geng* (更) and *more*, and *duo* (多)/*xuduo* (許多) and *many*/*most*. These cover epistemic, scalar and approximate stretchers. While the most-used general stretcher in Chinese is *deng*, the most frequently used general stretcher in English is *things*.

We identify eleven pragmatic functions of EL in the context of online health communication in Chinese and English. Six of them are first-order functions as they are interpreted based more on the propositional content of the elastic expression in the sentence: softening, avoiding, intensifying, deintensifying, approximating and shortening. Apart from the six first-order functions, five second-order functions are also identified: tendency describing, reporting research, correcting, advising gently and emotionally supporting. The second-order functions of EL are more interpersonal than referential and they are served particularly in the health context and especially when two elastic terms or more co-occur in the sentence. A first-order function (e.g., approximating) can have different second-order functions (e.g., tendency describing, reporting research, correcting) in different sentences, exemplifying different textual environments and conveying multiple facets of health communication. On the other hand, the ways a function is fulfilled vary in Chinese and English (see Table 6.1). For example, in Chinese, *duo* plus a suggested action has become a formulaic expression used to deliver advice. By contrast, the English near-equivalent of *duo*, whether it be *frequently* or *more*, may be used in an imperative to form advice, but based on our English data, it does not seem to have developed into a formulaic expression for advice. In English, the function of advising gently can be realised by a range of structural constructions beyond just imperatives (e.g., *If . . .* , *you need to . . .* ; *It is important to . . .*).

In terms of how the four categories of EL are distributed, the Chinese and English data exhibit two different patterns – that is, SC-AQ-GE-EP and EP-AQ-SC-GE, respectively. The least frequently used category in the Chinese corpus – epistemic stretchers – is the most used in the English corpus. The most-used category of EL in the Chinese data is scalar stretchers, which rank second-to-bottom in the English data. This striking difference might be underpinned by a deep-rooted conception regarding the online delivery of health communication to the public. In Chinese, when health information is delivered, elaborating on degree, extent and frequency is the priority, while in English modifying the truth condition of the health statement based on the known evidence is the main concern. In view of the highest frequency count in the Chinese data being scalar stretchers such as intensifiers and high-frequency adverbs, we call the Chinese tendency an *upward-looking, amplifying* style. By contrast, the tendency dominated by epistemic stretchers in the English data can be called an *inward-looking, attenuated* style as it is based on the health professional's reasoning as to whether the given statement completely matches medical knowledge.

A series of comparisons of the most-used stretchers of each of the four categories in the Chinese and English corpora yields some interesting findings (see Section 6.3). In terms of approximate stretchers, online health information in English utilises many more non-number stretchers (e.g., *some*, *most* and *many*) than number-based stretchers (e.g., *about*, *over*). In the Chinese data, there are more counts of non-number approximate stretchers than number-based ones *yue* ('about') and *yishang* ('more than') ranked first and third, respectively. In English, *some* tops the list while its Chinese counterpart, *yixie* ('some'), is ranked fifth, behind *duo* and *xuduo*. Health professionals' preference for *some* suggests that their emphasis is on details that suit a medium-range quantity, a phenomenon that seems to match the pervasive use of *may* in the English data, as both contribute to qualifying health statements by taking a riskless and commitment-less stance. As for general stretchers, three out of the top five items on the Chinese and English lists are similar in meaning – that is, *youshi* corresponding to *sometimes*, *mouxie* to qualitative *some*, and *youren* to *someone*. Nevertheless, the number-one general stretcher in Chinese and English is *deng* ('etc.') and *things*, respectively. We believe this difference can be attributed to certain rhetorical views concerning *things* or *deng*. In English writing, despite being a general noun, *things* contributes to creating cohesion as it can cohere with a number of nouns mentioned in the text. By contrast, in Chinese writing, *deng* ('etc.') is not considered an expression to be avoided as it appears across formal and informal genres. The established convention concerning the respective general stretcher encourages the use of *things* in English and *deng* in Chinese. The scalar stretchers in the Chinese data and those in the English data behave similarly in that high-end, rather than low-end, scalar stretchers are preferred in both corpora. Furthermore, four out of the top five scalar stretchers are similar across the lists: *hen*, *chang*, *tongchang* and *geng* in Chinese correspond to some extent in meaning to *very*, *often*, *usually* and *more* in English, respectively. Next, in both corpora, there is an enormous gap in the frequency count between the most commonly used epistemic stretcher and the next. Specifically, there is a clear preferred epistemic stretcher in online health information in Chinese and English, that is, *keneng* (可能) and *may* respectively.

7 Perceptions of and Attitudes Towards the Use of Elastic Language in Chinese

Previous studies concerned with Mandarin VL address issues such as whether the sensitivity of conversational topics affects the use of VL in form and frequency (Zhang and Feng, 2013), what forms of VL were used in spoken business negotiations (Zhao, 2010) and what functions a given elastic expression may fulfil in a specific context (Zhang, 2016). Building on previous studies of VL and taking them as a point of departure, a recent study by Tseng and Zhang (2018) explored how doctors employ EL in order to stretch both language and medical knowledge in their delivery of online medical consultations. This study further extends the line of enquiry to perceptions of and attitudes towards online health information written in Chinese.

Since how readers react to Chinese elastic expressions in online health information is little investigated, in the spirit of integrative pragmatics, this chapter tackles the issue.[1] It analyses Taiwanese university students' perceptions of and attitudes towards EL in the context of health communication to the public. Readers' comments on EL constitute metalanguage 'that reflects reflexive awareness on the part of users about their use of language' (Culpeper and Haugh, 2014: 240; cf. Caffi, 2009; Mey, 2001: 173–229; Silverstein, 1993). As such, understanding how elastic terms are perceived and interpreted contributes to revealing aspects of the metapragmatics of EL. Such understanding complements and enriches an analysis of language purely from the analyst's viewpoint and sheds light on how public health communication may improve due to its empirical nature.

Based on a total of 516 questionnaires collected, we report whether the participants had difficulty understanding health excerpts containing EL and whether they liked the information items with EL or their non-elastic counterparts or both. More importantly, we invited the participants to explain why they made the choices they did, thus using a combination of closed and open-ended questions. Although some did not give any reason for their responses, those who did provided valuable feedback that tells us about their attitudes towards EL. Among the 516 valid questionnaires and for each of the six health excerpts

[1] An earlier version of this chapter appears in Tseng and Zhang (2020).

in the questionnaire (see Chapter 3), an average of 46% – nearly 240 participants – provided reasons for their options. Those willing to do a follow-up one-on-one interview were later invited for further elaboration and clarification. The interview data is particularly useful in that some of the participants who considered EL difficult to understand explained why they felt that way.

7.1 Responses to Whether Elastic Language Is Difficult to Understand and Why

In this section, we focus on the elastic terms used in the Chinese-language health information excerpts selected, which cover the four categories, and examine whether they are understood by the participants. Some respondents to the questionnaire experienced difficulties, and we seek to explain why.

Figure 7.1 shows the percentages of the respondents who had or did not have difficulty understanding the EL marked in the excerpts used. As can be seen, the majority had no problem interpreting EL in the six excerpts in the questionnaire. We seek to explain the difficulty based on three perspectives: the severity of the disease, the number of elastic expressions in the excerpt, and participants' feedback as expressed in interviews with them.

Does the rate of difficulty relate to the severity of the health condition? This study supports an approximate correlation. As Table 7.1 suggests, with the exception of anxiety disorder, the rates of difficulty appear to increase with the severity of the health condition. Another way of interpreting Table 7.1 is to view the six health conditions in pairs. The difficulty level associated with the

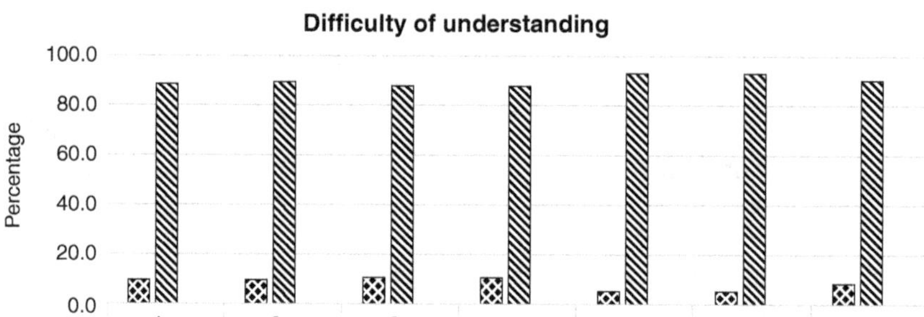

	1a	2a	3a	4a	5a	6a	Average
Yes	10.5	10.1	11.6	11.8	6.6	5.6	9.4
No	89.1	89.7	88.0	88.0	93.4	94.2	90.4
N/A	0.4	0.2	0.4	0.2	0.0	0.2	0.2

Figure 7.1 Summary of answers regarding difficulty in understanding all six excerpts (Chinese data)
Note: 1a stands for question 1a in the questionnaire.

Table 7.1 *Severity of disease and rate of difficulty*

Disease	Rate of difficulty	Excerpt #
Anxiety disorder	13.3	4
Pancreatic cancer	9.6	2
Thyroid cancer	7.5	3
Schizophrenia	5.8	1
Influenza	3.8	5
Cold	2.9	6

Table 7.2 *Number of elastic expressions and rate of difficulty*

Total # of elastic items (number of different elastic terms)	Rate of difficulty	Excerpt # (disease)
7 (6)	13.3	4 (anxiety disorder)
4	9.6	2 (pancreatic cancer)
4 (3)	7.5	3 (thyroid cancer)
3	5.8	1 (schizophrenia)
3 (2)	3.8	5 (influenza)
4 (2)	2.9	6 (cold)

excerpt about pancreatic cancer was indeed higher than that for thyroid cancer. Similarly, the rate derived from the excerpt concerning flu was higher than that for the one about colds. Schizophrenia is clinically regarded as more severe than anxiety disorder. Nevertheless, their relative severity does not correspond to the difference in the difficulty rates of understanding EL. This suggests that, in order to fully understand why the reader finds it hard to understand, considerations other than the severity of the health condition are needed.

Table 7.2 shows the rates of difficulty in relation to the numbers of elastic expressions in the six excerpts (labelled Excerpts 1–6).[2] The numbers in parentheses refer to the counts of different elastic terms in the excerpts. For example, in Excerpt 6, although four elastic terms are used, one of them is repeated three times. In other words, only two different terms of EL are actually used. The more varied the EL terms used, the more reported cases of difficulty there tended to be. Based on the responses from the university students in Taiwan, the increasing number of elastic terms correlated well with the level of difficulty in understanding EL. Apart from the number of elastic terms, we may

[2] Please refer to the Chinese questionnaire in Appendix 2 for the six health excerpts, which are not cited here.

also need to consider the types of EL used in the excerpt. For example, Excerpt 4 had the highest number of doubtful respondents, and this probably also relates to such approximate stretchers as *xuduo* (許多 'many') and *yixie* (一些 'some'), whose interpretations vary from person to person.

Among those who indicated having difficulty understanding EL, 19 respondents were interviewed. Based on the interviews, we identified six reasons for their difficulties.[3] First, a common reason is the expectation of more specific information, as interview examples 7.1–7.2 illustrate. When reading health information, the reader might not be content with the general information being delivered and s/he expects further clarification of whatever implied meaning can be deduced from the use of a vague expression. Should such expectation be unfulfilled by the text, the question that arises in the reading of the information could create the difficulty.

7.1 F61: (Female, #61 participant)
因為那時候這句話好像看了兩、三遍我才看懂在講什麼。
'[I had difficulty understanding about/over 100 cases] because I seemed to have read it two or three times before I knew what it was about.'

I: (Interviewer)
嗯嗯嗯。
'Uh-huh.'

F61:
就是它說累積了上百例, 然後我就在想說是百例以上還是已經快到百例。
'That is, the excerpt said accumulated about/over 100 cases, and I just wondered if it meant over 100 cases or about to reach 100 cases.'

7.2 I: OK, 好再來看一下三這邊, 你寫說有理解困難是指哪方面的理解困難?
'OK, Right, let's look at the third one. What did you refer to when you wrote you had difficulty understanding it?'

F44: 他說「例如碘過多」, 一樣可以是那個量, 也許是多幾 ml。
'He said "for example, too much iodine intake". The [necessary] amount of intake can be fixed, but perhaps several more ml [millilitre] [than the amount needed].'

I: 什麼多少要幾 ml? 多少量才叫過多?
'How many ml are needed? How much is too much?'

F44: 對。
'That's right.'

The second reason is a combination of the fuzziness of EL and insufficient health literacy. As interview example 7.3 suggests, older generations might misinterpret *duo he shui* ('drink water frequently' or 'drink more water') and drink as

[3] There are reasons mentioned in the interviews and questionnaires that are less relevant to this study, for example personal conditions, formatting of the excerpts in the questionnaire and suchlike. This applies to the English data in the next chapter as well.

much water as they can, possibly resulting in water intoxication – that is, a low sodium level in the blood due to excessive water intake. Specifically, EL could cause misinterpretations, and in the health context, it could lead to potential risk if it is interpreted incorrectly. Nevertheless, misinterpretation is the result, not the cause, of VL. The misinterpretation suggested in interview example 7.3 is caused partly by the ambiguity of EL and partly by insufficient health literacy.

7.3 I: OK, 好, 那看一下最後一個, 第六說有理解困難是指哪一方面呢?
'OK, let's look at the last one. You found the sixth hard to understand. What made it difficult to understand?'

F19: 嗯, 理解困難, 因爲他說多嘛、多嘛那可能會對於現在的民衆來講說, 可能阿公阿嬤[喝過]多, 可能會造成現在說的喝水中毒。
'Well, it's difficult to understand, because he said *duo*, and to people now, e.g., grandpas and grandmas, they [might drink] too much [water], and this could result in the so-called water poisoning.'

I: 噢噢, OK。
'Oh, OK.'

F19 就可能喝到 2000 或是短時間喝太多了, 對, 所以有具體的建議會比較好, 就像是每天喝六杯開水。
'It is possible to drink 2000 [cc] or too much in a short time, yes, so it is better to have specific suggestions, like drinking six glasses of boiled water every day.'

I: 所以你覺得說, 就是很明確的告訴你說要喝幾杯這樣子。
'So, you think it's better to tell you how many glasses to drink.'

The third reason is a heightened awareness of a patient's identity. As 7.4 demonstrates, when the reader is a patient or a member of the patient's family, precise information is desired and expected as general information with EL no longer fulfils their needs and they are concerned about possible risks, therefore finding it hard to understand EL.

7.4 I: 好, 我們再來看一下, 在第三題裡面, 你一樣說到說像「過多」啦、「可能」啦、「等等」啦, 都有造成理解上的困難, 那可以請你再稍微說明一下哪方面困難嗎?
'Right, let's take a look here. Regarding question 3, you also said terms such as *too much*, *possibly* and *etc.* cause difficulty in understanding. Could you please briefly explain what kind of difficulty you mean?'

M273: (Male, #273 participant) 因為像如果我是患者或是我是家屬, 我很在意他到底, 比如說這營養物要攝取多少或這個藥物不能吃太多免得會發生很嚴重的後果, 那我當然要很清楚的希望可以明白是到底是幾 percent, 或者是幾公升這樣或幾次, 很明確。
'It's because if I am a patient or a family member of the patient, I care very much about, say, what quantity of nutrients should be taken, or if a large dose of a drug causes a severe side effect, then I certainly want to be clearly informed of the right amount in terms of percentage, litres or the number of times.'

The fourth reason for the difficulty in understanding EL is intensive use of it. It can take the form of the repetitive use of one or more elastic expressions, as pointed out in 7.5. Presumably, such intensive use of VL may increase the vagueness of the text.

7.5 I: OK 好, 再來看一下第四題, 你這邊有理解困難指的是?
'OK. Well, let's look at question 4. Here, what did you refer to when you said you had difficulty understanding it?'
F61: 好像是後面這邊。就我覺得「一些」太多了, 就前面已經用「一些」, 然後後面又用「一些」。
'It seems to be this bit. I think there are too many uses of *some*; it is used in the first part of the excerpt and is reused again in the latter part.'

The fifth reason is the sentence in which the elastic term is embedded. This reason relates more to the sentence or clause in which the elastic term appears than the elastic expression itself. For example, the participant in 7.6 finds his understanding of the sentence challenged by its sentence structure, which reverses the normal verb–object order and involves the use of the particles *yi . . . lai* (*yi* + object + *lai* + verb; 以輕微腹痛或背痛來表現 'slight abdominal pain or back pain is shown'). The structure is permissible in Chinese, but possibly because the structure makes the sentence longer, the sentence is likely to take more time to process. In 7.7, the participant was puzzled by 'changing doctors instead of changing medication' in the case of the patient of schizophrenia not seeing any improvement. Such puzzlement may be further derived from the participant's not having a similar experience and from his unfamiliarity or disagreement with the presupposition behind the sentence – that is, a patient of schizophrenia may change his/her psychiatrist should no immediate improvement be made.

7.6 M66: 我覺得這一句「許多病人以輕微腹痛或背痛來表現」, 他的[. . . 動詞]受詞的倒裝, 不是那麼的直觀。
'I think this sentence 'Many patients with slight abdominal pain or back pain shown', with the reversal of the verb–object order, is not self-evident.'
I: 理解困難指的是這個句子句法上面的問題、結構上的問題這樣子?
'So, the difficulty lies in the syntactic, structural problem?'
M66: 對。對。
'That's right.'

7.7 M37: 我看不懂「太急著換醫師」是什麼意思。
'I did not quite understand what being "too eager to change doctors" means.'
I: 喔就是你對於這個「太急著」 . . .
'Oh, you mean you are unsure about "too eager"?'
M37: 不是, 我就是, 我有問題的地方不是你畫線的地方。
'No, I mean, the part that I find problematic is not theunderlined expression.'

I: 你有疑問的地方是 . . . ?
'The part that you have doubt with is . . . ?
M37: 藥物如果作用比較慢, 應該是換一個藥而不是換一個醫師。
'If the medicine is slow in its effect, what is to be changed should be medicine, not doctors.'
I: OK你覺得個題目邏輯上是有點怪怪的是不是?
'OK, you think the logic of the sentence is a bit odd, right?'
M37: 我覺得啦。對我覺得而已, 我不確定是不是這樣。
'I feel it that way. It's just what I think. I am not sure if this is the case.'

Finally, the sixth reason relates to an undesirable effect created by EL. For example, in response to the phrase 'some family issues (e.g., financial problems and children's educational problems)', the participant in 7.8 considered the use of *yixie* ('some') in the phrase redundant as two examples were already given in it. In 7.9, the redundancy takes the form of an epistemic term *keneng* ('may/possibly') combined with another expression *ruguo* (如果 'if') that also indicates uncertainty. The participant found it inappropriate to the reporting style of health information because the wording creates a far too uncertain tone. Therefore, in 7.8 and 7.9, what makes EL somewhat unclear or hard to understand seems to be an undesirable effect (e.g., redundancy or incompatibility between an uncertain tone and health information), as EL may interrupt information flow when the reader feels its use is unhelpful or unnecessary.

7.8 M99: 嗯 . . . 是因為, 這個「家庭的一些問題」感覺就是, 這「一些」的存在感覺就是不那麼明確的指出是哪些, 但是後面已經有寫出來, 所以這個「一些」其實是不需要的。
'Um . . . because the expression "some family problems" gives the impression that the problems are to be left unsaid, but then in the following segment the problems are spelt out, so the expression "some" is actually not needed.'
I: 所以你覺得「一些」是一種比較不明確的概念?
'So, you think "some" is a rather implicit concept?'
M99: 對。對對對對。
'Right, right, right, right, right.'

7.9 I: OK, 好再看一下第二題這, 你這邊有理解困難是指的是哪一部分?
'OK, let's take a look at the second excerpt. What part do you have difficulty understanding?'
M166: 最後一句話「則可能有因阻塞膽管所導致的黃膽產生」, 這個「可能」這邊, 因為前面已經表示「如果」了, 他已經有可能性在這裡了, 那加上這邊的文字, 這邊的文字是比較醫學的文字, 所以如果他有比較重複這種字彙的話會有點 . . . 對。
'The last sentence "there may be yellow bile caused by obstruction of the bile duct", the word "may" here. Because in the preceding sentence, "if" has been used and a possibility has already been indicated, adding the repeated "may" in the medical text would be a bit . . . you know.'

I: 所以你覺得這種醫學方面的, 你覺得是應該要更精確一點的意思嗎?
'So, you think a medical text like this should be a bit more precise. Is that what you mean?'

M166: 不一定要更精確, 但是因為這看起來是一個報導, 所以用字遣詞上面還可以再更精練一些。
'It doesn't necessarily have to be more precise, but because this seems to be a report, it could have been more refined and concise in word choice.'

In short, the cited interview examples suggest that difficulty of understanding VL/EL relates to the following: unfulfilled expectation of further clarification, semantic ambiguity combined with insufficient health literacy, unclear instructions not as anticipated and needed by the patient and family, increased vagueness due to intensive use of EL, the sentence in which the elastic term is embedded, and an undesirable effect that interrupts information without adding anything new.

Worthy of note is the fact that not all those who found EL problematic in interpretation necessarily preferred non-EL. In other words, understanding the precise meaning of a given expression is not the only determinant for participants' preference of EL or non-EL. One possible interpretation of this is that for some respondents, the benefit of EL outweighs the need to be precise. In a similar vein, those who did not find EL difficult to understand did not necessarily opt for EL or non-EL, as evidenced in greater variations in the distribution of respondents' preferences. While the overall no-difficulty rates were around 90%, neither the preference rate of EL nor of non-EL was that high. This suggests that the reasons for EL or non-EL preferences are complicated and, thus, are worth exploring.

7.2 Responses to Why Elastic Language or Non-elastic Language Is Preferred

Whether respondents preferred EL or non-EL varied from case to case (see Figure 7.2). In four of the six cases (i.e., Q1, Q2, Q5, Q6), the percentages of the respondents who favoured EL were about two to five times as many as the percentages of those who preferred non-EL. This shows that most respondents considered the use of EL positive. By contrast, Case 4 (i.e., responses to questions related to Excerpt 4 in the Chinese questionnaire) showed the reverse result.

Our survey shows that readers have different reactions to EL. Based on the responses collected, we have identified six frames that are operationalised in the perceptions of EL: communication (positive versus negative), trust–scepticism, folk–idiosyncratic, lay–professional, voluntary–involuntary action and difference–indifference. Each of the frames can be regarded as a higher-

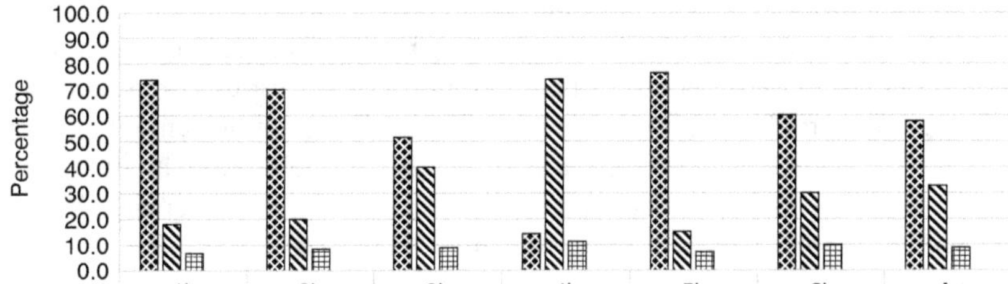

	1b	2b	3b	4b	5b	6b	Av
EL	74.0	70.3	51.4	14.5	76.6	59.9	57.8
Non-EL	18.2	20.3	39.5	74.0	15.1	29.7	32.8
Both	7.4	8.9	8.7	11.4	7.8	10.3	9.1
N/A	0.4	0.4	0.4	0.0	0.6	0.2	0.3

Figure 7.2 Preference for EL/non-EL in six excerpts (Chinese data)
Note: 1b stands for question 1b in the questionnaire.

order mechanism that affects the reception of EL. A frame, although organised around a theme, is not necessarily homogeneous but schematised in two directions or valences. Specifically, one and the same frame may generate contrastive reactions to a given elastic or non-elastic expression because individual readers may resort to different aspects of the activated frame (e.g., accuracy attached to professionals versus approximation associated with laypersons).

7.2.1 Communication Frame

This frame is theoretically underpinned by the Cooperative Principle (CP; Grice, 1975), which addresses the issue of interpreting utterances in communication. Many of the respondents' comments concern evaluations of what counts as effective or negative communication, thus constituting evidence of metapragmatic awareness being at work. We treat communication as a frame as it can explain a wide range of responses pertaining to the maxims of the CP (e.g., being informative enough, clear and truthful). It concerns the informativeness (see 7.10a–7.10e), clarity (7.11a–7.11e) and truthfulness of one's contribution (7.12a–7.12b), which correspond to the Maxims of Quantity, Manner and Quality, respectively (Grice, 1975). In a way, these examples reinforce the operation of the CP, as respondents' comments frequently refer to those aspects of communication compatible with the maxims of the CP. We do not mean the theoretical richness of the CP can be reduced to the aspects of the communication frame highlighted; instead, the frame is supported by the tenets of the principle.

If we regard the Maxim of Manner as affecting the overall effects of communication, then the maxim can be expanded to cover the needs to be fluent, persuasive and emphatic. This would explain various communicative effects associated with the communication frame. For example, among participants' responses regarding the use of EL or their non-elastic counterparts are the polarised effects such as fluency (7.14a–7.14c) versus non-fluency (7.14d), persuasion (7.15a) versus non-persuasion (7.15b–7.15c) and effectiveness (7.16a–7.16c) versus ineffectiveness (7.16d–7.16e). In the context of public health communication, of great significance is the effectiveness in communicating health and risk information and in leading the public to take the necessary precautions. It is worth exploring the role the communication frame plays in relation to EL versus non-EL used in health communication.

The communication frame consists of a variety of polarised effects, ranging from clear–unclear, through persuasive–unpersuasive, to effective–ineffective. Listed below are such effects illustrated with corresponding examples cited from the survey. They concern the uses of all six Chinese elastic terms investigated (and their non-elastic counterparts) in the questionnaire, covering the four categories of stretchers.

	Positive communicative effects		Negative communicative effects
	Informative enough		Too informative
7.10a	在這裡應該只要表現出經驗豐富的意思就好了。 'Here the expression [saying that psychiatrists have treated *over 100 cases* of schizophrenia patients] is fine so long as it indicates the meaning of rich experience.'	7.10c	4.94 [is] too trivial.
		7.10d	四點九四太冗長。 'The number 4.94 is unnecessarily long.'
7.10b	知道有很多經驗就好。 'Knowing it means much experience is good enough.'	7.10e	[5 and 4.94] 很接近了, 小數沒必要。 '[The number 5] is very close [to 4.94]; the decimal point is not necessary.'
	Clear		Unclear
7.11a	上百例比較好懂。 'Saying *over 100 cases* is easier to understand.'	7.11d	「上百例」的表達方式不明確。 'The expression *over 100 cases* is not clear.'
7.11b	清楚。 'Clear.'	7.11e	"許多"是多少要定義清楚, 否則太抽象, 也不客觀。[4] 'The expression *many* should be clearly defined; otherwise, it would be rather abstract and not objective.'

[4] The double quotation marks in this Chinese sentence and some other cited examples in this Chapter were originally used by the participants; therefore, we cite them in their original form.

7.11c	誇大化的指詞有時更能容易理解 'Using exaggerated expression is sometimes easier to understand . . . .'		
	Truthful/Evidence-based		Not based on reality
7.12a	沒有100%確定前用「可能」比較好。 'It is good to use *may* when one is not 100% certain.'		– –
7.12b	非實際數字, 較符合現實。 'Using a non-specific number is more in line with the real situation.'		– –
	Concise		Redundant
7.13a	較簡潔。 '[Not using *may* is] more concise.'	7.13b	「可能」有冗字感。 'Using *may* creates a sense of redundancy.'
	Fluent		Non-fluent
7.14a	[上百例]語意通順。 '[Using *over 100 cases* is] fluent.'	7.14d	100 太精準了, 邏輯上不順。 '*100* is far too accurate and is not logically sound.'
7.14b	[上百例]比較順 . . . '[The expression *over a hundred cases*] is more fluent . . . '		
7.14c	[多喝水]語意整體較流暢。 '*Drink water frequently* sounds more fluent.'		
	Persuasive		Unpersuasive
7.15a	用上百例表示感覺累積經驗較多, 較有說服力。 'Using *over 100 cases* sounds like having more experience, hence it is more convincing.'	7.15b	太多數量的形容詞, 沒說服力。 'Using too many adjectives is unpersuasive.'
		7.15c	如果為「可能」較沒說服力。 'If *possibly*/*may* is used, the statement will become less persuasive.'

	Effective/Emphatic		Ineffective/Non-emphatic
7.16a	確定還有其他傳染方式，過於侷限於1、2種方式可能導致民眾疏於防範。 '[I am] sure that there are other ways of contagion [hence the use of *etc.* here]; simply listing one or two ways [without the use of etc.] could cause the public to neglect prevention.'	7.16d	流感是負面的，列舉出所有可能才能有效預防。 'Flu has a negative impact; only by listing all the possible ways of contagion can it be prevented effectively.'
7.16b	上百例的範圍較廣，有誇大的效果，較一百例好。 '*Over 100* cases indicates a broader range than *100 cases* and has a maximising effect, so it is better than *100 cases.*'	7.16e	一百例感覺太限制，不能是一百零一例或一百零二例，只能是一百例。 'Saying *100 cases* feels rather constrained as it cannot be 101 or 102 cases and can be just 100.'
7.16c	感覺經驗豐富。 '[The expression *over 100 cases*] creates the feeling of much experience.'		

As can be seen from the examples, when commenting on a given expression, whether elastic or not, the participants drew on the communication frame. While most of these participants viewed the elastic expression positively (e.g., 7.10a–7.10b, 7.11a–7.11c, 7.12a–7.12b, 7.14a–7.14c, 7.15a, 7.16a–7.16c), some saw it negatively (e.g., 7.11d–7.11e, 7.13b, 7.15b–7.15c, 7.16d). Relevance theory (RT) (Sperber and Wilson, 1995) may generally explain why a given response receives a more positive or more negative comment. Specifically, when the given information generates optimal relevance to the reader at the point of communication, s/he is likely to accept it. For example, when the reader only wants to know that the medical doctor is rather experienced, an elastic expression such as *shang bai li* ('over 100 cases') is relevant enough to do the job (7.15a). Nevertheless, when the reader wants to know more than that, a rough estimate does not generate the anticipated optimal relevance (7.11d). Or when the reader wants to be informed of all the possible ways one contracts influenza (7.16d), a list of possibilities would be more relevant than simply saying *coughing, sneezing, etc*. Apart from using the communication frame underpinned by the CP and RT in providing a general explanation, we can further enquire into other patterns of thought that people resort to when reacting to general health information. This will provide a fuller understanding of how EL is perceived. We illustrate below the possible activation of five more frames other than communication.

7.2.2 *Trust–Scepticism Frame*

Also worthy of attention is a frame which affects people's attitudes towards the credibility of the information being processed – that is, the trust–scepticism frame. This frame relates to the Maxim of Quality, which requires one's contribution to be truthful or evidence-based. Nevertheless, the Maxim of Quality is posited more from the viewpoint of the speaker or production, and less from that of the listener or reception. Even a statement predicated on the true situation may not be regarded as credible by the listener/reader. The trust–scepticism frame is cast more from the perspective of reception.

As has been pointed out in previous studies of health communication (cf. Borah and Xiao, 2018; Paige et al., 2017; Thon and Jucks, 2017), readers' attitudes towards the credibility of online information may be subject to their level of health literacy and the authenticity of the information from the site source. Nevertheless, how EL affects people's perceptions of health information remains under-explored. Our survey shows that certain uses of EL or non-EL could lower participants' trust of the health information they read. Cited below are responses that showcase this phenomenon. We use the upward-pointing arrow to indicate trust while the downward-pointing arrow denotes scepticism.

	Elastic language
7.17a	上百例直覺上有誇大成分 . . . (↓) 'Intuitively speaking, saying *over 100 cases* is exaggerating . . . '
7.17b	以「約」來表達真實性。(↑) 'Using *about* expresses the truthfulness.'
7.17c	上百例會比較接近真實數據。(↑) '*Over 100 cases* is closer to the real number.'
7.17d	模糊的敘述感覺較真實。(↑) 'Vague expressions feel more realistic.'
7.17e	整數較易有真實感。 (F101) (↑) 'An integer increases authenticity.'
7.17f	不大可能那麼剛好 100 例, 就算真的, 也只是那時如此, 用比較模糊的上百例較好。(↑) 'It's unlikely that it happened to be exactly 100 cases; even if it's true, it happened just then, it's still better to use the vague expression *over 100 cases*.'
	Non-elastic language
7.17g	要考慮前後文, 若以此篇第一年來看, 一百例感覺較真實。(↑) ' . . . considering the context of the first year of training, *100 cases* feels more realistic.'

7.17h [一百例]對於醫生的專業技術指數偏向較不誇大。(↑)
'Saying *100 cases* makes the doctor's professional index less exaggerating.'

7.17i 一百例太過精準, 感覺不太真實。(↓)
'*100 cases* seems too precise and does not feel true.'

7.17j 直接說一百, 過度精確反而不真實。(↓)
'Directly saying *100 cases* is too exact and makes the statement untruthful.'

7.17k 因太精確的說一百例反而會讓人質疑真實性。(↓)
'Saying exactly *100 cases* causes people to doubt its authenticity.'

7.17l 不可能精準到真的 4.94。(↓)
'It's impossible to be really exactly 4.94.'

7.17m 一百例有很假的感覺。(↓)
'*100 cases* feels unreal.'

7.17n 一百例過於精確, 看起來假假的。(↓)
'The expression *100 cases* is too accurate and looks somewhat suspicious.'

The comments above all concern quantification. As they show, while a specific number without any approximator could cast doubt over the statement (e.g., 7.17i–7.17n), using elastic approximators could make statements credible (e.g., 7.17b–7.17f). Nevertheless, the opposite could also occur (e.g., 7.17a, 7.17g–7.17h). The ambivalent attitudes towards numbers reinforce and are reinforced by the tricky nature of quantification in health and risk communication. Jones identified quantification as one of the features of modern health communication and as 'a *rhetorical device* that is used to make some aspects of reality criterial and obscure others' (2013: 40, emphasis original; see also Potter et al., 1991). In our survey, comments implying a statement felt fake were concentrated on cases involving a specific number, with or without an approximator. This suggests that, in the Chinese-speaking context, the trust–scepticism frame is likely to be activated when numbers are used.

7.2.3 Folk–Idiosyncratic Frame

A frame concerning the activation of folk knowledge or of idiosyncratic views is also operationalised, and we call it the folk–idiosyncratic frame. It works in two directions. It may be more folk-oriented, that is, geared towards common sense (e.g., *People are counted in integers*), widely held beliefs or assumptions (e.g., *The public prefers* ...) and formulaic expressions shared among users of the same language (see 7.18h, below). When motivated by the folk-oriented end, the option of EL or non-EL usually matches that of the majority of the participants, although the frames activated in their responses may differ. In contrast to being folk-oriented, the activated end of the frame may be more idiosyncratic and personalised – that is, more oriented towards individuals' considerations (e.g., 7.18k) or individuals' stances (7.18n). An example motivated by the idiosyncratic polarity of the frame is typically marked by *geren renwei* (個人認為, 'I personally think') or *wo juede* (我覺得, 'I think') followed by a somewhat less shared view, but the marker is not always present. The idiosyncratic end of the frame may indicate the participant's personality trait (e.g., a tendency to dislike precise numbers) and/or the concern (e.g., a panic) s/he associates with a given expression (e.g., 7.18k). The idiosyncratic end of the frame does not necessarily mean the view is peculiar; instead, it explains a variety of responses that may be less common than those activated by the folk-oriented end.

The comments 7.18a–7.18i are motivated by the folk-oriented end of the frame, while 7.18j–7.18n are more motivated by the idiosyncratic-oriented end.

	Folk-oriented
7.18a	4.94 聽起來很奇怪, 就像人可以切割一樣。 'It sounds very strange to hear 4.94, as if a person can be cut up.'
7.18b	不會有四點九四人存在, 這是平均下的算術, 可用大約描述。 'There is no such thing as *4.94 persons* as this is based on an average calculation and could have been replaced by *about 5 persons*.'
7.18c	人數不應該有小數點。 'The number of people should not contain a fraction.'
7.18d	人是整數計算, 不需因統計上的計算刻意出現小數點以示真實性。 'People are counted in integers, and it is unnecessary to show authenticity by deliberately using decimal points based on statistical calculations.'
7.18e	4.94 人太過精準, 一般大眾只要瞭解大約有幾人即可。 'Saying *4.94 persons* is unnecessarily precise; the general public needs to know only about how many people.'
7.18f	民眾較喜歡此說 [許多]。 'The public prefers the use of *many*.'
7.18g	可能大家都會說多喝水, 講一天 6 杯有點奇怪。 'It's possible that because most people say *Drink water frequently*, saying *Drink six glasses of water* sounds somewhat odd.'
7.18h	[上百例]為一般說法。 '[*Over 100 cases* is] a common expression.'
7.18i	[上百例]慣[用語]。 '[*Over 100 cases* is] a formulaic [expression].'
	Idiosyncratic-oriented
7.18j	個人認為 30% 以上有此症狀就算「許多」。 'I personally think so long as over 30% of people have the symptom, then it means *many*.'
7.18k	用於病症時, 有精確的調查數據較不易造成社會恐慌。 'In the context of delivering health information, having a precise figure based on a survey is less likely to cause societal panic.'

7.18l 愈少人死於胰臟癌愈好。
'The fewer people die of pancreatic cancer, the better.'

7.18m 作為一個科學人, 習慣確切數字。
'As a scientist, I am used to precise statistics.'

7.18n 我覺得這種統計不用寫得太清楚。
'I think a statistical figure like this [i.e., about death rates] does not need to be precise.'

The similar comments against the use of decimals in describing human death rates (7.18a–7.18e) are motivated by the common-sense observation that people are not counted using decimal places. The folk-oriented end of the frame makes some participants consider it strange to present a death rate with a decimal point. In a similar vein, the comments in 7.18g–7.18i are motivated by a shared awareness of formulaic expressions in Chinese, the awareness being part of a folk-oriented frame. When the stretcher *duo* (多 'frequently' or 'more') or *shang* (上 'over/about') was replaced by a number (6 glasses or 100 cases), some participants found it odd.

By contrast, comments 7.18j–7.18m all prefer the use of precise numbers and are more motivated by the idiosyncratic end owing to their personal considerations and/or somewhat diverse ways of thinking – for example, a personal definition of *many* (7.18j), avoidance of rounding up a death rate (7.18l), a scientist's habit (7.18m) and an association of a rough number with potential societal panic (7.18k). Example 7.18n shows a preference for an elastic expression but is also characterised by the personalised end. These examples suggest that the idiosyncratic end may give rise to diverse responses.

7.2.4 Lay–Professional Frame

This frame concerns the evocation of an identity either as a layperson interested in basic information or as a professional anticipating certain features associated with professionalism (e.g., accurate statistics, strong confidence, scientific research). Because respondents are not medical professionals, when they stress the knowledge gap between medical professionals and laypersons, the lay end is likely to be activated. By contrast, those who anticipate a strong identity projection of professionalism are likely to employ the opposite end, associated with a professional identity. While the lay end is used in 7.19f–7.19g, the professional end is implemented in 7.19a–7.19e.

Professional

7.19a [4.94] 比較精準, 比較專業。
'[The number 4.94] is precise and shows a professional approach.'

7.19b 數據精準的數目更顯專業。
'Accurate statistics demonstrate professionalism.'
7.19c 統計的詞較專業。
'Using statistics is more professional.'
7.19d「可能」表達不太專業。
'Using *may* makes the statement somewhat unprofessional.'
7.19e ...「約」一字會使文章專業性降低。
'... the expression *yue* ['about'] would reduce the professional quality of the article.'

Lay

7.19f 我們不是專家, 可以說得更彈性。
'We are not experts; delivering information in more elastic ways is fine.'
7.19g 傳達科普之文章不需以如此精確之數值表達。
'In an article delivering popular science, it's unnecessary to use such a precise number.'

Associating statistics with professionalism is understandable as our society increasingly views health sciences in terms of quantification, which is accredited with 'an epistemological authority' (Danisch and Mudry, 2008: 130). Those who subscribe to the idea of numbers representing authority prefer a more accurate number, while those who do not, find a rough calculation sufficient. Nevertheless, the extent to which readers activate the frame in their perceptions of EL may vary from society to society.

7.2.5 *Voluntary–Involuntary Action Frame*

This frame involves the imposition of an action, usually in the form of advice or suggestions. While some like to be informed of exactly what to do, others prefer to be given freedom and flexibility. As for the above frames, the action frame has two possible orientations. It may be oriented towards voluntary action – that is, the reader would feel like following an action out of his/her volition; s/he is keen to know the points and steps to follow. By contrast, it may be oriented towards the involuntary side – that is, the reader would like to know about a rough direction, not an exact path. S/he would feel less willing to follow order-like advice or advice that could make the reader feel pressured.

Cited below are examples showing the two ends of the frame. Comments 7.20a–7.20e are motivated by the voluntary end, while 7.20f–7.20i are shaped by the involuntary end.

Voluntary

7.20a [說每天喝六杯水]可明確知道該怎麼做才是對方想要的。
'[Saying *Drink six glasses of water every day*] can clearly inform the reader of what to do, and this is what the addressee anticipates.'

7.20b	有個實際數字就比較能督促是否符合要求。 'If there is an actual number, it is more likely someone will check whether the requirements are met.'
7.20c	[說每天喝六杯水]有目標去執行。 '[Saying *Drink six glasses of water every day*] provides a goal to be achieved.'
7.20d	雖多喝會因不知該喝多少而補充更多水份, 但若有一個確切數字執行上較能持久不懈。 'Although saying *drink water frequently* may lead to drinking much more water, nevertheless it does not say how much to drink. So, if there is an exact number, the advice can be carried out more assiduously.'
7.20e	有一個明確的準則 (醫療方面) 容易使人有安全感。 'A clear rule regarding medical advice makes people feel safe.'
	Involuntary
7.20f	"多"可由自己決定。 'It's up to each individual to decide on the meaning of *more*.'
7.20g	被規定反而不太容易做到。 'To feel obliged to do something makes it hard to actually do it.'
7.20h	六杯太限制, 覺得不必要。 '*Six glasses* is unnecessarily restrictive, and I do not feel it is needed.'
7.20i	後者感覺很受限制、有壓力。 'The latter [i.e., drink *six glasses of water a day*] makes one feel very constrained and under pressure.'

These responses also show that a non-elastic expression can generate two clashing types of reaction depending on the focus-end of the frame. It would be interesting to know the general distribution of how the public reacts to health advice delivered in EL as opposed to non-EL in a given society (see Figure 7.3 in Section 7.2.9).

7.2.6 Difference–Indifference Frame

This frame is concerned with perceiving a difference in meaning versus not being interested in the difference. For example, while 7.21a–7.21b show an interest in differentiating elastic versus non-elastic terms, 7.21c–7.21g signal a lack of interest in the move. The two ends of the frame explain why some participants ticked both elastic and non-elastic expressions and considered them both equally acceptable. Interestingly, 7.21b and 7.21e, the latter of which shifts to English, are cited from a response by the same participant. This suggests that although making a difference and lacking an interest in it appear to be opposite, they can both be activated in a given response.

	Difference
7.21a	兩者意思不全然相同。 'The two do not mean exactly the same.'
7.21b	在病例上, 不需太過精確字眼, 且於寫報告時上百例似乎更有說服力; 但以實際了解, "一百例" 較準確。 'In the context of the health record, there is no need to be precise, and *over 100 cases* seems more persuasive in a report, but *one hundred cases* conveys a more precise meaning in reality.'
	Indifference
7.21c	. . . 2 個敘述都滿合理的。 ' . . . The two versions are both reasonable.'
7.21d	都可。 'Both are OK.'
7.21e	. . . Who care[s!] [the original utterance was in English]
7.21f	. . . 4.94 我也會直接解讀成 5。 ' . . . I would interpret 4.94 as 5.'
7.21g	個人覺得數據的精準度在本篇文中作用不大, 但也沒有壞處。 'I personally feel a precise number makes little difference in the text, but it doesn't have a bad effect either.'

7.2.7 No Relevance

If a comment is irrelevant or insufficient, or it amounts to saying nothing about the reason why an elastic or a non-elastic expression is preferred, e.g. *wu* (無 'No comment'), then it will be coded as 'no relevance'.

7.2.8 A Glance at the Bipolar Ends of the Six Frames

For convenience of reference, the analysis refers to the ends of each of the six frames by a code (Table 7.3) when presenting coding results. An irrelevant or insufficient response is coded as G, though it is not a frame.

7.2.9 A Hierarchy of Frames

In order to further investigate what motivated respondents' preferences, we analyse their explanations based on the coding of their answers in the questionnaires.

Table 7.3 *Notes on the codes used in the coding of respondents' comments*

Code	The end of a frame	Code	The end of a frame
A1	Positive communicative effect	A2	Negative communicative effect
B1	Trust	B2	Scepticism
C1	Folk	C2	Idiosyncratic
D1	Lay	D2	Professional
E1	Voluntary	E2	Involuntary
F1	Difference	F2	Indifference
G	Insufficient and irrelevant information		

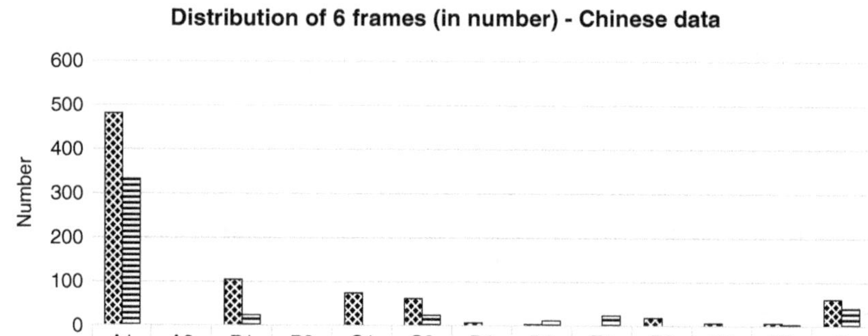

	A1	A2	B1	B2	C1	C2	D1	D2	E1	E2	F1	F2	G
EL	479	0	106	0	72	62	5	6	0	18	6	8	59
non-EL	333	0	27	0	0	30	0	11	21	0	2	4	43

Figure 7.3 Distribution of six frames (in number; Chinese data)

Figure 7.3 reveals a hierarchy of frames that explain the choices of EL or non-EL. The top four frames accounting for preferences of EL are the positive effects of communication, both ends of the folk–idiosyncratic frame, the trust end of the trust–scepticism frame and the involuntary end of the action frame. At times a participant may explain why a given expression is preferred by saying the negative aspect of the expression s/he did not choose. For example, a participant in favour of *shang bai li* wrote 'I feel that *100 cases* sounds far too precise to be believable, lowering its credibility' (覺得一百例太精確, 讓我不太相信, 可信度反而降低). Here, the comment evokes the scepticism end of the trust–scepticism frame, but the evoked end of the frame does not directly explain the participant's option for the elastic term. Instead, it is the opposite end of the frame – trust – that is used when doing the coding of this comment as it implicitly explains the option for *shang bai li*. Because Figure 7.3 lists the results of the coded ends, not those of the evoked ends, it does not show the numbers for negative communication effects or for the scepticism end. Nevertheless, in the coding process, we found it not uncommon for respondents to explain a preference not in terms of its advantage but due to a drawback of the non-preferred option. This phenomenon is found especially in the activation of communication and trust–scepticism frames.

The top four frames motivating non-EL preferences are communication, the idiosyncratic end, the trust end and the voluntary end. As can be seen, both EL and non-EL preferences are overwhelmingly navigated by the communication frame. While both folk- and idiosyncratic-oriented ends are operationalised in the EL preferences, only the idiosyncratic-oriented end is activated by those selecting non-EL. The trust end is used much more frequently in EL cases than in their non-EL counterparts. While the involuntary end is associated with EL, the voluntary end is activated by non-EL preferences. In other words, the coding results reveal differences in the focus ends of the folk-idiosyncratic and action frames and in the frequency of the trust end. Importantly, there emerges a hierarchical ordering of frames that explains respondents' attitudes towards EL and non-EL: communication, followed by the folk–idiosyncratic, trust–scepticism and action frames. The order may have been shaped by the health excerpts used. If more cases that involve the delivery of health advice had been used in the survey, there may have been more responses associated with the voluntary–involuntary action frame. Furthermore, responses that accepted both EL and non-EL are mainly activated by the difference–indifference frame.

In order to further understand how the frames relate to EL and non-EL in different health contexts, we next examine the distribution of the key frames in each case and cite responses exemplifying the frames used.

7.2.10 Why Is Elastic Language or Non-elastic Language Preferred in Each Case?

We further examine respondents' attitudes towards the four types of EL versus non-EL in terms of frame. Figure 7.4 shows the most-used frames and ends in the three cases involving approximators (*shang*, *yue*, *xuduo*) or quantification.[5]

In Cases 1 and 2 (i.e., responses to questions related to Excerpts 1 and 2 in the Chinese questionnaire), while EL and non-EL responses are both motivated by a concentration of the communication frame, the second common frame differs: the trust end in Case 1 versus the folk end in Case 2. By contrast, in Case 4, most respondents preferred non-EL, although they were also motivated by a concentration of the communication frame. Two issues arise: why an approximator (e.g., *shang* 'over/about' or *yue* 'about') is sometimes preferred and at other

[5] Only the counts of the most common three frames in these cases are presented. The total numbers in the right square cover the counts for all of the six frames plus the 'no relevance' code.

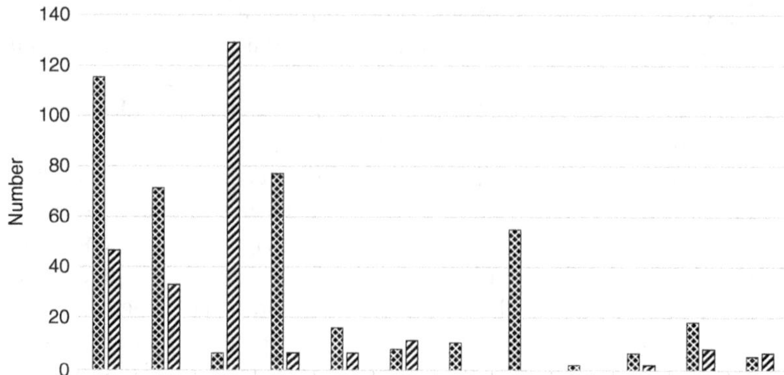

	Q1	Q2	Q4	Q1	Q2	Q4	Q1	Q2	Q4	Q1	Q2	Q4
		A1			B1			C1			C2	
Elastic	116	71	6	78	17	7	11	55	1	6	19	5
non-Elastic	46	33	129	6	6	12	0	0	0	1	8	6

Figure 7.4 Most frequently used frames in three cases (Cases 1, 2 and 4)

times rejected, and why the second frame activated in each case differs. The difference could be attributed to the nature or topic of the excerpts in these cases. The excerpt in Case 1 is aimed at persuading patients not to change their psychiatrists frequently because a qualified one must be very experienced, as indicated by *over 100 cases*. Should the approximate stretcher be replaced by an exact number, the reader's scepticism could be generated, with the accuracy of the figure being questioned, thus indirectly explaining why the trust end of the trust–scepticism is attached to the EL *over* in *over 100 cases*. Using *over* is emphatic in the context of Excerpt 1 (see the Chinese questionnaire in Appendix 2) as the stretcher functions well to stress the considerable experience of a psychiatrist. *Shang* (上) in Chinese is literally a term indicating an upward position. Like English and other languages, Chinese also conceptualises UP as MORE. This is a common cognitive metaphor based on our embodied experience of quantity – for example, the more something piles up, the higher it becomes (Lakoff and Johnson, 1980). It is therefore unsurprising that *shang* in Chinese carries the meanings of 'about' and 'over'.

In Case 2, the excerpt concerns an average death rate of pancreatic cancer of 4.94 per 100,000 people. While most viewed *about 5* as informative enough or clearer (7.25), apparently due to the communication frame, a significant number of responses were also motivated by the folk end of the folk–idiosyncratic frame – that is, people should be counted using integers (7.26). Unlike Cases 1 and 2, Case 4 involves an excerpt concerned with the symptoms of anxiety disorders. This case suggests that a difference in the nature of health information (e.g., topic) may lead to a contrast in respondents' preferences. Most respondents preferred the relatively less elastic *80%* to *many*, presumably because readers anticipate more or clearer information than is communicated by *many* when the message being delivered concerns the symptoms of a health condition or when the interpretation of a stretcher is likely to vary considerably. This also explains that although it is the most salient frame in all the three cases, communication is far more important than any other frame in Case 4 (e.g., 7.35–7.36). Cited below are some responses featuring the frequently activated frames (with their codes; see Table 7.3).

Preference for EL

Case 1

7.22 如果是給病患看的, 上百例會覺得醫師比較有經驗。(A1)
'If the excerpt is for the patient to read, *over 100 cases* would create the impression that the doctor is quite experienced.'

7.23 上百例可信度較高。(B1)
'*Over 100 cases* is more trustworthy.'

7.24 作為一個科學人, 習慣確切數字。(C2)
'As a scientist, I am used to precise figures.'

Case 2

7.25 很接近了, 小數沒必要。(A1)
'[The number *5* is] very close [to 4.94]; the decimal point is not necessary.'

7.26 . . . 人應是整數的。(C1)
'. . . people should be counted in integers.'

7.27 模糊的敘述感覺較真實。(B1)
'Vague language feels more realistic.'

Case 4

7.28 有未受試者, 不能準確說明是 80%。(B1)
'Without information about subjects, it's impossible to justify how the figure 80% is derived.'

7.29 知道是大多數就好。(A1)
'It is enough to know *many* [patients have problems with insomnia].'

Preference for non-EL

Case 1

7.30 100 跟 900 個例子的經驗應該相差很多。(A1)
'A huge difference is expected between 100 and 900 cases.'

7.31 上百例非實數不明確, 可信度低。(B1)
'*Over 100 cases* is a vague number, with a low trustworthiness.'

Case 2

7.32 較為明確的數字。(A1)
'[4.94 is] a clearer figure.'

7.33 有明確的統計的話, 希望能告知準確的數據。(C2)
'If a precise statistical figure is available, I would like to be informed of it.'

7.34 有分析過的數據→可信度高。(B1)
'A number based on an analysis is trustworthy.'

Case 4

7.35 若此數據非胡謅, 數字會讓人覺得更有說服力。(A1)
'If the figure [80%] is not unfounded, it is more convincing.'

7.36 估計值較具體可信。(B1)
'A calculation [such as 80%] is more concrete and trustworthy.'

Next, let us turn to Case 3, where the key elastic expression is the epistemic stretcher *keneng* (可能 'possibly/may'), used in describing the potential causes for thyroid cancer: environmental pollution and physical and mental stress. Although slightly more respondents preferred EL to non-EL, responses in this case were relatively divided (see Figure 7.5). The uncertainty indicated by the epistemic stretcher protects the writer (Prince et al., 1982; Zhang, 2015), and some respondents aligned with the writer in their support for the used strength of a claim compatible with the limited evidence (see 7.38 below). By contrast, the uncertainty may be viewed as redundant (7.40) or ineffective (7.39) as it does not help prevent the disease, a perspective more oriented towards the reader or patient expecting medical professionals to be more certain in their delivery of health information – especially regarding the causes of a health condition – and to provide more effective information in combatting the health problem. The communication frame motivating both EL and non-EL preferences suggests a tug of war among different aspects of communication – for example, between being truthful and being informative, between being concise and being effective.

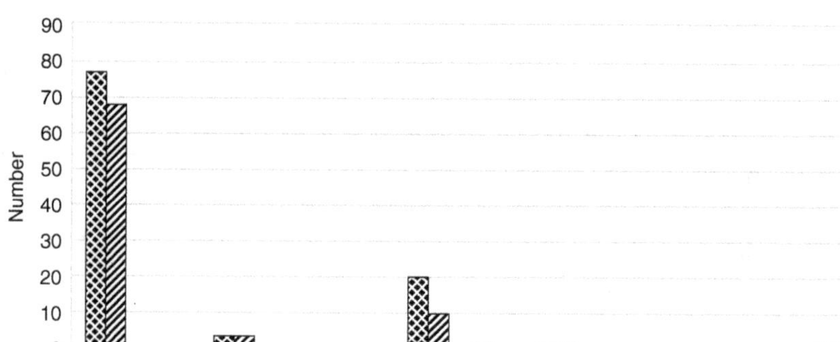

	A1	A2	B1	B2	C1	C2	D1	D2	E1	E2	F1	F2
EL	77	0	3	0	0	20	1	1	0	0	0	0
non-EL	68	0	3	0	0	9	0	2	0	0	0	1

Figure 7.5 Coding results of Case 3

Preference for EL

7.37 文中提到目前確認的因子僅有遺傳和輻射曝露, 其餘因子應準確告知閱讀者其尚未被證實的狀[況]。(A1)
'The excerpt mentions that the currently confirmed factors are genes and radiation exposure, and regarding the remaining factors, the reader should be accurately informed of their unconfirmed status.'

7.38 每個人症狀不同, 病因也就不同, 在個體確診之前一切本就只是"可能"而已。 (C2)
'Everyone has different symptoms and causes. Before the individual is diagnosed, everything is just possible.'

Preference for non-EL

7.39 希望知道近事實的原因才可加以防範。(A1)
'I hope to know close-to-fact causes, as this would help with prevention.'

7.40 贅字。
'[The expression *possibly/may* is] a redundant word.'

7.41 不喜歡不清楚的表達方式。(C2)
'I don't like vague expressions.'

Figure 7.6 shows the coding results of Case 5, which uses an excerpt concerning how the flu virus spreads. The key elastic expression is the general extender *deng* (等 'etc.'). Using the stretcher adds fluency and aligns more with the reality that there are more methods of transmission than those on the list, as comments 7.43–7.44 point out. This explains why the communication frame largely motivates EL responses. Non-EL preferences are also mainly based on the communication frame but for different aspects – for example, wanting to know the omitted information (7.46) and to make the prevention of contagion

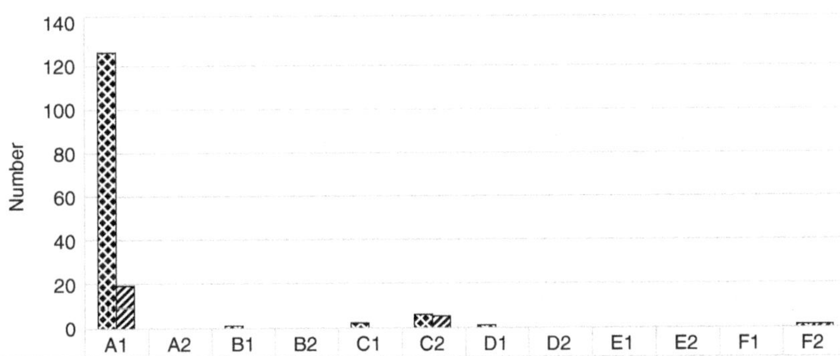

	A1	A2	B1	B2	C1	C2	D1	D2	E1	E2	F1	F2
EL	125	0	1	0	2	6	1	0	0	0	0	1
non-EL	19	0	0	0	0	5	0	0	0	0	0	1

Figure 7.6 Coding results of Case 5

as effective as possible (7.47–7.48). This seeming paradox of having contrasting preferences motivated by the same frame suggests, again, a potential tug of war among different aspects of communication (e.g., truthfulness, informativeness and effectiveness). For example, by listing more possible means of contagion instead of providing merely two common ways followed by *etc.* would be more effective in combating the flu, as 7.48 points out. Nevertheless, whether informativeness (i.e., the right amount of information) or preventive effectiveness is more important is subject to each individual's situation, knowledge and concern when reading the health information.

Preference for EL

7.42 文句通暢。(A1)
'The sentence [with *etc.*] is smooth and fluent.'

7.43 飛沫傳染方式並非只有咳嗽、打噴嚏兩種。(A1)
'The modes of droplet infection are not restricted to coughing and sneezing.'

7.44 流感傳染方式無法確定只有咳嗽、打噴嚏才會傳染, 考慮到可能有未知飛沫傳染方式, 應加入[等]。(A1)
'It's uncertain whether the ways flu is spread are by contact with fluids from coughs and sneezes only. In view of the possibility of unknown droplet infection, the expression *etc.* should be used.'

7.45 習慣會使用"等"在句子中。(C2)
'I am used to using *etc.* in sentences.'

Preference for non-EL

7.46 不知道等方式還有哪些。(A1)
'By the expression *etc.* I do not know what other modes of infection there are.'

7.47 等字會不知道還需避免什麼。(A1)
'The expression *etc.* does not tell us what other precautions are needed.'

7.48 流感是負面的, 列舉出所有可能才能有效預防。(A1)
'Flu has a negative impact; only by listing all the possible ways of contagion can it be prevented effectively.'

7.49 會希望知道所有情況。(C2)
'I would like to know all the details [about possible ways of getting the flu].'

The above analysis can be reinterpreted in terms of interactional meanings characterised by integrative pragmatics (Haugh and Culpeper, 2018). They accumulate by the interactions of three layers of meaning. First, the general stretcher *etc.*, like other stretchers, has a pragmatic meaning – for example, its implicature that the mentioned items preceding it are not comprehensive. Second, this pragmatic meaning is embedded within the pragmatic act of delivering health information about the flu. Third, evaluations (e.g., likes and dislikes) are initiated by the respondents in response to the pragmatic meaning couched in the pragmatic act of explaining or providing health information.

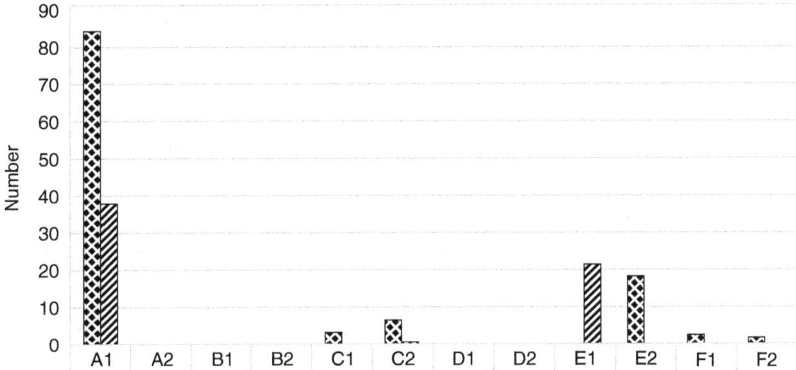

	A1	A2	B1	B2	C1	C2	D1	D2	E1	E2	F1	F2
EL	84	0	0	0	3	6	0	0	0	18	2	1
non-EL	38	0	0	0	0	1	0	0	21	0	0	0

Figure 7.7 Coding results of Case 6

From all these meanings emerge interactional meanings identified by the observer/analyst and based on the production and reception of discourse.

Figure 7.7 demonstrates the results of responses to Excerpt 6, which contains an excerpt offering advice to patients contracting a cold. The elastic term here is the scalar stretcher *duo* (多 'frequently/more') functioning as an adverb intensifying the extent of the suggested action (e.g., drinking water). The communication frame, again, mainly motivates EL and non-EL responses. Nevertheless, over twice as many respondents preferred EL in this case. It is worth highlighting at this point the use of the voluntary–involuntary frame, which is activated only in Case 6. This is attributed to the context in which the scalar stretcher is used – that is, in the excerpt providing advice. The delivery of advice is inevitably accompanied by some weight of imposition, and how respondents feel about it varies. In this case, among those who activated the action frame, slightly more respondents used the voluntary end (E1) than the involuntary one (E2). Specifically, when the action frame is activated, more respondents preferred non-EL to EL, in contrast to the situation when the communication frame is activated. This has an implication for the presentation of advice. While EL may help generate an appropriate weight of imposition for a significant number of readers, non-EL may be more suitable to some others. Some responses are cited in 7.50–7.57.

Preference for EL

7.50 已達提醒作用。(A1)
'[Using *frequently*] has achieved the function of a reminder.'

7.51 "多"應該只是表達"次數頻繁"的概念, 而非數量。(A1)
'The expression *duo* should mean 'high frequency', not quantity.'

7.52 比較輕鬆的表達方式患者要多喝水。(E2)
'This is a less imposing way of telling the patient to drink more water.'

7.53 有時候過於精確的數字較難達成, 鼓勵語氣較合適。(E2)
'Sometimes using a precise number makes it hard to achieve the target; an encouraging tone of voice is more appropriate.'

Preference for non-EL

7.54 醫療上明確點好。(A1)
'In medicine, clear information is better.'

7.55 有明確的範圍。(A1)
'[*Six glasses of water* provides] a clear target.'

7.56 有明確數據較容易去實行。(E1)
'A precise number makes it easier to achieve the target.'

7.57 我會試圖達成指定的量。(E1)
'I will try to achieve the set target.'

7.3 Social Factors

This section discusses two social factors (gender and age) that may influence participants' understanding of or attitudes towards the use of EL.

7.3.1 Gender Attitudes

Figure 7.8 showcases the gender factor in relation to whether elastic items cause difficulty in understanding. A Chi-square test of the raw data in the 'yes' group generated the following result: χ^2 [d.f. 1, n = 291] = 0.345, $p = 0.5570$ (> 0.05), which reveals no statistical significance of difference between males and females as the *p*-value is larger than 0.05. The average rate for females indicating a comprehension difficulty was approximately 0.5% higher than that for their male counterparts. If we look at the cases where the difference gap was larger than 0.5%, we can see an interesting contrast. Regarding Chinese Excerpt 5 (see the fifth health excerpt in Appendix 2), almost 8% of male Chinese-speaking participants found the EL in it hard to understand, while less than 5.5% of female participants felt the same way. Excerpt 5 concerns how the flu virus spreads, and a larger percentage of males expected to be more clearly informed rather than be given two means plus the use of the general extender *deng* (等 'etc.'). Excerpt 6 concerns advice to those with a cold. The fact that a larger percentage of female participants than their male counterparts found elastic expressions such as *duo* problematic may suggest that

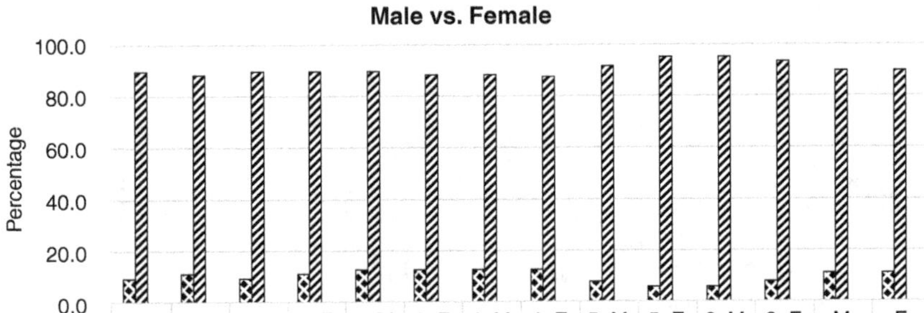

	1aM	1aF	2aM	2aF	3aM	3aF	4aM	4aF	5aM	5aF	6aM	6aF	M	F
Yes	9.5	11.5	9.5	10.7	11.7	11.5	11.4	12.3	7.7	5.3	4.8	7.0	9.1	9.7
No	90.1	88.1	90.1	89.3	88.3	87.7	88.6	87.2	92.3	94.7	94.9	93.0	90.7	90.0
N/A	0.4	0.4	0.4	0.0	0.0	0.8	0.0	0.4	0.0	0.0	0.4	0.0	0.2	0.3

Figure 7.8 Male versus female responses to Type A questions
Note: 1aM = Excerpt 1, Type A question, male participant; 1aF = 1aM's female counterpart.
Yes = having difficulty, No = no difficulty. The last two columns are averaged figures for the two gender groups.

females might be more willing to follow specific steps while males prefer more autonomy and, therefore, would not find EL hard to understand.

We next bring the gender factor into the landscape of preferences over elastic versus non-EL by looking at the overall gender distribution in relation to how Chinese-speaking participants reacted to Type B questions (see Figure 7.9, below). For example, in response to Excerpt 5, a larger percentage of male participants in fact preferred non-EL than their female counterparts, thus echoing a larger proportion of males having difficulty with EL in this case. In response to Excerpt 6, the percentage of males choosing EL was not very different from that of their female counterparts. In this case, a larger percentage of females accepted either EL or non-EL. This seems to reinforce the relative flexibility that more females than males demonstrated. In other words, there are different types of EL, and they are used for different purposes in various contexts. We need to be cautious over gender generalisations in relation to EL.

Within the no-difficulty group, a larger percentage of males than females indicated no difficulty in understanding EL across five of the six cases. Based on the data pertaining to the 'no' group, a Chi-square test was conducted. The result, χ^2 [d.f. 1, n = 2798] = 0.052, p = 0.8202, confirmed that the difference between males and females in the group was not statistically significant. In other words, although slightly more males than females consistently showed no difficulty in their perceptions of EL except for Case 5, the gender difference was not significant enough to render gender a crucial factor that would

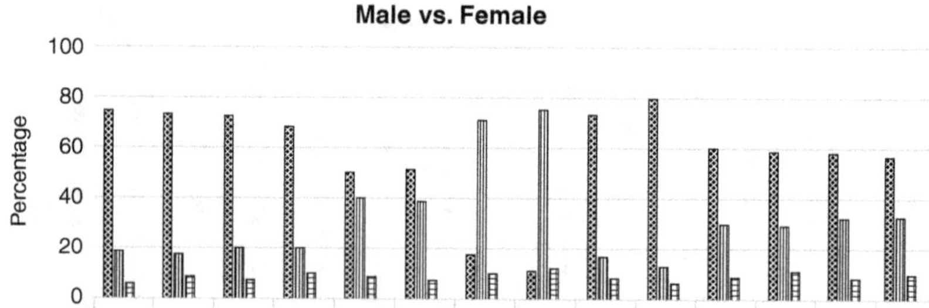

	1bM	1bF	2bM	2bF	3bM	3bF	4bM	4bF	5bM	5bF	6bM	6bF	M	F
EL	74.4	73.7	72.2	68.3	50.9	51.9	17.6	11.1	74.0	79.4	60.4	59.3	58.2	57.3
Non-EL	18.7	17.7	19.4	21.4	39.9	39.1	71.8	76.5	16.8	13.2	29.7	29.6	32.7	32.9
Both	6.2	8.6	7.7	10.3	9.2	8.2	10.6	12.3	8.4	7.0	9.5	11.1	8.6	9.6
N/A	0.7	0.0	0.7	0.0	0.0	0.8	0.0	0.0	0.7	0.4	0.4	0.0	0.4	0.2

Figure 7.9 Male versus female responses to Type B questions
Note: 1bM = Excerpt 1, Type B question, male participant, 1bF = 1aM's female counterpart.
EL = prefer EL, Non-EL = prefer non-EL, Both = both EL and non-EL are fine, N/A = no available information. The last two columns are averaged figures for the two gender groups.

necessarily mark an important distinction between males' and females' perceptions of understanding EL.

Figure 7.9 presents the results of responses to Type B questions in relation to gender. The average percentage of male participants preferring EL is almost 1% higher than that of their female counterparts. Why the participants preferred EL or non-EL has been expounded in Sections 7.2.1–7.2.9. Here, let us briefly consider whether gender has an impact on the participants' preferences.

Concerning preferences over EL or non-EL, gender did not seem to make much difference as male and female participants' respective percentages of preferences over EL and non-EL did not differ significantly. Based on the raw data in Figure 7.9, a Chi-square test was conducted, and three categories (EL, Non-EL and Both) were used. The test result, χ^2 [d.f. 2, n = 3086] = 0.971, p = 0.6153 (> 0.05), verifies that there was no statistically significant difference between males and females. The result supports Guan's (2010) study of whether gender affects the use of VL. The similarities-across-gender observation also supports previous research into gender differences in online interactions (Blank and Adams-Blodnieks, 2007; Gooden and Winefield, 2007; Musambira et al., 2006; Ravert et al., 2004). For example, according to Mo et al. (2009), gender differences were less evident in communication patterns in mixed-gender online health support groups than in single-sex online support groups.

7.3.2 Age Factor

Responses to Type A questions in relation to four age groups are summarised in Figure 7.10. Although 516 people participated in the survey conducted in Taiwan, two of them did not specify their age; therefore, Figure 7.10 is based on a total of 514 participants' information about their age. The numbers of participants in the group aged between 26 and 29 and the group aged 30 or above are smaller than those of the younger groups aged 18–21 and 22–25. The 22–25-year-old group, who were third- and fourth-year undergraduates or postgraduate students, had greater difficulty in understanding EL than the younger group, who were first- and second-year undergraduates. This might be due to them being more critical and expecting to know more, hence being more doubtful over EL. The rate of people indicating difficulty in the 26–29-year-old group was not as high as that of the 22–25-year-old group. However, compared to the group aged 22–25, the rate of difficulty was twice as high in the group aged 30 or above. This may be attributed to the maturity of the oldest group, who could expect more specific health information than the younger groups. On the other hand, the huge fluctuation could suggest that the age of 30 might be a good cut-off in differentiating how age relates to participants' understanding of EL. Because the sample of the most mature group was small, more evidence is needed to support the observation.

Figure 7.11 summarises the results of the answers to Type B questions in relation to age. Here, a very interesting pattern can be identified if Figures 7.10

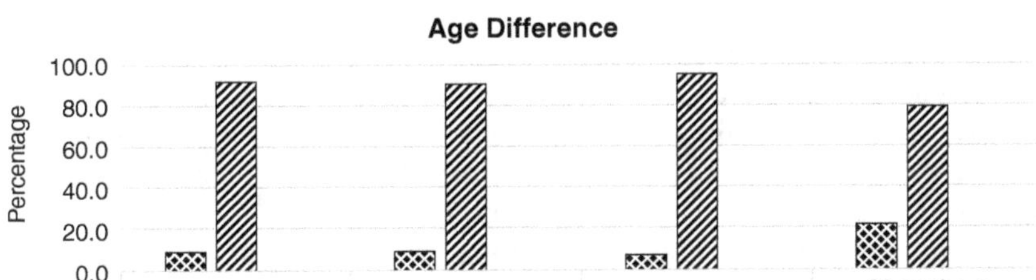

	18–21 (n = 343)	22–25 (n = 154)	26–29 (n = 8)	30 or above (n = 9)
Yes	8.7	10.3	6.3	22.2
No	91.0	89.6	93.8	77.8
N/A	0.3	0.1	0.0	0.0

Figure 7.10 Age difference in understanding EL

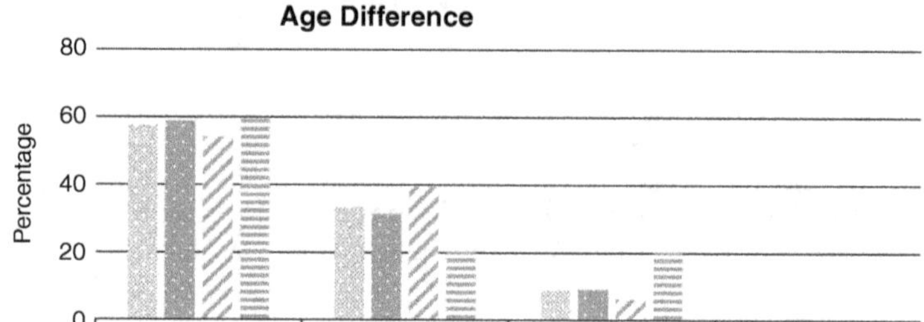

	EL	Non-EL	Both	N/A
18–21 (n = 343)	57.4	33.5	8.8	0.3
22–25 (n = 154)	58.9	31.5	9.2	0.4
26–29 (n = 8)	54.2	39.6	6.3	0.0
30 or above (n = 9)	59.3	20.4	20.4	0.0

Figure 7.11 Age difference in EL/non-EL preference (%)

and 7.11 are juxtaposed. Although the percentages of those preferring EL were much higher than the rates of those indicating difficulty understanding EL, the sequence of the four groups from the highest to the lowest rate of difficulty completely matches the order of the groups from the highest to the lowest percentage of people in favour of EL: those aged 30 or above, 22–25 year olds, 18–21 year olds, followed by those aged between 26 and 29. Specifically, the higher the rate of difficulty in understanding EL in an age group, the larger the percentage of people who prefer EL. If we are aware that participants who experienced no difficulty in understanding EL did not necessarily prefer it and that those who found it difficult did not always reject it, the relation between Figures 7.10 and 7.11 can be meaningful in two ways. First, as has been illustrated, having difficulty in understanding EL in health contexts can have different causes – for example, the complex nature of EL, unfamiliarity with the health information in which EL is used, a mismatch between the health professional's delivery of health information to the general public and the diverse expectations of the heterogeneous public, the reader's need to grapple with EL's tentative meaning, and the reader's lack of health literacy. The extent to which these different causes affect participants' preferences regarding EL varies among individuals. Age by itself is probably not a crucial variable in interpreting the whole landscape concerning participants' perceptions of and attitudes towards EL. Instead, it is the causes of difficulty and the reasons for preferences and the interaction between them that are more significant than age. Age may assist in demarcating the pattern emerging out of the interaction but on its own does not necessarily produce the pattern itself. Second, having difficulty understanding EL does not mean EL is always ineffective. For

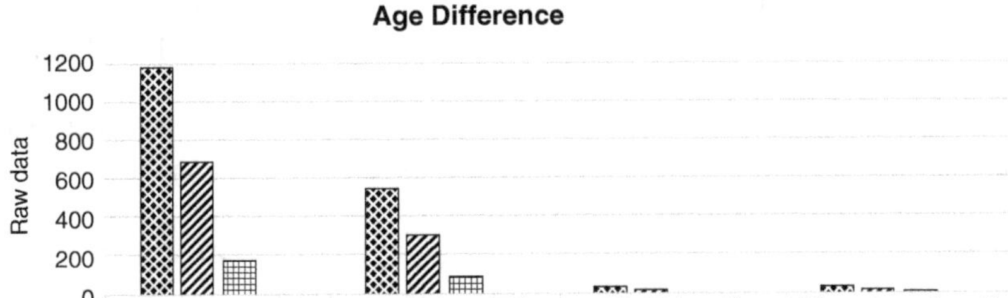

	18–21 (n = 343)	22–25 (n = 154)	26–29 (n = 8)	30 or above (n = 9)
EL	1181	544	26	32
Non-EL	689	291	19	11
Both	182	85	3	11
N/A	6	4	0	0

Figure 7.12 Age difference in EL/non-EL preference (raw data)

example, we sometimes enjoy a statement that requires a bit more thought or prefer a commercial whose target product is not self-evident until we have almost got to the end. To some extent, the matched order reinforces the paradoxical nature of EL, which may hinder and facilitate communication at the same time. The result supports Cheshire's (2007) view that expressions of VL are highly context-dependent, making any generalisations about VL in relation to age somewhat tentative.

The percentages listed in Figure 7.11 are based on raw data shown in Figure 7.12. Using the statistics in it, a Chi-square test was conducted, with only two categories (EL and Non-EL) used. The other two categories (Both and N/A) were excluded because they both have more than 20% of their cells consisting of a less-than-5 expected frequency, which would render a Chi-square test invalid. The test result, χ^2 [d.f. 3, n = 2793] = 3.801, $p = 0.283$ (> 0.05), confirms that the difference among the four age groups is not statistically significant.

7.4 Concluding Remarks

This chapter investigates whether Taiwanese university students find EL in health information difficult. On average, approximately 90% of them did not have any difficulty understanding EL while about 10% of them did. The rates of difficulty appear to increase with the severity of the health condition being described. Furthermore, the higher the number of different elastic terms intensively used in the excerpt, the more difficulty the participants experienced in understanding EL.

Based on interviews with approximately 20 participants, we address what may cause the difficulty and identify six reasons: unfulfilled expectation of specific information, semantic fuzziness combined with insufficient health literacy, unclear instructions that do not match the need of the patient and family, increased vagueness caused by the intensive use of EL, the structure of the sentence in which the elastic term is embedded or the presupposition behind the sentence, and an undesirable effect (e.g., redundancy or strong uncertainty) that interrupts information without adding anything new.

Regarding whether Taiwanese respondents preferred EL or non-EL, in five of the six cases (i.e., Q1, Q2, Q3, Q5, Q6), there were many more participants who preferred EL than those who were in favour of relatively precise language. By contrast, only one of the six cases showed a higher percentage of participants preferring non-EL, the case involving the use of the elastic term *many* in the description of a symptom: *Many patients [of anxiety disorder] have insomnia.* In order to understand participants' attitudes towards EL and non-EL, we analysed the participants' written feedback as to why they preferred EL or non-EL in the health context. Based on the analysis, six sets of frames were identified, each with two orientations. The operation of the communication frame may be latent in each act of communication as participants often react to discourse in terms of being clear, fluent, effective, convincing or the opposite. The frame can be superseded or modified by the folk–idiosyncratic frame as participants can be more similar or diverse in their knowledge and in their expectations of the content or expression of discourse. Interpretations are 'sensitive to social expectations about the situation in which the utterance to be interpreted is embedded' (Capone, 2005: 1357). The trust end of the trust–scepticism frame may be built or assumed by the build-up of positive communication effects, while the scepticism end may be activated by negative communication effects. The voluntary–involuntary action frame is associated with the discourse segment of offering advice and suggestions. The lay–professional frame plays only a marginal role in the results of the survey; it tended to be employed when participants were reading discourse segments regarding the causes of a disease and its symptoms. The difference–indifference frame explains the responses that selected both EL and non-EL.

Based on the coding of Taiwanese participants' written feedback, the analysis suggests that four frames play a relatively significant role, as they are activated more frequently than the other two frames. A hierarchy of frames that explains respondents' attitudes towards EL and non-EL is identified in the questionnaire data in Chinese: communication, folk–idiosyncratic, trust–

scepticism, followed by the action frame. Whether this pattern is culturally significant is discussed further in Chapter 9.

As regards whether gender significantly affects participants' understanding of EL, there was no striking difference between males and females in the group having difficulty in interpreting EL. In the no-difficulty group, there were significantly more males than females, but this may be due to a higher number of male participants in the survey. Concerning preferences over EL or non-EL, gender did not seem to make much difference either.

Concerning how age relates to the difficulty rate, there were fluctuations among the four age groups: 18–21, 22–25, 26–29 and 30 or above. There appeared to be a huge increase between the last two groups, a finding that seems to support the idea that 30 years of age may be a good cut-off in evaluating the relationship between age and perception of difficulty as regards EL. One interesting pattern is that the order of the four age groups from the highest to the lowest rate of difficulty matches the order of the groups from the highest to the lowest percentage of people favouring EL. This suggests that the causes of difficulty and the reasons for preferences regarding EL are more important than age itself. The matching order reveals and reinforces the paradoxical, unsettling nature of EL, which hinders and simultaneously facilitates communication.

8 Perceptions of and Attitudes towards the Use of Elastic Language in English

The focus here is on people's perception of and attitude towards EL, which is a less explored area in EL research.[1] One of the few studies in this respect is Cutting's (2015) work, where she investigated Germans' beliefs about German VL. Her findings revealed positive as well as negative views on VL. For example, on the one hand, VL may create an informal tone and closeness, but, at the same time, it gives an impression of laziness and incompetence.

Following the principles and criteria adopted in Chapter 7's analysis for the Chinese data, this chapter conducts comparable analyses based on the English data to reveal the perceptions and attitudes of participants towards the English corpus (questionnaire and interview data). For the questionnaire survey, there were altogether six excerpts extracted from the data in this study. Participants answered two types of questions for each excerpt: Type A questions concerned whether they had difficulty in understanding the content of an excerpt, while Type B questions addressed their preference over a precise or elastic expression. How they responded depended on several factors, including participants' 'personality and expectation', and the discourse environment also played a role in affecting their perceptions (Tseng and Zhang, 2018: 42).

There was a total of 541 questionnaires in the English corpus, of which 265 participants filled in both closed- and open-ended questions. The remaining 276 participants answered the closed questions only. There was a total of 112 participants who came back for follow-up interviews, where they then elaborated on their choices in the questionnaires. Typical questions asked in the interview were as follows: (1) *Could you please let me know why you had difficulty in understanding EL in the text?* and (2) *Could you please elaborate on the reasons you preferred EL/non-EL?*

[1] An earlier version of some parts of this chapter appears in Zhang and Tseng (2020).

8.1 Responses to Whether Elastic Language Is Difficult to Understand and Why

It is generally assumed that people have no problem in understanding EL or VL (Channell, 1994; Dines, 1980; Jucker et al., 2003), particularly when used appropriately (Parvaresh, 2015, 2017a). However, little empirical evidence has been presented to verify this assumption, and this study puts it to the test by examining the evaluation of native English speakers in terms of their own ability to understand EL used on Australian healthcare websites.

Medical diagnoses and prognoses are often underspecified – that is, they are not clear-cut. How to convey this kind of elasticity is a challenge to health professionals but is a skill that they must master in order to convey medical information effectively. To help them present online health information to the public effectively, a greater understanding of the public's ability to understand EL may be beneficial. This research is a start, an account based on participant feedback that suggests better ways of communicating elasticity.

8.1.1 Analysis of Questionnaire Responses

In the questionnaire (see the English questionnaire in Appendix 1) and follow-up interview, the participants were asked whether they found elastic items used in the text problematic. What follows is the data analysis for the six excerpts. In each case, the following question was asked: Do you have difficulty understanding the above paragraph due to the underlined expressions?

8.1 In schizophrenia, these experiences last for **more than** a month – even for six months **or longer**. Other common symptoms of schizophrenia are problems with low mood and motivation, isolation from family and friends, and feeling cold or emotionless. People with schizophrenia **may** also have trouble with thoughts, concentration, speaking and memory.

Response to Excerpt 8.1 (Schizophrenia)

Q1a	Yes	No	N/A
	5.2	94.3	0.5

In Excerpt 8.1, the underlined items are *more than*, *or longer*, and *may*. They do not convey an exact amount. A total of 5.2% of participants (28 of 541) expressed difficulty in understanding the expressions, and 0.5% (3 participants) marked 'not applicable'. The vast majority of participants (510) had no problem in understanding the text. This trend carries through all six excerpts, suggesting that people generally have no difficulty in understanding EL.

8.2 **Some** risk factors are modifiable, such as lifestyle or environmental risk factors, and others cannot be modified, such as inherited factors and whether **someone** in the family has had pancreatic cancer. Having 1 **or more** risk factors does not mean that you will develop cancer. **Many** people have at least 1 risk factor but will never develop cancer, while others with cancer **may** have had no known risk factors.

Responses to Excerpt 8.2 (Pancreatic cancer)			
Q2a	Yes	No	N/A
	10.9	88.7	0.4

Excerpt 8.2 discusses the risk factors of pancreatic cancer. In the 'yes' minority group, more people encountered problems in understanding the language used – twice as many as for Excerpt 8.1. It could be that the difficulty was because of more elastic expressions (5 in total) in this excerpt, the longer text and a wider range of EL types: approximate (*some*, *many*, *or more*), general (*someone*) and epistemic (*may*).

8.3 **Many** people today have ultrasounds and other scans for totally unrelated health issues, and those tests **sometimes** end up picking up **very** small thyroid nodules. Even if they turn out to be cancerous, **many** of these are **so** tiny and slow-growing that they **might** not ever cause problems during your lifetime.

Responses to Excerpt 8.3 (Thyroid cancer)			
Q3a	Yes	No	N/A
	9.1	90.8	0.1

In response to Excerpt 8.3, 9.1% of participants did not understand the EL well, which could again be caused by the number of elastic expressions used (6 in total).

8.4 Anxiety disorders are the most common mental disorders, affecting one in four Australians at **some** stage in their life. Women are **more likely** to develop anxiety than men, but it is not clear why. There are **many** forms of anxiety disorder, but the one thing they have in common is their impact on day-to-day activities.

Responses to Excerpt 8.4 (Anxiety)			
Q4a	Yes	No	N/A
	3.7	96.1	0.2

Fewer people found it difficult to understand the elastic expressions in Excerpt 8.4. This can perhaps be attributed to the fewer elastic expressions used (only 3).

8.5 Influenza viruses can survive an hour **or more** in enclosed environments or surfaces, which means we can pick up the virus even without **someone** coughing or sneezing near us. Even before we display the virus symptoms, we can be spreading the influenza viruses, which **may** infect people around us.

Influenza viruses are characterised by constant evolution, which can change their characteristics. Influenza type A, Influenza type B flu (**and so on**) are constantly changing.

Responses to Excerpt 8.5 (Influenza)			
Q5a	Yes	No	N/A
	7.2	92.4	0.4

In Excerpt 8.5, elastic expressions such as *and so on* can convey the speaker's perspective on 'the newsworthiness of a proposition and their evaluation of its desirability' (Jucker et al., 2003: 1763). It contains four elastic expressions, and the rate of difficulty is relatively higher than in those with three (1a, 4a, 6a). However, we must not forget that the majority had no problem interpreting the elastic expressions here, which supports Clark's (1996) findings that people rarely have a problem understanding VL.

8.6 There is no need for bed rest if your child has a cold – let the child decide **how much** activity they want to take part in. Although children are **unlikely** to be hungry, make sure they drink **lots of** fluids. Appetite will return as the child starts to feel better.

Responses to Excerpt 8.6 (Cold)			
Q6a	Yes	No	N/A
	4.4	94.8	0.8

As regards Excerpt 8.6, 94.8% of respondents reported no problem interpreting the language of this extract: as before, with only three elastic expressions in the excerpt to consider, respondents reported a low rate of incomprehensibility.

Figure 8.1 is a summary and graphic representation of the results based on the answers to the six questions.

Figure 8.1 shows the responses to the question of whether the participants had difficulty in understanding the EL used in the six excerpts. 'Yes' means that participants had some problems in understanding the EL in question, 'No' means the opposite, and N/A means 'not applicable'. The numbers in the figure are percentages.

The Chi-square test of independence was used to test the association among responses to the questionnaire questions (Smith et al., 2009). The overall difference between Yes, No and N/A categories was statistically significant, χ^2 [d.f. 5, n = 3233] = 34.239, $p < 0.05$. A $p = 0.05$ level of significance was used as the criterion for statistical significance in this study. The calculation was performed using an online tool provided by Preacher (2001).

According to the data, on average 6.8% had difficulty understanding EL, but 92.9% had no problem, and 0.4% did not find either of the answers applicable.

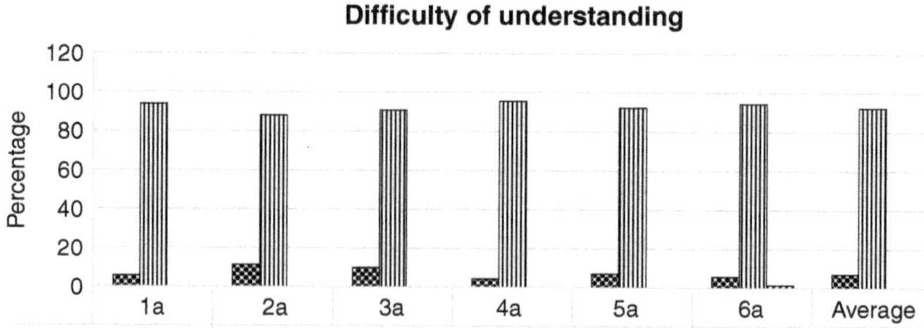

	1a	2a	3a	4a	5a	6a	Average
Yes	5.2	10.9	9.1	3.7	7.2	4.4	6.8
No	94.3	88.7	90.8	96.1	92.4	94.8	92.9
N/A	0.5	0.4	0.1	0.2	0.4	0.8	0.4

Figure 8.1 Summary of answers regarding difficulty in understanding all six excerpts (English data)
Notes: 1a stands for the Type A question in the questionnaire.
After rounding, the total percentage for the 'average' column is 100.1%. This also applies in a few other cases in this study.

This finding is consistent with Zhang's (2020) study of conversations between Australian customs officers and passengers, which found that people accepted the use of VL with no problem 92% of the time. However, VL was challenged in 8% of cases. The two studies involved different groups of people and discourses, yet the findings are similar. Zhang (2020) also found a correlation between the severity of the situation (e.g., suspicion of drug trafficking versus carrying prohibited food) and the frequency of the challenged cases of EL: the more severe the situation, the more VL challenges occurred. In this study, a difference in the severity of diseases is also noted, although its correlation with the understanding of VL is not very clear-cut, as Table 8.1 shows.

Table 8.1 shows a ranking of understanding difficulty from the highest to the lowest. The top level of difficulty is in the pancreatic cancer category, which is the most severe disease (the five-year survival rate for pancreatic cancer is only 8.7%); the second is thyroid cancer (with a five-year survival rate of 97%; www.cancer.org.au), much less severe. The third is influenza, which can be severe; the fourth one is schizophrenia; the fifth is cold; and, finally, anxiety takes the bottom place. Among the last four, influenza is indeed more severe than a cold, while schizophrenia is more severe than anxiety, but determining whether influenza is worse than schizophrenia is problematic. Therefore, the correlation of the severity of a disease with the level of understanding difficulty is only valid to a certain extent. The severity of a health condition is not always clear-cut – for example, whether a cold should rank above anxiety. This is because mental illness could be something 'beyond an individual's control' and is unlike

Table 8.1 *Severity of disease and rate of difficulty*

Severity of disease	Rate of difficulty	Excerpt #
Pancreatic cancer	10.9	8.2
Thyroid cancer	9.1	8.3
Influenza	7.2	8.5
Schizophrenia	5.2	8.1
Cold	4.4	8.6
Anxiety	3.7	8.4

Table 8.2 *Number of elastic expressions and rate of difficulty*

Total # of elastic items (number of different elastic terms)	Rate of difficulty	Excerpt # (disease)
5	10.9	2 (pancreatic cancer)
5(6)*	9.1	3 (thyroid cancer)
4	7.2	5 (influenza)
3	5.2	1 (schizophrenia)
3	4.4	6 (cold)
3	3.7	4 (anxiety disorder)

Note: * 5 excluding a repeated item, 6 including the repeated item.

other illnesses such as the flu or cancer (Barry et al., 2013; Major, 2009). The correlation in Table 8.1 should be viewed as approximate, rather than absolute. There is another possible correlation in the data, shown in Table 8.2.

Table 8.2 shows a downward trend in terms of difficulty as the number of elastic terms decreases. The correlation, therefore, is the more elastic items used in an excerpt, the higher the rate of difficulty.

8.1.2 Reasons for Problems in Understanding Vague Language

As shown above, 6.8% of participants on average indicated having difficulty in understanding EL. Among them, 18 volunteered to be interviewed. Based on their interviews, we identified the following four reasons for the difficulty in understanding, illustrated by examples from the interview data.

Vague information: Vagueness conveyed by the EL in the online healthcare information caused confusion in understanding the meaning of the text.

8.7 I (Interviewer): Okay. Number four is on anxiety. Again, difficulty understanding the text. Is there anything different from what you mentioned about two or three, the difficulties?

C17: Yes, it just seemed more vague. So, it was harder to understand. I guess I prefer more statistics than 'women are more likely to develop anxiety'. So, if it gave me a percentage of how more likely women are, it would be more easier for me to grasp what it's trying to talk about, I guess.

This participant, C17, clearly had problems making sense of the EL that occurred in the text. Precise language is what C17 wanted to see, which would ensure the delivery of successful communication.

8.8 I: What was the difficulty understanding the text?

A5: It wasn't very detailed.

I: Okay, it wasn't very detailed?

A5: It said many people today have ultrasounds, but not how many, and those tests sometimes end up picking up very small thyroid nodules, so sometimes it does, but what happens when it doesn't? It's just, like, yes, going into detail.

A5 attributed their difficulty understanding the text to a lack of detail, indicating that vagueness causes the problem here. A5 preferred to be provided with an exact number of people or number of times, rather than VL. Details, namely precise information, is needed for A5 to understand the text without problems.

Disease-related factors: The nature of diseases can be taken into consideration when participants try to interpret the medical information with EL in it.

8.9 I: You have some difficulty understanding the text. Can you tell us what it is?

C17: I feel like with things like cancer I want more definite information so I can actually understand what's happening as it is quite a serious issue. So, if there were more definite terms, I would have a better grasp of what's actually happening.

The participant indicates that cancer is a serious disease and that they need to know precise information to be confident in dealing with it. It suggests that vagueness does not bring clarity in understanding cancer, but precise language would help him/her to see the situation clearly.

Unnecessary information: EL is considered something unnecessary in the text, as adding it to the text makes understanding of the text problematic.

8.10 I: In this one, you had some difficulty understanding. Can you tell me?

C18: Yes, because all the highlighted words were making it, like, uncertain, like they were doubting themselves. It's like might or many people, where you can just say 'people today' instead. It was unnecessary in my opinion. That's why I found it annoying and made it more difficult to understand.

In this case, C18 thinks that EL creates uncertainty, something one can do without. EL in the text is considered annoying and confusing and, therefore, should not be used in medical information.

8.11 I: Any particular words, or all of them, are quite distracting, is it?
A16: Yes, I think because, like, initially, I didn't really understand, like, thyroid nodules and all that sort of thing – that was intimidating. But then having these words, again, didn't really seem as necessary.

Participant A16 feels that talking about thyroid issues was a challenge, and the use of elastic words makes things worse for them. A16 thinks that EL was not necessary, that it hindered their understanding of the text.

Personal experience: The understanding difficulty lies in a conflict between one's experience and the medical information provided in the questionnaire.

8.12 I: Number four, anxiety disorders – again, you have difficulty understanding the text with the highlighted words.
C13: Yes, and I was stuck on the whole women are more likely to develop anxiety than men.

During the interview, C13 explained why she felt stuck when reading *Women are more likely to develop anxiety than men*. She said that the information went against her past work experience, which involved being around soldiers affected by post-traumatic stress syndrome. Based on her experience, man might be just as likely, if not more likely, to develop some mental conditions.

8.2 Responses to Why Elastic Language or Non-elastic Language Is Preferred

In this section, two issues are discussed: (1) the results of participants' preferences in terms of precise or elastic expression, and (2) the reasons for their choices. The discussion is based again on the 541 English questionnaires collected for this study and is elaborated on in 112 follow-up interviews. The interview data provides clarification around the answers in the questionnaires.

8.2.1 Frequency Distributions of Participants' Choices over Elastic or Non-elastic Language

This section discusses the answers to the Type B questions, exemplified by the following excerpt from the data.

Excerpt 8.1: In schizophrenia, these experiences last for **more than a month** – even for six months **or longer**. Other common symptoms of schizophrenia are problems with low mood and motivation, isolation from family and friends, and feeling cold or emotionless. People with schizophrenia **may** also have trouble with thoughts, concentration, speaking and memory.

1b. Which of the following expressions do you prefer? (Multiple choices allowed)
□ In schizophrenia, these experiences last for a month.
□ In schizophrenia, these experiences last for **more than a month**.

Please briefly explain why you prefer such expression/s:

There are four categories of responses: EL (e.g., *more than a month* was chosen), non-EL (e.g., *a month* was chosen), both (e.g., both were chosen) and N/A (e.g., neither was chosen). Figure 8.2 shows there are different attitudes towards EL in the six excerpts. In Excerpts 8.1 and 8.3, EL was chosen by a large majority, but in Excerpt 8.2, non-EL was strongly preferred. In Excerpt 8.4, EL was preferred slightly to non-EL, and in Excerpts 8.5 and 8.6, non-EL was favourite. Specifically, in three cases, EL was preferred, and in the other three, non-EL was preferred. The final column of Figure 8.2 shows that, on average, EL and non-EL were liked almost equally, while 3.5% of the participants were indifferent, and 1.1% provided irrelevant answers.

Figure 8.3 presents the results in raw-data form, which enables statistical tests to be conducted. The Chi-square test shows that the overall difference among the four categories (EL, non-El, both and N/A) is statistically significant, χ^2 [d.f. 15, n = 3247] = 516.08, $p < 0.05$. Another test conducted on the two major categories (EL and non-EL) also showed that the difference among the six excerpts is statistically significant, χ^2 [d.f. 5, n = 3098] = 496.189, $p < 0.05$. While there is a verified difference among the six excerpts, on average, a similar total number occurs between the category of EL and non-EL: 1,563 (EL) versus 1,535 (non-EL).

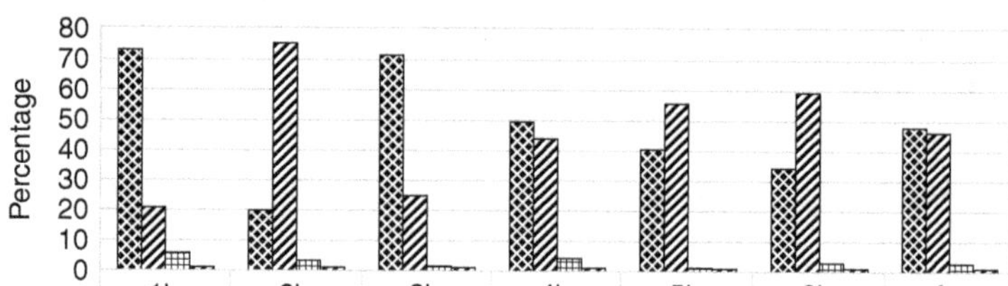

	1b	2b	3b	4b	5b	6b	Av
EL	72.7	20.1	71.2	49.4	40.6	34.9	48.2
Non-EL	20.8	76	25.7	44.9	56.1	60	47.3
Both	5.6	2.8	1.7	4.6	2.1	4	3.5
N/A	0.9	1.1	1.4	1.1	1.2	1.1	1.1

Figure 8.2 Preference for EL/non-EL in six excerpts (%)

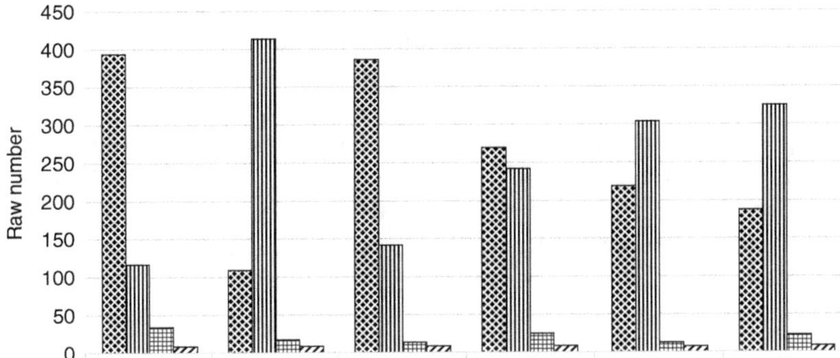

	1b	2b	3b	4b	5b	6b
EL	393	109	385	267	220	189
Non-EL	113	411	139	243	304	325
Both	30	15	9	25	11	35
N/A	5	6	8	6	6	6

Figure 8.3 Preference for EL/non-EL in six excerpts (raw data)

8.2.2 Participants' Reasons for Their Choices

The previous section presented an overall picture of whether participants preferred EL or non-EL, and this section discusses why they chose one over the other. The data were collected from the open-ended questions in the questionnaire: 'Please briefly explain why you prefer such expression/s' at the end of each of the six questions, and 'Do you have any additional comments about this questionnaire?' at the end of the whole questionnaire. The questionnaire data was cross-checked with the interview data for clarity and accuracy. The interview data were used for further elaboration and clarification of the questionnaire data.

Based on the data, three groupings of frames can be observed: language-focused, language-user-focused and disease-focused. The comments across the six excerpts are discussed together because they recur or are repeated (although not always using the same wording) from one question to another. There is a total of 12 frames in the English corpus, seven of them are adopted from Tseng and Zhang (2020): informativeness, trustfulness, clarity, folk–individual, lay–professional, voluntary–involuntary, and indifference. The other five frames based on the data are fluidity, accuracy, relevance, discourse management and disease-focus The criterion for presenting data for analysis here is at least 30 answers for the total of six disease categories and five for each on average, as fewer than five answers is insufficient for a detailed analysis. Some participants did not adequately provide reasons for why they chose a particular answer, in which case the answers are considered 'insufficient information'. There are also cases where participants did not provide reasons at all, where no words were given. Neither of these two cases, insufficient information cases (1.8% on average) and no information (10.3% on average) cases, is counted in the English corpus.

In general, comments appear in two opposite groups: positive or negative. The positive frame, according to Tseng and Zhang (2020), indicates a maximum cognitive effect and optimal relevance of the use of EL in the data, while the negative frame implies a minimum cognitive effect and minimal relevance. These two frames represent positive or negative responses by the participants, which can lead to acceptance or rejection of EL used in the data.

8.2.2.1 Language-Focused Frames This frame focuses on the language itself. For example, whether the language used in the online medical information is fluid, informative, relevant, accurate or clear. This frame consists of six sub-frames: fluidity, informativeness, relevance, accuracy, clarity and discourse management.

Fluidity Frame (FL) The fluidity frame can be triggered when participants' motivation relates to fluidity and under-specification of the EL in question. In Table 8.3 and the tables that follow, the left column contains extracted responses from the participants who chose EL as their preference, and the right column contains comments from the participants who chose non-EL as their preference. (E1) stands for comments in relation to Excerpt 8.1, and so forth. Each frame is illustrated by ten samples from the data, and #1 stands for Example 1 in that frame, and so on.

In Table 8.3, #1 correctly observes that *lots of* indicates an emphasis of 'more than usual', which does not necessarily refer to a number (Moxey and Sanford, 1993). The EL group highlights the usefulness of elastic expressions with a positive tone: it is open to interpretation and is more inclusive. However, #6 insists that EL must be eradicated in medical advice, owing to its subjectivity. The non-EL group tended to emphasise the unhelpfulness of EL and viewed EL negatively, saying it was too general and uncertain. Exact information was promoted for better-informed parents as well (#8).

Informativeness Frame (IN) This frame adheres to Grice's (1975) conversational maxim of being informative. As shown in Table 8.4, the EL side argued that more detailed and optional information is informative, while the non-EL side disagreed, presenting the counterargument that more specific information brings a good understanding and is thus more informative. For example, #1 explains that the reason for choosing EL is its informativeness, but #6 argues for the opposite: non-EL is more informative than EL.

Table 8.3 *Fluidity frame*

EL (pro-EL group hereafter)	Non-EL (pro non-EL group hereafter)
1. Amount of fluid needed may vary per child. *Lots of* encourages 'more than usual' levels of fluids should be consumed. (E6) 2. It allows for more fluid interpretation as recognition of disorders change. (E4) 3. The statement is flexible. (E3) 4. *Might* is a lot more accommodating for possibilities that could be expected. (E3) 5. *10 forms* seems too definitive. (E4)	6. Medical advice must eradicate subjectivity, as *lots of* is such a subjective term. (E6) 7. If we know how many are defined, why not say '10 known' or '10 diagnosed' – *many* is too generic. (E4) 8. It is specific and I know exactly what I would need to do. The term *lots of* leaves me unsure. (E6) 9. Leaves less room for questioning. (E5) 10. Specific – better for worried parents, gives parents stricter and more direct guidelines to adhere to. (E6)

Table 8.4 *Informativeness frame*

EL	Non-EL
1. Sentence seems to be more informative and intelligent when the *more than* is included. (E1) 2. *And so on* shows you that there are more than 2 types of flu. (E5) 3. Informative plus clear. (E5) 4. Includes more information, indicates that there are more types, therefore I feel more informed. (E5) 5. Encompassing detail is more helpful in this scenario. (E5)	6. A more specific sentence is more informative. (E1) 7. More informative. (E6) 8. The use of the word *ten* is far more specific and allows better and more thorough understanding. (E4) 9. (EL) too open, EL sentence is too ambiguous – they need to be concise and informative. (E1) 10. Specific information can lead to a more effective treatment, as everyone may have different perceptions of *lots of*. (E6)

Relevance Frame (RE) This frame relates to Grice's (1975) maxim of relation, where one tries to be relevant and says things that are pertinent to the discussion. This conversational principle was later developed into relevance theory (Sperber and Wilson, 1995 [1986]). One of its core principles is that relevant communication is to achieve maximum cognitive effects using minimal processing effort. In Table 8.5, #1 commented that an exact number might not be relevant in the case under consideration, and, therefore, EL is good enough to fit the context (Zhang, 2015). Most comments in the EL camp mentioned that non-EL is not necessary and not relevant. #5 states that EL makes it easier – in

Table 8.5 *Relevance frame*

EL	Non-EL
1. Unless the 10 forms are relevant, I don't need to know exactly how many there are, at least in this statement. (E4) 2. The other line is too specific and I think the number being included is a little unnecessary. (E6) 3. 10 is not elaborated, and an unnecessary specificity. (E4) 4. I don't think the specifying of 6 glasses is necessary. (E6) 5. The extra 0.2 of 7.2 is unnecessary. No such thing as 0.2 of a female; does not affect perception. Simplifying it to *about* makes it easier. (E2)	6. I don't need to know the rest unless relevant. (E5) 7. Irrelevant information. (E5) 8. Elastic expressions are not necessary. (E1) 9. The second expression is far more specific and easily interpreted as a whole rather than singling out pointless words that I find irrelevant. (E6) 10. *And so on* seems unnecessary. (E5)

other words, it requires 'less processing effort'. The quotes from the non-EL camp, however, consider EL negatively – for example, #6 considers EL to be pointless and irrelevant.

Accuracy Frame (AC) The accuracy frame tends to be employed when participants' motivation relates to exactness, correctness, truthfulness and verisimilitude. In Table 8.6, participants who prefer EL argue that general and elastic information is actually more accurate (#1 and #2). EL is also true to life (#3) and reflects the dynamics of the real world (#4). Participants also point out that non-EL is unrealistic (#5). On the other hand, participants who prefer non-EL interpret the data differently. The reasons for them choosing non-EL include that non-EL is more specific (#6), more concise (#7) and gives the desired non-guessing impression (#8). Non-EL is desired for its objectiveness and non-ambiguity (#9 and #10). The same set of data generates contrastive perceptions and comments, as shown in Table 8.6.

Clarity Frame (CL) This frame adheres to Grice's (1975) maxim of manner: speak clearly, briefly and in an orderly way, and avoid obscurity and ambiguity. For clarity, more comments were made by the non-EL group; few in the EL camp mentioned them. This suggests that clarity may be seen as more non-EL features than EL. Support for non-EL was also asserted by the mention of the negative aspect of EL – for example, #5, #6, #9 and #10 in Table 8.7. This group considered non-EL easy to understand, and EL rambling and confusing.

Table 8.6 *Accuracy frame*

EL	Non-EL
1. More general – an exact time frame is less accurate. (E1) 2. More precise – leaving the possibility open. (E3) 3. More realistic to life. (E4) 4. It provides more specific info, saying other types of flu (not just A and B) are constantly changing. (E5) 5. It's unrealistic to expect a sick child to drink 6 glasses of water. (E6)	6. It's more specific and more than a month can mean 10 years or anything > a month. (E1) 7. 'Might' seems redundant in this case, less concise. (E3) 8. Definite number suggests you have correct information and not guesses. (E4) 9. Concise language giving straightforward information. (E5) 10. Provides an actual number that isn't subjective. (E6)

Table 8.7 *Clarity frame*

EL	Non-EL
1. It is more clear. (E2) 2. Lots of fluid is clear. (E6) 3. Informative plus clear. (E5)	4. Clear, more brief, to the point. (E1) 5. It is a more certain and leaves less up to guessing, far more to the point. (E3) 6. Many could mean 20 or 100 forms, isn't clear. (E4) 7. (6 glasses of water) more clarity to what lots of fluid means. (E6) 8. More specific to parents with no experience. (E6) 9. It gives an exact measurement/number which is easier to understand. (E6) 10. 7.2 is easy and quick, about stops and makes me re-phrase. (E2)

Discourse-Management Frame (DM) This frame represents participants who express their reasons relating to discourse management. For example, they mention that EL or non-EL makes the content 'flow better' (#1) or is 'more cohesive' (#6) in Table 8.8. This type of frame focuses on how well the text itself flows, paying attention to the consistency and structure of the text.

8.2.2.2 Language-User-Focused Frames This frame differs from the above-mentioned language-focused frame in that this frame does not so much concern the language itself as the language users' beliefs about and feelings towards the language used. This frame consists of five subframes: trustfulness, folk–individual, lay–professional, voluntary–involuntary and indifference.

Trustfulness Frame (TR) Table 8.9 shows that when participants consider some information true or untrue, or when they view healthcare professionals as trustworthy or unreliable, the frame of trustfulness is activated.

Table 8.8 *Discourse-management frame*

EL	Non-EL
1. Provides more variety, flows better. (E1) 2. Better flow and cohesion. (E2) 3. Makes the wording follow a better pattern. (E2) 4. Stating there are 10 forms will need to be followed by describing each type. (E4) 5. It sounds better as if there is only A and B, the use of 'and' instead of a comma would be more appropriate. (E5)	6. More cohesive. (E1) 7. Consistency, why use a rounded figure for females and not for the other decimals in the same sentence? (E2) 8. 'Might not ever' doesn't sound quite right, second option flows better and still makes sense. (E3) 9. 'Might not ever' sounds chunkier than 'will never' and the meaning of the sentence does not change. (E3) 10. There are other decimals in the paragraph, so it should be taken to the same number of significant figures, not just left at 'about'. (E2)

Table 8.9 *Trustfulness frame*

EL	Non-EL
1. *A month* can be dangerous; if someone happens to last longer, they may question the integrity of the text. (E1) 2. *Never* doesn't appear to be true; *may* would be better. (E3) 3. The first one does not imply that there are more not listed, whereas there is. The second one is more truthful. (E5) 4. Don't say something is absolute when it isn't. (E3) 5. Saying *never* makes a promise that can be broken, which makes it seem like a lie. It seems more truthful and accurate to use *might*. (E3)	6. If it is expressed that schizophrenia lasts for more than 1 month, it might imply that if you exhibit symptoms of this condition for only 1 month, you do not have schizophrenia, which may not be true. (E1) 7. More specific leading to more trust in health professional. (E2) 8. *About* makes stats seem less reliable. (E2) 9. Seems specific, so I would more than likely trust information rather than the vague term *lots of*. (E6) 10. If true, then it gives more validity to the article – more accurate and precise. (E4)

Uncertainty characterises sources of medical information and leads to issues of credibility and trustworthiness. Trust between the medical information giver and receiver is something that both parties need to work on to minimise the doubt and uncertainty of the receivers towards the information sources (Babrow et al.,1998: 3). The trustfulness frame corresponds especially to Grice's (1975) maxim of quality: the speaker tries to be truthful and does not give false or unsubstantiated information. This frame includes feedback on the credibility of the EL or non-EL used, in particular whether participants thought the EL or non-EL was trustworthy or not; it relates to online users' level of health literacy and trust in the source of the information (Borah and Xiao, 2018; Paige et al., 2017; Thon and Jucks, 2017). Tseng and Zhang (2020) argue that the trustfulness frame may be activated when numbers are involved, and trustfulness is brought up only when a specific number, with or without an approximator, occurred in the data. This claim is not supported by the data here. For example, #2 and #5 in Table 8.9 do not refer to numbers. This means that a trustfulness frame can be activated whether numbers are mentioned or not.

The pro-EL group explained trustfulness in terms of the language user's sense of reality: elasticity is a matter of fact, saying otherwise is untrue. Those who chose non-EL argued that precision and exactness lead to trustfulness and reliability – for example, #7. Comment #10 seemed unsure whether the non-EL expression ('There are *10* forms of anxiety disorder') was true, but if it was true, the precise form was preferred. The data highlights a trust issue involving medical information.

Folk–Individual Frame (FI) This frame includes the comments relating to folk knowledge or individual views. According to Tseng and Zhang (2020), folk knowledge refers to common sense and common beliefs or assumptions; the individual frame refers to individuals' considerations, stance and personality traits (e.g., a personal like/dislike of EL or non-EL). The individual frame is triggered more often than the folk-knowledge frame in the English data. In the EL group, as shown in Table 8.10, the common-sense frame was evoked from #1 to #3. For example, #1 states that his/her reason for choosing EL was that it is known that a person is a whole person, not a segment of one. Furthermore, #3 makes the point that parents always know best for their children. Both the EL

Table 8.10 *Folk–individual frame*

EL	Non-EL
1. It is clearer to keep it in whole numbers, because you can't have 0.2 of a person. (E2)	6. (I don't like) vague. (E5)
2. Common knowledge of what means to drink *lots of* fluids. (E6)	7. I didn't even know there were more types of flu, I guess I liked the clarification. (E5)
3. Leave interpretation open to parents who know child best. (E6)	8. I like it more specific. (E6)
4. Statistics confuse me. (E2)	9. I prefer knowing the exact number. (E4)
5. I feel that 6 glasses is a tad unrealistic to give kids who are feeling unwell. (E6)	10. I personally prefer solid numbers. *About 7* could be anywhere from 6.5% to 7.4%. (E2)

and non-EL groups were also motivated by individual viewpoints. For example, #4 makes it clear he or she does not like exact numbers, while #6 and #8 do not personally like vague numbers.

Lay–Professional Frame (LP) According to Tseng and Zhang (2020), this frame includes comments in relation to the views of a layperson versus a professional. For example, when commenting on a professional issue, a non-medical participant might mitigate their tone by evoking the layman frame. There were generally two groups in the English corpus: humanities students and health-science students. Some students from health science suggested they had medical knowledge, but other students tended to consider themselves laypersons. This gap in professional knowledge evokes the lay–professional frame.

As shown in Table 8.11, examples from the EL group were hard to come by, and there were more examples from the non-EL group. #1 is a layman frame, where the participant is positioned as a non-professional. In contrast, #2 evokes the professional frame, with the writer of the website information presented as an authoritative figure. *And so on* is a general extender, and its interpretation needs shared knowledge (Overstreet, 1999), which all evoke the layman frame

Table 8.11 *Lay–professional frame*

EL	Non-EL
1. I don't need to know the different forms of anxiety. (E4)	2. It gives the impression that the writer knows what they are talking about. (E1) 3. *And so on* requires prior knowledge and educated assumption, not all of us do. (E5) 4. *And so on* doesn't mean anything to me, I don't know the other types. (E5) 5. I don't know enough about the different types to know what *so on* refers to. (E5) 6. Setting a minimum or a number could be more beneficial as parents' and doctor's point of view could be different. (E6) 7. Tells us exactly how many drinks they need. We can't gauge how many drinks *lots of* is. (E6) 8. It's better to provide explicit instructions. (E6) 9. Gives exact amount, also gives a goal for treating cold. (E6) 10. Better to be specific when giving health/medical advice. (E6)

(e.g., #3, #4, #5). From #6 to #10, a major point made is that non-EL is needed as most of us need precise medical advice, given our lay backgrounds.

Voluntary–Involuntary Frame (VI) According to Tseng and Zhang (2020), this frame is evoked in comments expressing how the advice and suggestions sound to the participants. Participants may or may not like being informed about what to do. Thus, some were happy to follow the advice (voluntary frame), but others were not so willing (involuntary frame). All examples in this frame, as shown in Table 8.12, are specifically from Excerpt 6. There is a trend: the EL group tends to be motivated by the involuntary frame, while the non-EL group leans towards the voluntary frame. The former argues that freedom and flexibility for patients are crucial if they are to make the best decisions in their different situations; the latter group are happy to follow authorised instruction/guidance, which in their view is more beneficial to patients.

Indifference Frame (ID) According to Tseng and Zhang (2020), this frame is evoked when participants show indifference to the use of EL by ticking both EL and non-EL, or neither, as their preference. In Table 8.13, #3 points out that the register of EL fits the context, though both EL and non-EL are fine in principle. #4 highlights the role of context, which can sort out which form of language is better suited. #5 argues that there is a difference between someone who suffers anxiety and someone who just generally browses

Table 8.12 *Voluntary–involuntary frame*

EL	Non-EL
1. No restrictions as every child is different, allows for flexibility and less pressure to have 6 glasses. (E6) 2. Some children may not want 6 glasses, because I am drawing on prior knowledge and that's what I've been told. (E6) 3. *6 glasses* is too specific, *lots of fluid* is subjective – it's up to what person needs. (E6) 4. Second sentence sounds too specific and regimented, it [EL] doesn't force them to consume, just suggests. (E6) 5. *6 glasses* is too prescriptive. You cannot force a child to drink 6 glasses daily, so *lots of fluid* is a more understanding and achievable approach. (E6)	6. More direct, better instructions for potentially nervous parents. (E6) 7. Gives the reader more guidance. (E6) 8. I couldn't really decide here, but the specific instructions are less arbitrary. (E6) 9. *Lots of fluids* is not a good description. *6 glasses* is a set guideline helpful to caregivers who may be unsure. 10. Gives clear guidance on expectation when taking direction, not up for debate. (E6)

Table 8.13 *Indifference frame*

Excerpts from the data
1. Neither/both expressions are fine, they have different meanings though and this is important. I don't feel like these have to be specific in the context of the excerpt, but it could be needed. (E1)
2. They are both fine, but *more than* implies more time for the symptoms to be experienced, whereas *a month* by itself assumes it ends right then. It depends what you want to say. (E1)
3. Both are OK, the 2nd (*about*) should not be used in formal academic writing though. (E2)
4. I would use both, however if there was absolutely no chance I would say *never*. It would depend on the situation. (E3)
5. It depends on the context a bit as if I was suffering from anxiety I would like to know specifics to potentially diagnose, but if just looking at general info the top one (EL, author notes) is okay. (E4)
6. Both make sense, depends how many flu [*sic*] the paper is referencing. (E5)
7. I really prefer neither. (E5)
8. The first doesn't include all varieties, and the second is unprofessionally worded. (E5)
9. Depending on the facts, the sentence should reflect correct facts. If it's just A and B, then first option is right, and if it's more than two, second option [*and* so on, author notes] is right. (E5)
10. Both work well. If someone wants to know an exact amount, they have it, but they can also assume that from *lots of*. They both make sense and are to the point and equally informative. (E6)

online. There are two attitudes here: both are fine (e.g., #6), or neither is to my liking (e.g., #7). One point made clear is that context plays a dominant role in deciding whether to use EL or non-EL in a given situation.

8.2.2.3 Disease-Focused Frame (DI) This frame is operationalised when aspects of a particular disease are mentioned. In the questionnaire, the six excerpts cover six diseases, each of which exhibits its own features. For example, mental illness can be seen as something beyond an individual's control, unlike other illnesses (Barry et al., 2013; Major, 2009). In Table 8.14, pro-EL participants argue that elastic expressions suit the nature of the diseases in question, as reinforced by #2 and #3, both of which highlight the positive side of *might*. Participants favouring non-EL think exact information is needed to address the specific qualities of the diseases.

As shown by the examples in Table 8.3–8.12, when participants explain their choices, two approaches are taken: positive about the choice, negative about the alternative. For example, as Table 8.12 shows, when one chose EL, one of the positive answers was '(EL) No restrictions as every child is different, allows for flexibility and less pressure to have 6 glasses. (E6)', and the negative answer was '6 glasses is too prescriptive. You cannot force a child to drink 6 glasses daily .... (E6)'. The ranking of negative answers is as follows: Excerpt 8.6

Table 8.14 *Disease-related frame*

EL	Non-EL
E1 (schizophrenia) 1. Due to the nature of schizophrenia, I feel *more than* is more appropriate as it's ongoing. (E1) *E3* (thyroid cancer) 2. The emphasis on *might* shows that the small thyroid nodules may cause problems, but it is unlikely which makes me feel better. (E3) 3. The use of *might* is more accurate as there is still a possibility of cancer development, it would be problematic to claim these growths definitely won't cause harm if even a slight possibility exists. (E3) *E4* (anxiety) 4. Anxiety disorder seems too complex to categorize into such specific forms. *Many* rather than the set number *10*, makes anxiety a bit more serious, as if given a strict rule of *10* people will categorise and self-diagnose, most likely incorrect. (E4) *E5* (influenza) 5. I have gotten the point that flu types are forever changing and I don't need each one listed out. (E5) 6. (*And so on*) acknowledges there are other types of flu, provides more info. Possibility of flu evolving to type C, wider range of influenza embodies flu family. (E5)	*E2* (pancreatic cancer) 7. Mortality rate should be a specific figure. (E2) *E3* (thyroid cancer) 8. Although there might be a risk, it might never happen. (E3) *E4* (anxiety) 9. Anxiety disorders are clearly classified as being *10*, thus an exact number is preferred, which can be helpful for those with anxiety. (E4) *E6* (cold) 10. Cold is so common that people should know how much fluid to drink to get better. (E6)

(cold) 24%, Excerpt 8.5 (influenza) 23.8%, Excerpt 8.3 (thyroid) 19.6%, Excerpt 8.2 (pancreatic cancer) 17.9%, Excerpt 8.1 (schizophrenia) 12.6% and Excerpt 8.4 (anxiety) 12%. The average percentage was 18.3%. This means that for approximately every five answers, one was in the negative form. When participants talked about cold and influenza, they tended to use the negative form more than when they talked about anxiety and schizophrenia. It appears that they avoided using a negative form in mental illness discussion. It could be the sensitivity around communicating mental illness affecting this.

The above twelve frames illustrate varied reasons from the opposing camps. For example, whether they preferred EL or not, the participants agreed that the use of language should be truthful, informative, clear, relevant and accurate – all these adhere to the cooperative principle (Grice, 1975) and the principles of relevance theory (Sperber and Wilson, 1986). A general trend shown is that the same elastic expression in the survey generates opposing perceptions. For example, some found *lots of* informative, others found it confusing. These views echo the findings in the existing literature. VL is traditionally described as something to be avoided, as it seems misleading and muddy (Channell, 1994; Jucker et al., 2003). Cutting (2015: 108, 118) confirms respondents (in her survey of their views on VL) also showed both positive (e.g., an informal tone, closeness) and negative (e.g., impressions of laziness, incompetence, impatience, hurried speech, indifference and unreliable/ill-informed responses) attitudes towards the use of VL.

8.2.3 Frequency Distributions of the 12 Frames

This section discusses the quantitative data of the 12 frames, revealing the patterns that emerged in terms of how the frames were employed to explain reasons for choosing EL over non-EL, or vice versa.

There are three groups in Figure 8.4: Group 1 (language-focused) – FL, IN, RE, AC, CL, DM; Group 2 (language-user-focused) – TR, FI, LP, VI, ID; and Group 3 (disease-focused). In total, participants presented 2,800 frames: 1,350 concerning EL, 1,375 concerning non-EL and 75 concerning indifference. There is an even frame distribution between EL and non-EL. Most frames occurred in Group 1, with the fluidity frame almost all for the EL preference. The majority of the accuracy frames were for the non-EL preference. This pattern suggests that EL is chosen primarily for its fluidity, which provides flexibility and space for healthcare information to be conveyed. On the other hand, the accuracy frame is chosen primarily for its exactness, which provides certainty and precision for healthcare information to be conveyed. The focuses differ between the two camps, a situation which is attributed to the differing nature of EL and non-EL.

Figure 8.4 shows that the top three frames are AC (754), FI(I) 646) and FL (619), while the bottom three frames are LP(P) (29), DM (52) and TR (63). This suggests that when people decide whether EL or non-EL is preferred, they are mostly concerned about accuracy, individual/personal opinion and fluidity. They are least concerned about professional opinion, discourse management and trustfulness. To elaborate further, in terms of the dual folk–individual frame, it is primarily used for the 'individual' side of the sub-frame. Participants from both sides (EL or non-EL) explained that they preferred EL or non-EL based on their own views, highlighting individuality as opposed to collective/community/folk views. The issue of trust is also shared almost equally between EL and non-EL groups – both sides employed this frame at a similar rate. When coming to the clarity frame, the non-EL group activated this frame five times more than the EL group, indicating that clarity is associated more with non-EL. As far as the disease-focused frame is concerned, the EL group picked it about 10 times more than the non-EL group, suggesting that elasticity is needed in describing

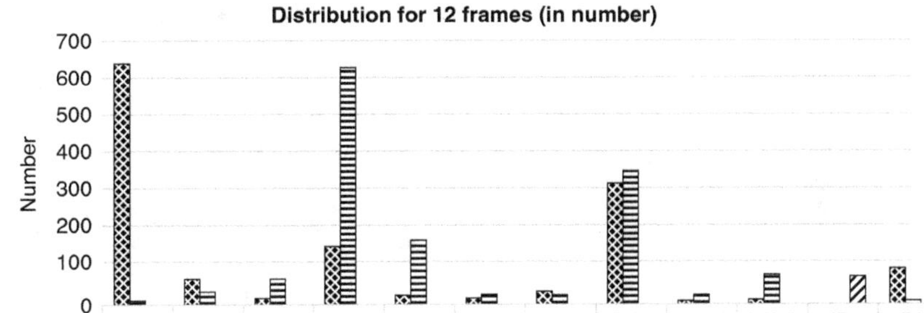

	FL	IN	RE	AC	CL	DM	TR	FI(I)	LP(P)	VI(V)	ID	DI
EL	608	73	20	150	29	21	33	309	5	7	0	95
non-EL	11	35	56	604	163	31	30	337	24	75	0	9
ID											75	

Figure 8.4 Distribution of 12 frames (in number; English data)
Note: Fluidity (FL), informativeness (IN), relevance (RE), accuracy (AC), clarity (CL), discourse-management (DM), trustfulness (TR), folk–individual (individual, FI(I)), lay–professional (professional, LP(P)), voluntary–involuntary (voluntary, VI(V)), indifference (ID) and disease-focused (DI). Due to a limited occurrence, the folk, lay and involuntary frames were omitted.

diseases. The indifference frame was independent, belonging neither to EL nor to non-EL.

Overall, the frames used to argue more for EL choices are fluidity, informativeness, trustfulness and disease-focused. On the other hand, those used to argue more for non-EL are relevance, accuracy, clarity, discourse-management, folk–individual (individual), lay–professional (professional) and involuntary–voluntary (voluntary). According to the results, EL is perceived as more fluid, informative, trustful and good enough to communicate disease information; and non-EL is more relevant, accurate, clear, useful for discourse management, professional and more helpful. The findings brought to light in the data feature EL and non-EL in this way.

Figure 8.5 shows that the 2,800 individual frames are evenly distributed among the six diseases, with between 435 and 468 frames each. However, the type of frame varies across the six diseases. The fluidity frame is used most in the thyroid excerpt, the informativeness frame most for schizophrenia, the relevance frame most for influenza, the accuracy frame most for pancreatic cancer, the clarity frame most for pancreatic cancer, the discourse-management frame most for influenza, the trustfulness frame most for thyroid, the folk–individual (individual) frame most for pancreatic cancer, the lay–professional (professional) frame most for influenza, the voluntary–involuntary (voluntary) frame most for colds, the indifference frame most for schizophrenia and the disease-focused frame most for influenza. The pattern that emerges here is the

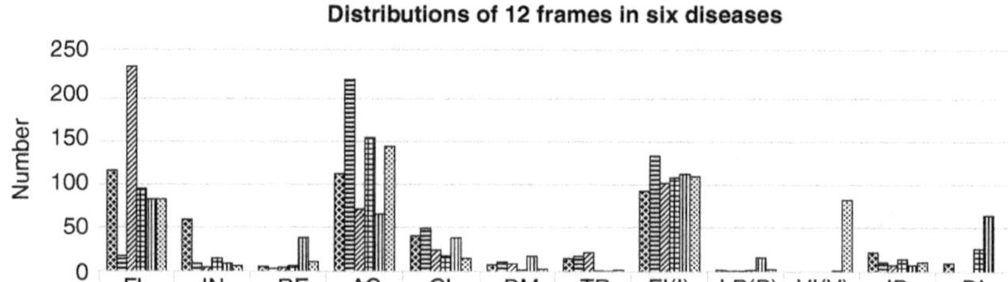

	FL	IN	RE	AC	CL	DM	TR	FI(I)	LP(P)	VI(V)	ID	DI
SCHI	113	59	7	109	42	7	16	91	3	0	23	12
PANC	18	9	5	216	49	11	20	132	2	0	12	0
THYR	229	4	6	71	24	11	21	100	2	0	8	0
ANXI	97	17	7	153	20	2	1	106	3	0	16	28
INFL	80	12	39	64	40	18	2	110	17	1	5	64
COLD	82	7	12	141	17	3	3	107	2	81	11	0

Figure 8.5 Distribution of 12 frames across six diseases

following: thyroid tops the frames of fluidity and trustfulness; schizophrenia tops the frames of informativeness and indifference; influenza tops the frames of relevance, discourse management, lay–professional (professional) and disease focused; pancreatic cancer tops the frames of accuracy, clarity and folk–individual (individual); and colds tops the frame of voluntary–involuntary (voluntary). Two diseases, influenza and pancreatic cancer, generate a wider range of frames – four each – than the other four diseases. Colds generates the least number of frames in the data.

Table 8.15 shows the different frame focuses of each of the six diseases. For example, four of the six – schizophrenia, thyroid cancer, anxiety and colds – all have the same three frames for their top three, though in different orders. By juxtaposing Table 8.15 and Figure 8.4, we can see that, when responding to the data related to the four diseases, EL/non-EL groups anticipated elasticity (most for EL) or accuracy (most for non-EL), respectively, as well as individual views collectively. For pancreatic cancer, the non-EL group has the majority, because the accuracy and clarity frames tend to be employed to support the non-EL preference. For influenza, the EL group comes out on top, as the fluidity and disease-focused frames are used more and, in particular, used more to support EL preference. Folk–individual (individual) is in the top three for all six diseases, indicating that the choice of EL or non-EL is often a matter of individual preference.

8.3 Social Factors

This section considers two social factors, gender and age. VL is seen conventionally as less powerful language (Channell, 1994) and women's language has

Table 8.15 *Top three frames for six diseases*

Disease	Top 1	Top 2	Top 3
SCHI	FL	AC	FI(I)
PANC	AC	FI(I)	CL
THYR	FL	FI(I)	AC
ANXI	AC	FI(I)	FL
INFL	FI(I)	FL	AC/DI
COLD	AC	FI(I)	FL

a 'high degree of unspecificity' (Carter, 1980: 232). Does gender, then, have an impact on people's preference for EL?[2] There is no consensus on this: some researchers find that VL is not influenced by gender (e.g., Aijmer, 1997; Cheshire, 2007), while others disagree. For example, men have been found to use fewer boosters such as *very* (Murphy, 2010) and fewer general extenders such as *something like that* (Levey, 2012). However, other studies have found that men use more VL (e.g., *very*) than women (Parvaresh, 2018; Pichler and Levey, 2011). Such contradictory findings suggest that gender differences in the use of EL are not absolute but act more like 'tendencies' or 'variations' (Sunderland, 2004: 14).

Similar conflicting results appear when considering the age factor. Some studies have found that adults use VL more than teenagers, although the teenagers love it for its coolness and because they 'cannot be bothered to be precise', as in 'they, like, wanna see, like, how we talk an' all that, you know' (Stenström et al., 2002: 86–88). Others have found the opposite (e.g., Pichler and Levey, 2011; Tagliamonte and Denis, 2010), that teenagers use VL more than or as much as adults (e.g., Palacios Martínez, 2011). One thing is relatively clear: older people tend to be more formal and traditional than younger people, preferring to use such vague expressions (e.g., *and things*) (Tagliamonte and Denis, 2010) *and so on and so forth* (Palacios Martínez, 2011), while younger individuals use vague phrases such as *and stuff* (Tagliamonte and Denis, 2010), *and blah blah blah, and stuff like that, and crap, and junk like this* and *shit like that* (Stenström et al., 2002).

This section investigates whether gender and age have an influence on the ability to understand EL and how EL is preferred, an approach that has not been taken in the literature up to now. The findings may contribute to making a link between specific social factors and the understanding of EL and preference for EL/non-EL.

[2] The term 'preference' in this study refers to whether a participant in the survey likes health information to be delivered using EL or non-EL.

8.3.1 *Gender Attitudes*

Of the 541 participants, 378 (70%) were female and 163 (30%) were male. In the 6.8% group who had problems with the use of EL, women were found to have a greater level of difficulty in understanding EL.

In Figure 8.6, on average, 8.3% females had difficulty understanding EL, twice as many as the men (3.4%). The gap between the two groups is particularly wide in answers to question 2 (more than three times), question 5 (close to 4 times) and question 6 (5 times). The finding that women had more difficulty in understanding EL, coupled with the finding that women actually preferred EL less than man (Figure 8.7), is not in line with the stereotypical theory that women prefer to use VL more than men do (Channell, 1994) and that women's language has a 'high degree of unspecificity' (Carter, 1980: 232). Female participants in this study preferred EL less than the male participants, perhaps because some of them found difficulty in dealing with vagueness in language.

While Figure 8.6 shows some differences between male and female participants, their differences within the yes-category and the no-category, respectively, are not statistically significant: for the 'Yes' group χ^2[d.f. 5, n = 220] = 4.808, p = 0.44, and for the 'No' group, χ^2[d.f. 5, n = 2914] = 8.247, p = 0.143 (p = 0.05). From a statistics point of view, this similarities-across-gender result supports, in principle, findings by Cheshire (2007), Aijmer (1997) and Zhang (2015) in that they did not always find a gender influence in language use. For example, Zhang (2015) found no statistical significance between men and women in using boosters, but there

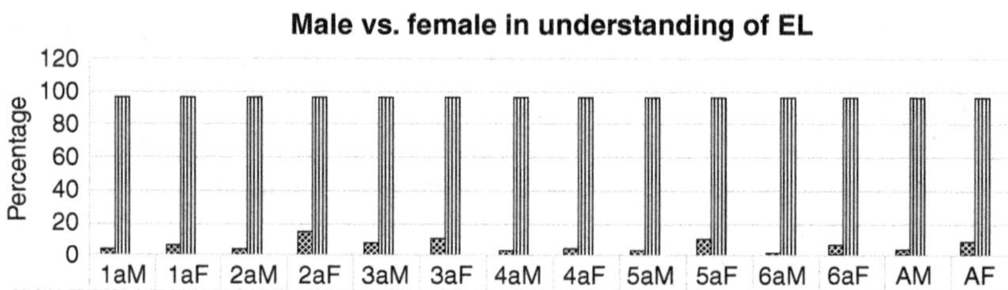

	1aM	1aF	2aM	2aF	3aM	3aF	4aM	4aF	5aM	5aF	6aM	6aF	AM	AF
Yes	3.1	6.1	4.3	13.8	6.7	10.1	2.5	4.2	2.5	9.3	1.2	6.1	3.4	8.3
No	96.3	93.4	95.1	86	93.3	89.7	97.5	95.5	96.9	90.5	98.2	93.4	96.2	91.4
N/A	0.6	0.5	0.6	0.2	0	0.2	0	0.3	0.6	0.2	0.6	0.5	0.4	0.3

Figure 8.6 Male versus female responses to Type A questions
Note: 1aM = Excerpt 1, Type A question, male participant; 1aF = 1aM's female counterpart. The last two columns (i.e., AM and AF) are the averages for the male and female participants.

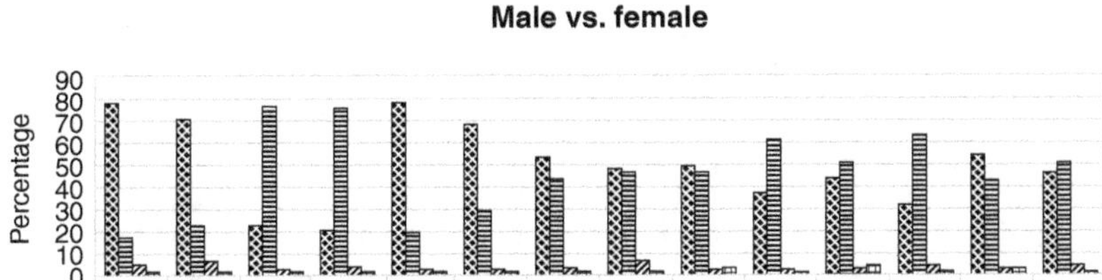

	1bM	1bF	2bM	2bF	3bM	3bF	4bM	4bF	5bM	5bF	6bM	6bF	AM	AF
EL	77.3	70.6	22.1	19.3	77.3	68.5	52.8	47.9	49.1	36.8	43.6	31	53.7	45.7
Non-EL	16.6	22.5	75.5	76.2	19.6	28.3	42.9	45.8	46	60.3	49.7	64.3	41.7	49.6
Both	4.9	5.8	1.8	3.7	1.2	1.9	3.1	5.3	1.8	2.1	2.5	4.5	2.6	3.9
N/A	1.2	1.1	0.6	0.8	1.9	1.3	1.2	1	3.1	0.8	4.2	0.2	2	0.9

Figure 8.7 Male versus female responses to Type B questions
Note: 1bM = Excerpt 1, Type B question, male participant; 1bF = 1bM's female counterpart. The last two columns (i.e., AM and AF) are the averages for the male and female participants.

was a significant difference in using hedges, which men actually used more. Women were found to use more intensifiers (e.g., *very*), bringing more interactivity to communication (Wright and Hosman, 1983), as the use of intensifiers may signify the speaker's power over others (Zhang, 2015). There have been discrepancies in terms of gender difference in using EL, owing to the studies being conducted in different discourses and their use of different methodologies.

Figure 8.7 shows that women preferred less EL than men, especially in Excerpt 3, concerning whether very small thyroid nodules would 'never' or 'might' not ever cause problems during one's lifetime; and in Excerpt 6, concerning whether children with a cold should 'drink six glasses of water' or 'drink lots of fluids' each day. The conventional assumption that women are likely to prefer and use VL as it is less powerful language (Channell, 1994; Carter, 1980) is not supported here. Cutting (2007) also reports a sevenfold greater use of EL in conversations by females than males.

Based on the raw data in Figure 8.8, a Chi-square test was conducted, but this time only three categories (EL, Non-EL and Both) were included, with no category for N/A. This is because it is inappropriate to include a category with more than 20% of its cells consisting of a less-than-5 expected frequency, and N/A is such a case. The test result, χ^2 [d.f. 20, n = 3206] = 499.746, p <0.05, verifies that the difference between males and females is statistically significant.

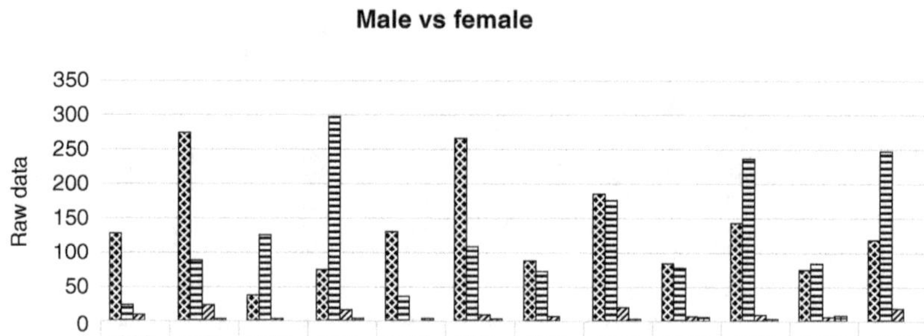

	1bM	1bF	2bM	2bF	3bM	3bF	4bM	4bF	5bM	5bF	6bM	6bF
EL	126	267	36	73	126	259	86	181	80	139	71	117
Non-EL	27	85	123	288	32	107	70	173	75	228	81	243
Both	8	22	3	14	2	7	5	20	3	8	4	17
N/A	2	4	1	3	3	5	2	4	5	3	7	1

Figure 8.8 Impact of gender factor (raw data)

8.3.2 Age Factor

Almost all participants were 17–29 years-old, divided as follows: 17-year-olds (mostly foundation-year students), 18–21 year-olds (mostly undergraduates, with a four-year range), 22–25-year-olds (undergraduates and postgraduates, with a four-year range) and 26–29-year-olds (mostly postgraduates, with a four-year range). The criteria for the four categories are age and their study stages: the 17-year-olds were quite a young and special group – they were not quite adults yet. The remainder of the three categories were divided equally, four years apart, making the data comparable. They were also at different stages of their studies, possibly with changed perceptions of language use.

The total number of participants in the English corpus was 541, but the total number included in Figure 8.9 is 515, as the remaining 26 participants were between 30 and 50 years old. They are not included in this analysis due to their small number in groupings – that is, their grouping covered 20 years instead of one or four years, which makes a clear diagram difficult to construct.

Figure 8.9 shows an approximate correlation: the younger the participants, the greater the level of difficulty in understanding EL. This makes sense in that older participants will have had more linguistic experience. The 17-year-old group shows the highest rate of difficulty, and the 26–29-year-olds show the lowest. However, the 22–25-year-old group show a higher level of difficulty compared with the 18–21-year-old group, so the correlation is an approximate one rather than absolute.

The findings support what is stated in the literature. For example, Parvaresh (2015: 129) confirms that usually 'vague expressions are used appropriately, interpreted normally and thus do not cause any problem for the hearer'. Other

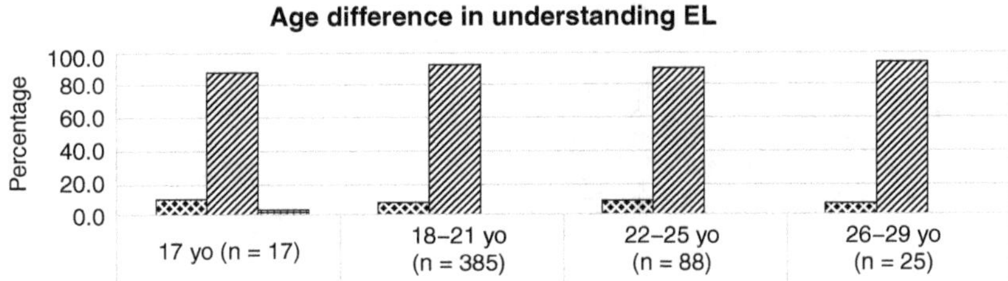

	17 yo (n = 17)	18–21 yo (n = 385)	22–25 yo (n = 88)	26–29 yo (n = 25)
Yes	8.8	6.6	7.8	5.3
No	89.2	93.2	91.7	94.7
N/A	2.0	0.2	0.6	0.0

Figure 8.9 Age difference in understanding EL

studies have found that an estimated 80–90% of patients are satisfied with the information they find online and would use the Internet again for health information (Lagan et al., 2010; Neelapala et al., 2008). The English data collected for this study found approximately 93% of participants had no trouble dealing with the use of EL in online information. People can use EL to communicate without difficulty when they share 'common ground' (Jucker et al., 2003: 1737). The findings demonstrate that when EL is used, the vast majority of recipients can understand its meaning because of the common ground they share with the authors of the online medical information.

The pattern in Figure 8.10 indicates that the older the respondents were, the more they preferred EL and that the younger they were, the more they preferred non-EL, except in the case of the 22–25-year-old cohort – therefore, the trend is an approximate one. This group also shows the highest rate of responses that are 'both' (indifference) and 'N/A' (irrelevant) results. This finding aligns with the findings from Tseng and Zhang (2020) regarding their Chinese data, in that the younger the respondents were, the lower their level of preference for EL, except among 22–25-year-olds.

The English data show that the younger respondents had greater difficulty understanding EL, a tendency which fits with their lower preference for it. Another possible reason is that young people may not use the same style of EL that the creators of the websites used. For example, the younger ones use *and stuff* (Tagliamonte and Denis, 2010), *and blah blah blah*, *and stuff like that*, *and crap*, *and junk like this*, and *shit like that* (Stenström et al., 2002), which are all different from the style of the EL examples in the six excerpts used in the questionnaire for this study. The above different uses might be due to different contexts explored in different studies.

Figure 8.10 generally supports studies confirming that adults use more VL than teenagers (Stenström et al., 2002: 86–88) and not those that find that young

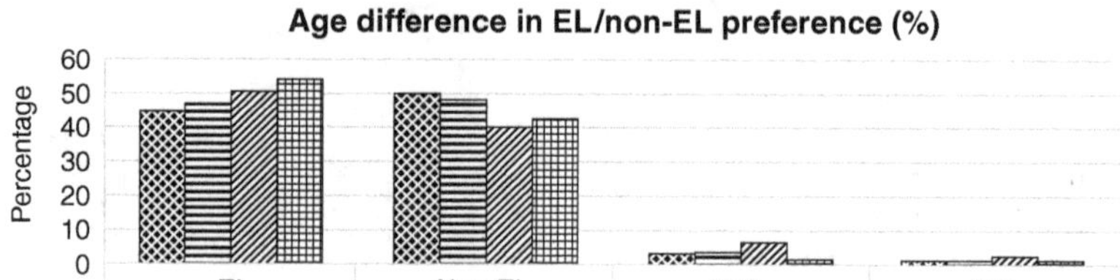

	EL	Non-EL	Both	N/A
17 yo	45.1	51.0	2.9	1.0
18–21 yo	47.0	49.2	2.9	0.9
22–25 yo	51.3	40.5	6.1	2.1
26–29 yo	54.7	44.0	0.7	0.7

Figure 8.10 Age difference in EL/non-EL preference (%)

people use just as much VL as adults (Palacios Martínez, 2011) or even more (Tagliamonte and Denis, 2010; Pichler and Levey, 2011). 'Generally' is used here because the English corpus in this study investigates the preference for EL rather than actual use of it, although the two are linked in that those who dislike it are unlikely to use it.

Based on the raw data in Figure 8.11, a Chi-square test was conducted. The test result, χ^2 [d.f. 3, n = 2953] = 9.937, $p < 0.05$, confirms that the difference among the four age groups is statistically significant.

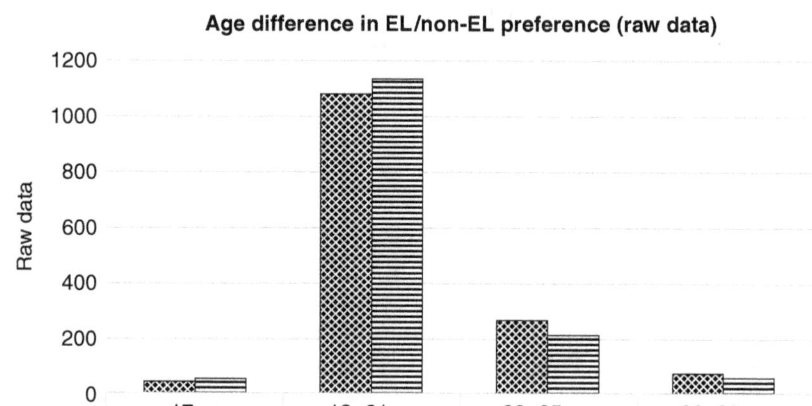

	17 yo	18–21 yo	22–25 yo	26–29 yo
EL	46	1085	271	82
Non-EL	52	1137	214	66

Figure 8.11 Age difference in EL/non-EL preference (raw data)

The findings regarding the age factor on the use of EL raise an interesting question: is there a standard EL for all ages, or should medical writing online offer different versions with EL for different age groups? This is beyond the scope of this study but would be something worth investigating in future research.

8.4 Concluding Remarks

It is important to determine how EL is evaluated in terms of its understandability. It not only contributes to the conceptualisation of EL but also benefits communities (especially the medical community) by suggesting ways to achieve a better understanding of information receivers' ability to comprehend what they are being told. Future research could include a more elaborate study of age factors across a wider range (e.g., from teenage to elderly groups) to provide a more comprehensive account of how age influences the understanding of EL. In the meantime, this study makes a start in helping medical professionals consider a more effective use of EL in their dissemination of online health information to the public.

On average, only 6.8% of participants found it difficult to understand the meaning of EL used in online medical texts constructed for the public. The reasons for having problems in understanding EL are vagueness in language, disease-related factors, unnecessary information and personal experience. In the English corpus, EL empirically proves to be an effective way of communicating general healthcare information, based on the evidence that most participants had not reported incomprehension with the use of EL. This is consistent with the common assumption in the existing literature that people can understand EL.

The findings show that participants' attitudes towards the use of EL in online medical information differ across the six excerpts: while three excerpts with EL were preferred by most, the other three with non-EL were also favoured by some. On average, a neutral attitude emerged: close to half of the participants preferred EL, and the other half, non-EL. What this means is that it is unnecessary to deliberately promote or avoid the use of EL, or to use more or less EL without a specific purpose in mind. EL should be treated just like other types of language, to be utilised when and where it fits. This supports the point made by Channel (1994: 3) that vagueness in language is not a matter of all 'bad' or all 'good'; what matters is the appropriate use of it.

Twelve frames generated from the data explain why the participants made their choices as regards EL, non-EL, both or neither. The frames are categorised into three groups: language-focused, language-user-focused and diseased-focused. The first grouping consists of six frames: fluidity, informativeness, relevance, accuracy, clarity and discourse management. They all adhere closely to cooperative principles and the relevance theory framework, as EL or non-EL was chosen due to its being fluid, informative, relevant, accurate, clear and discourse-required. The second grouping consists of five frames: trustfulness, folk–individual, lay–professional, voluntary–involuntary and indifference, all of which further elaborate the beliefs and feelings of participants in making their choices. The third grouping is disease-focused; namely, the choices that were made closely linked to the nature of the six diseases listed on the questionnaire. This grouping of frames is specific to medical communication.

The patterns emerging from the data suggest that participants tend to employ both positive and negative framing in explaining their preferences, with no clear indication as to whether one is weightier than the other. Often the same expression generated two opposite types of frames (e.g., clear or not clear) depending on participants' viewpoints. Moreover, the pro-EL group tended towards the use of the involuntary frame, and the pro-non-EL group preferred the voluntary frame; it may be that the former appreciated the freedom, flexibility and elasticity of VL while the latter preferred precision and certainty. While this conclusion relates to the context of EL in online medical writing, it could also be a general conclusion based on further research.

In terms of the FI frame in the English corpus, it is the individual views that are emphasised, rather than the folk knowledge. This contrasts with the Chinese corpus, where the folk knowledge is in focus. Of the six pairs of sentences (one original and the other invented) used in the questionnaire, most participants chose original sentences in four cases (1b, 2b, 3b, 4b), which constituted two-thirds of the six cases. There were only two cases (5b, 6b) – one third of the six cases – where most participants chose the invented sentences. This shows that participants preferred original sentences to invented ones, possibly suggesting that the original versions were written in ways the majority of the public accept and expect.

A line of future research could be an inquiry into the positive-versus-negative framing in other discourses, as such a framing is not unique in online medical interactions and can be applied to all kinds of interaction. A comparison between a face-to-face consultation with the doctor and being in front of the computer screen, or between medical and non-medical discourse may also yield interesting findings.

9 Comparison between Chinese and English Regarding Participants' Feedback

Attempts to compare how VL/EL is perceived by its speakers in different languages are rare. One recent study by Cutting (2019) investigates how German, Spanish and Mandarin speakers perceive VL in their languages. One shared attitude towards VL among these speakers, especially in conversations, is the sense of friendliness or closeness it creates, but negative perceptions such as laziness were also reported. Informed by integrative pragmatics, elasticity theory and framing theory, Chapter 7 attempts to understand how Chinese EL in the online health context is perceived, and Chapter 8 explores how Australian university students perceive English EL in a similar online health context. This chapter compares the results presented in the previous two chapters, with a view to rendering a cross-cultural perspective.

9.1 Responses to Whether Elastic Language Is Difficult to Understand and Why

Table 9.1 presents differences between Chinese and English corpora regarding the rates of difficulty in understanding EL, the numbers of elastic items in the health excerpts used and the corresponding diseases. Based on the Chinese and English questionnaire data, the information in Table 9.1 is presented in descending order, from the highest to lowest rate of difficulty. Apart from schizophrenia, the order of the health conditions and their difficulty rates in the Chinese data do not match that of their English counterparts.

Nevertheless, in the seeming disparity lie three similarities. First, the rate of difficulty highly correlates with the number of different elastic items. In the feedback on the Chinese data, the excerpt about anxiety disorder was ranked top in terms of difficulty level, while its counterpart in English received the lowest difficulty rating. The key difference can be attributed to the number of different elastic items used in the respective excerpts: six versus three – that is, there were twice as many in the Chinese excerpt. Second, if we view Table 9.1 in terms of the three disease clusters – cancer, common diseases and mental health conditions – then the excerpt concerning the more severe disease in each cluster tended to attract a higher rate of difficulty in understanding the EL in it,

Table 9.1 *A comparison: Rates of difficulty, numbers of elastic items and diseases*

Chinese data			English data		
Rate of difficulty	# of elastic items	Disease	Rate of difficulty	# of elastic items	Disease
13.3	7 (6)	Anxiety	10.9	5	Pancreatic cancer
9.6	4	Pancreatic cancer	9.1	6(5)	Thyroid cancer
7.5	4 (3)	Thyroid cancer	7.2	4	Influenza
5.8	3	Schizophrenia	5.2	3	Schizophrenia
3.8	3 (2)	Influenza	4.4	3	Cold
2.9	4 (2)	Cold	3.7	3	Anxiety

Note: The number in parenthesis indicates the number of elastic items in the excerpt excluding those that are repeated.

with the exception of the Chinese excerpt regarding anxiety disorder, which was rated more difficult than the excerpt about schizophrenia. This exception may be due to the intensive use of elastic items in the excerpt, and it might suggest that the intensity of EL in the excerpt has a stronger impact on the perception of difficulty than, say, the severity of the disease under discussion.

Third, if we look closely at the Chinese and English excerpts that received the highest difficulty ratings, both have three types of stretchers (see Appendix for the fourth health excerpt in the Chinese questionnaire and the second health excerpt in the English questionnaire). The Chinese excerpt contains three approximate stretchers (*xuduo* 許多 'many', *yixie* 一些 'some' and *jida* 極大 'considerable'), two scalar stretchers (*shifen* 十分 'extremely' and *bushao* 不少 'not a little bit') and one epistemic stretcher (*keneng* 可能 'possibly/ may'). The English excerpt uses two general stretchers (*some*, *someone*), two approximate stretchers (*many*, *or more*) and one epistemic stretcher (*may*). The participants' perceptions of difficulty in understanding EL in the texts seem to support the observation that an intensive use of different types of EL in a text is likely to increase its difficulty.

Apart from the health excerpts and written feedback collected from the questionnaires, interviews with some of the participants provide additional explanations that further clarify the issue. In Chapters 7 and 8, we have identified what makes EL difficult to understand in the Chinese and English corpora, respectively. Because the reasons were identified separately based on interviews conducted in Taiwan and Australia, and the coding for each reason is inevitably affected by the wording used by the interviewees, the six reasons identified in the Chinese-medium interviews (see Section 7.1) and the four reasons derived from English-medium interviews (see Section 8.1.2) may look different. Nevertheless, certain similarities exist. For example, the reasons found in the English interviews such as vagueness and unnecessary information match one of the two reasons identified in the Chinese interview data: 'unfulfilled expectation of more specific information' and 'an undesirable effect created by EL' inasmuch as vagueness or unnecessary information may be perceived as undesirable effects when the expectation for precise information is not met. Furthermore, a disease-related reason corresponds to the reason based on the level of health literacy.

We believe it is equally important to establish the key generic components that affect the perception of EL as difficult to understand. In general terms, three factors that influence potential difficulty caused or evoked by EL/VL are the reader, the health topic and the text. We believe any aspect pertaining to each of the three key components may evoke a difficult-to-understand-EL response. The reader stands for the reader's expectation activated when reading, the identity being constructed (e.g., as a general reader or as a patient looking for specific information), his/her past experience and level of health literacy. The health topic refers to the knowledge being delivered, and this also forms a situational context in which a specific health issue is under discussion. The text concerns language features such as sentence length, structure and the number of elastic terms used. The three key factors – the reader, the health topic and the text – pertain to elements that affect discourse comprehension. As van Dijk and Kintsch (1983: 73) put it, '[p]roduction and understanding require not only linguistic or grammatical information, but other information as well – for example, information about the context, episodic memories, knowledge of the world, intentions, plans and goals, and so on'. We may treat episodic memories (i.e., memories that can be retrieved from the long-term memory) and intentions or expectations as pertaining to the reader's experience and need. Knowledge of the world may be narrowed down to knowledge of health topics. Linguistic and grammatical knowledge corresponds to the text. Viewed in the light of discourse comprehension, the difficulties around understanding EL can be attributed to difficulties in one or more aspects pertaining to any of the three configurations, or a combination thereof, that affect discourse comprehension. A difficulty may arise when EL, or the discourse segment in which EL is used, is considered detrimental to or in conflict with any of the three configurations that constitute discourse comprehension factors. For example, one Australian participant said she felt 'stuck' when reading '*Women are* ***more likely*** *to develop anxiety than men*' because the stated information goes against her past work experience, which involved being around male soldiers affected by post-traumatic stress disorder. In other words, her difficulty with the elastic expression arises from a contradiction between the information delivered by the discourse segment and her episodic memory of working with male soldiers. For other examples, in our interview data, Taiwanese participants highlighted sentence structure and unfamiliarity with the presupposition behind the sentence, and Australian participants referred to the long length of the sentence and the technical terms (e.g., thyroid nodules). These issues concern both a heavy demand on lexico-grammatical knowledge and a lack of health knowledge. The interaction between one discourse comprehension factor and another also explains some cases of difficulty. For example, difficulty with understanding the presupposition of a sentence that uses an elastic term (see Example 7.7 in Chapter 7) may be explained by the reader's not being familiar with the health condition and episodic memories that fail to help him/her understand the sentence.

Because the investigation into what makes EL difficult to understand is based on the interviews with a limited number of participants, it is hard to claim that a cross-cultural difference is explicitly manifested in their stated reasons for difficulty. Furthermore, it seems unjustified to say that a specific reason stated in one culture cannot be applicable to another culture. Nevertheless, each language and each individual's experience with the language and with health are embedded in a cultural context, which may help explain striking differences. For example, in the Taiwanese interview data, the mention of the public ('they [grandpas and grandmas] might drink much water, and this could result in the so-called water poisoning [due to their misinterpretation of *duo* (多 'much/frequently)]'; see Example 7.3) and the reference to one's identity as the patient's family member (see Example 7.4) are manifestations of a more collectivist culture, as it is more oriented towards a collective group and benevolence instead of individual concerns and self-interest (Hofstede, 1983; Triandis, 1989). According to Hofstede's model of cultural dimensions, Taiwan is indeed much less individualistic than Australia, at 17 versus 90 on the scale.[1] The difference, as with other dimensions of culture (e.g., uncertainty, avoidance), is not absolute but, rather, is a matter of degree (Schwartz, 1990). According to Gudykunst and Matsumoto (1996), people from collectivistic cultures tend to use higher-context communication while members of individualistic cultures tend to adopt lower-context communication. This view is reinforced by the present study as a larger percentage of participants in Taiwan prefer EL than in Australia, the issue we turn to next.

9.2 Responses to Whether Elastic Language or Non-elastic Language Is Preferred and Why

The average of participants' preferences for EL is near 60% in Taiwan and less than 50% in Australia. To some extent, this reinforces the difference in terms of high- versus low-context communication (Hall, 1976). Taiwan is oriented

[1] These figures were retrieved on 17 April 2020 from www.hofstede-insights.com/product/compare-countries/.

towards a high-context culture, in which meanings rely more on the context, while Australia is a lower-context culture, in which specific and less ambiguous communication is preferred.

Despite the abovementioned tendency, there are cases that go against the pattern and where a striking difference between participants in Taiwan and those in Australia can be identified. Responses to questions 3b and 4b are such cases, in which EL was preferred by approximately 20% more and almost 35% more Australian participants, respectively, than their Taiwanese counterparts (see Figures 7.2 and 8.2). Chinese Excerpt 3 and English Excerpt 3 both concern thyroid cancer, and the key elastic terms in them express an epistemic stance: *keneng* (可能 'possibly/may') and *might* (see Appendix for the Chinese and English questionnaires). Using *keneng* or *might* in a way makes the statement more evidence-based, and thus, it is viewed as more truthful. Without it, the statement would be more certain. For example, the Chinese sentence is about the causes of thyroid cancer. A strongly certain statement could make prevention appear more effective, but the effectiveness of prevention would contest the need to be evidence-based. The key sentence in the English excerpt concerns whether small thyroid nodules *might* ever cause problems in one's lifetime. An overwhelming majority of the Australian participants preferred the elastic version. This may support the view that an evidence-based perspective could be more deeply rooted in Australian culture than Taiwanese culture. Furthermore, the difference in content could also affect whether EL or non-EL is preferred. Therefore, it might be an oversimplification to interpret the difference merely in cultural terms.

Chinese Excerpt 4 and English Excerpt 4 both concern anxiety disorder, and the key elastic term in each of them is an approximate stretcher: *duo* (多 'many') and *many*. In the Chinese excerpt, the two options in Question 4b concern the number of anxiety patients who have insomnia: *many* versus *eighty percent*. In the English excerpt, the two options relate to the number of anxiety types: *many* forms versus *10* forms. Among the Taiwanese students, the gap between those who favoured EL and those who preferred non-EL was almost 60%, while the gap in the Australian setting was less than 5%. In other words, Australian participants were rather divided in this case, with fewer than 5% more of the participants preferring non-EL than choosing EL, while an overwhelming majority of the Taiwanese participants preferred the non-EL option. The difference in content – one more related to patients and the other concerning the disease itself – might cause the difference in participants' preferences over *many* or a more specific number because if the information is of greater concern to someone, they might expect it to be more precise.

In Chapters 7 and 8, based on participants' written explanations for their preferences for EL or non-EL in six health excerpts in Chinese and English, respectively, we have provided a variety of frames that underpinned their comments. Except for two cases (3b and 4b) in the Taiwanese and Australian questionnaire data, Taiwanese participants preferred EL to a larger extent than did their Australian counterparts. Take, for example, Chinese Excerpt 2 and English Excerpt 2, both of which mention death rates among patients who suffered from pancreatic cancer. While only approximately 20% of the Australian participants preferred EL, more than 70% of the Taiwanese participants preferred EL. This difference can be explained in multiple ways. To begin, it might be due to a different attitude towards death. Taiwan is a culture where death is absolutely a taboo topic and talking about it – including talking about death rates – is expected to be vague, whereas Australia might not see the topic of death (rates) in the same way and people might expect the mention of a death rate to be in precise language. The participants' preference for how a death rate should best be presented is also reflected in their explanations of why they preferred EL or non-EL. In the questionnaire responses collected in Taiwan, a large proportion of respondents activated the folk frame that people should be counted in whole numbers, while more than half of the Australian participants who chose non-EL activated the accuracy frame as they expected information regarding death rates to be precise.

The comparison shows that whether participants prefer EL or non-EL in the health excerpt results from a combination of factors – for example, whether the participant is concerned about the health topic, whether the topic is deemed serious, whether the use of the elastic term may cause misunderstanding, and what frame is activated when s/he reads the excerpt. As regards the frames utilised by Taiwanese and Australian participants, similarities and differences emerge. The top four frames in the Chinese data are communication, folk-idiosyncrasy, trust and the voluntary–involuntary action frames (see Figure 7.3). The top four frames in the English data are accuracy, idiosyncrasy, fluidity and clarity (see Figure 8.4). As accuracy, fluidity and the other frames in the language-related group concern language and they may be regarded as desirable communication features, they can be grouped as one mega frame. Viewed this way, the distribution of frames in the two datasets has at least two similarities. The communication frame is number one in both datasets, and the second-ranked frame is the same (i.e., the folk–idiosyncratic frame). Nevertheless, within this similarity exists a difference as both the folk and the idiosyncratic sides of the frame were almost equally activated to explain the preference over EL in the Chinese data (72 and 62 times, respectively; see Figure 7.3). By contrast, in the English data, the idiosyncratic frame far outweighed the folk frame, as the idiosyncratic frame was activated more than 300 times to explain the preference of EL or non-EL. The folk frame was used only to explain why EL was preferred, and it occurred fewer than 20 times. While the frame ranked third in the Chinese data is the trust frame, it is the fluidity frame in the English data. The fourth-ranked frame in Chinese is the voluntary–involuntary action frame, but it is clarity in English. In the Chinese data, the two sides of the voluntary–involuntary action frame were approximately equally distributed, but in the English data, there was a tendency towards the voluntary side of the voluntary–involuntary frame. This finding in the English dataset may relate to the frame used most frequently: accuracy. If the expectation of accurate health information is met, participants are likely to follow the given health suggestion, hence the relatively frequent activation of the voluntary end of the voluntary–involuntary frame (see Figure 8.4). The disease-focused frame was identified only in the English data, and this may be due to the presence of students studying health sciences among the Australian participants only.

A hierarchical ordering of frames seems to emerge from the Taiwanese questionnaire dataset and from the Australian one. Of particular interest in the frame comparison are the similarities that conceal the differences and the differences that exist alongside the similarities. Based on the above comparison, the most frequently used frames in the Taiwanese and Australian data were, in decreasing order, as follows: communication, folk–idiosyncrasy/–individual, trust–scepticism, and voluntary–involuntary action/clarity frame.[2] Based on this order, a model for health communication, particularly as regards the use of EL, is developed (see Section 11.2 in Chapter 11).

9.3 Social Factors

Social factors cover gender and age in this study.

9.3.1 Gender Attitudes

From a cross-cultural perspective, the results of both the Chinese and English questionnaires showed that larger percentages of females found EL difficult to understand than their male counterparts. In the results of the Chinese feedback, the difference was small (9.7% versus 9.1%), while in the results of the English feedback, more than twice as many females as males reported difficulty in understanding EL (8.3% versus 3.4%). The result of a respective Chi-square test of the Chinese and English data showed no significant difference in terms of gender. As a whole, gender does not play any crucial role in terms of perceptions of understanding EL. The no-gender-difference finding offers an

[2] We do not use an exactly identical set of terms for the identified frames when coding Taiwanese and Australian participants' responses to their questionnaires. This is due to the consideration that even a similar frame does not always mean the same in different languages and cultures. Therefore, while a frame called folk–idiosyncrasy is used for the coding of data collected in Taiwan (see Chapter 7), a similar frame termed folk–individual is adopted for the coding of the Australian data.

interesting contrast with previous studies of VL and gender. Channell (1994: 192) stated that her participants had the impression that females used VL more frequently than males. According to her, this might be due to the stereotype that vagueness is more associated with females and could relate to power relations and politeness, as vagueness is a way of showing deference (Channell, 1994: 190). Nevertheless, online health information differs from mixed-sex interactions, on which previous studies of gender and VL were based. Our study supports a no-gender-difference view in terms of understanding EL in online health information.

Regarding feedback in response to Type B questions, both the results of the Chinese questionnaires and those of the English ones showed that, on average, larger percentages of males than females preferred EL: 58.2% versus 57.3% in Taiwan, and 53.7% versus 45.7% in Australia. We see a difference of more than 10% between Taiwanese female participants and their Australian counterparts, with a larger percentage of females in Taiwan preferring EL than in Australia. Whilst the gender difference was not huge among the Taiwanese participants, the gender difference in the Australian feedback was larger, at almost 8%. The significance of the statistical difference in terms of Australian participants' preferences for EL or non-EL in relation to gender is confirmed by the result of the Chi-square test based on the collected feedback (see Section 8.3.1 in Chapter 8).

Hofstede's cultural theory sheds light on the difference between Taiwan and Australia. According to Hofstede et al. (2010: 140), cultural masculinity/femininity is one of the key dimensions that distinguish cultures: 'A society is called masculine when emotional gender roles are clearly distinct: men are supposed to be assertive, tough, and focused on material success, whereas women are supposed to be more modest, tender, and concerned with the quality of life'. By contrast, a feminine society does not have such a clear-cut distinction in gender roles. A masculine society is more driven by success and competition, while a feminine society cares more for consideration of others and quality of life. Australia is more oriented towards a masculine society, while Taiwan leans more towards being feminine, but the difference is not huge as their scores regarding the dimension of cultural masculinity are 61 and 45, respectively.[3] This contrast in cultural masculinity versus femininity correlates with the difference in preferences for EL as found in the Australian and Taiwanese questionnaire data. Specifically, the lower the percentage of preference for EL, the more masculine the society. Indeed, a larger percentage of Taiwanese participants prefer EL than their Australian counterparts, echoing the comparison between Taiwan and Australia in terms of cultural masculinity

[3] These scores are based on information retrieved on 17 April 2020 from www.hofstede-insights.com/product/compare-countries/.

or femininity. If we accept the view that effects such as mitigation, rapport or evasiveness, all of which can be created by EL (Zhang, 2015), can counter assertiveness to some extent, then preferences for EL may be compatible with cultural femininity. In this light, the fact that a much smaller proportion of Australian females prefer EL than Taiwanese females may suggest that the smaller count of Australian females' preferences for EL reinforces the characterisation of Australia as a more masculine as opposed to feminine society, while the larger count of their Taiwanese female counterparts reinforces Taiwan more as a more feminine than masculine society. Of course, cultural masculinity or femininity does not equate to assertiveness or vagueness. Rather, this cultural dimension may help account for how gender relates to the attitudes towards EL in different cultures. Instead of being merely a demographic variable, gender is metaphorically interpreted, generating meanings associated with gender roles in specific societies and, thus, shaping cultural differences.

9.3.2 Age Factor

In comparing Taiwanese and Australian responses to Type A questions – whether EL is difficult to understand – in relation to age, we have two observations. First, while the group in Taiwan who found EL most problematic was the oldest group, aged 30 or above, their Australian counterparts were the youngest group, aged 17. Because the numbers of the two groups were relatively small, 7 in Taiwan and 17 in Australia, their 'difficulty' may not be one and the same. Second, if we exclude the age groups that were small (i.e., had fewer than 20 participants), then the group that showed the highest rate of difficulty in both Taiwan and Australia shared the same age range (i.e., between 22 and 25). This might be attributed to the group being largely third- and fourth-year undergraduates and postgraduates who had been trained to develop a more critical view than first- or second-year undergraduates.

Regarding how age relates to Taiwanese and Australian responses to Type B questions (i.e., whether EL or non-EL is preferred), three interesting points are highlighted here. First, in Australia, the order of the four age groups from the highest to the lowest percentages of participants preferring EL generally reflects the sequence of the groups from the lowest to the highest percentage of participants who found EL difficult. Specifically, the group aged between 26 and 29, who had the lowest proportion of participants finding EL difficult, had the highest proportion of people preferring EL. The 17-year-old group, who had the largest percentage of respondents considering EL difficult, had the smallest proportion of people favouring EL. The two groups in between did not reflect the above relationship between the high/low rate of difficulty and the low/high rate of preferences over EL. By contrast, in Taiwan, the four age groups exhibited a very different pattern: the order of the groups from the highest to the lowest percentages of participants preferring EL completely matched the order by percentage of the groups from the highest to the lowest difficulty. In the Australian questionnaire data, a similar pattern was found only in the two in-between groups (18–21 and 22–25 year-olds). Furthermore, if the age groups comprising fewer than 20 participants are excluded, then the age group with the highest percentages of participants preferring EL in Taiwan and in Australia is the same, that is, those aged between 22 and 25. The similarities and the somewhat conflicting patterns in Australia and Taiwan may reveal less about strong correlations between EL and age and more about the complicated nature of EL and about the role of age in health communication. Specifically, age does not play a determining role in participants' perceptions of and attitudes towards EL in the health context. The distribution patterns regarding whether EL is difficult and whether EL is preferred are more the result of various factors (e.g., reasons for difficulty and aspects of activated experience) and less determined by age. In other words, age may assist in demarcating the pattern emerging out of the interaction of diverse contributing factors, but on its own it does not necessarily produce the pattern itself. For example, in Taiwan, across the four age groups, more than half of the participants in each age group preferred EL, between approximately 55% and 60% (see Figure 7.11). By contrast, in Australia, only in two age groups – the two most mature ones (22–25 and 26–29 year-olds) – did more than half of the participants prefer EL (see Figure 8.10). Age on its own may not be held accountable for the pattern; instead, age-related factors (e.g., work experience and health experience) and factors beyond age are likely to interact to co-produce the results.

As a whole, our comparison of the results in relation to age reinforces previous studies that have viewed age as more than a 'variable' in research into health communication. For example, as Lippincott (2004: 160) put it, 'age alone is a meaningless demographic'. Southwell (2010: 525) suggests that age should be treated as 'a potentially valuable moderator of measure validity and campaign effects' when we evaluate health campaigns. By distinguishing between chronological age and age-related factors, Bol et al. (2018) argue for a new conception of age that consists of such age-related factors as *ability* and *motivation*, each of which has its own set of personal and message-experience characteristics. Take recall of online information, for example. An individual's ability covers personal characteristics, including education, level of health literacy and message-experience characteristics (e.g., perceived cognitive load and required resources), while a person's motivation comprises personal characteristics (e.g., future-time perspective and need for cognition) and his/her message-experience characteristics, including website involvement and level of satisfaction with the emotional support provided by the site (Bol et al., 2018:

11). While age may not be a determinant factor, it is a relevant and reinforcing factor.

9.4 Concluding Remarks

This chapter has revealed various similarities and differences between the Taiwanese and Australian data. In the Taiwanese and Australian questionnaire data, an approximate correlation was found between the severity of a disease and difficulty understanding EL. The intensity of items of EL in a given excerpt also affects the perception of difficulty with EL. The more different elastic expressions there are in the excerpt, the higher the rate of difficulty the excerpt is likely to have. Our interview data further explain what makes it hard to understand EL. Although the responses from Chinese-medium interviews looked different from those of the English-medium interviews, we believe some of the interview responses in Chinese correspond to those in English. Nevertheless, a striking difference was also identified, as one response in the Taiwanese interview data was more oriented towards a perspective that considers society as a collective group or community, a phenomenon not found in the Australian data. Culture may also play a role, but culture cannot be simplified and reduced to one determinant held accountable for any given cultural differences. In line with van Dijk and Kintsch (1983), we suggest three broad factors that affect discourse comprehension difficulty caused by EL/VL: the reader, the health topic and the text. In the health context, and in more specific terms, the three factors refer to linguistic knowledge, health knowledge and the reader's intention or expectation. A difficulty understanding EL can be attributed to one or more difficulties arising from any of the three factors or a combination of them.

A stronger overall tendency to favour EL is found in the Taiwanese questionnaire data than in the Australian data, thus reinforcing a contrast between a high- and low-context communication style. Nevertheless, there are counterexamples, suggesting that a variety of other factors are also involved.

The respective cultural tendency in terms of high or low context may conflict with other considerations, thus contributing to variability in attitudes towards EL. The variation may be seen as resulting from differences in the activation of different frames and opposing ends of frame continua (e.g., folk versus idiosyncrasy) and in their frequencies when participants evaluate EL or non-EL in the context of each health excerpt. The top four frames in the Taiwanese and Australian questionnaire data have two striking similarities as both utilised the communication frame(s) most frequently as well as the voluntary–involuntary action frame. Two differences are also identified, as Taiwanese participants utilised the folk-oriented end much more frequently than the idiosyncrasy-oriented one, but their Australian counterparts used the individual-oriented end much more frequently than the folk-oriented one. This difference echoes the cultural difference in terms of collectivism versus individualism (Hofstede 1980, 1983). Furthermore, while the trust–scepticism frame was the third-most-common frame in the Taiwanese data, the fluidity frame was the third most common in the Australian data. What has emerged from the explanations of participants in Taiwan and Australia is a similar pattern which also admits differences, one which we term *hierarchical ordering*. We further elaborate on its potential for the development of a model for the use of EL in delivering health information to the public in Chapter 11.

As regards whether it is difficult to understand EL in online health information, this study supports a no-gender-difference view based on the questionnaire feedback. By contrast, feedback in response to whether EL or non-EL is preferred showed that larger percentages of males than females preferred EL both in Taiwan and Australia. This differs from the gender stereotype that more females use VL, suggesting that generalisations concerning EL in relation to gender cannot be made easily without considering the context and type of VL being used. This study reveals that more females than males, both in Taiwan and Australia, prefer non-EL to EL when reading online health information. This suggests that females tend to expect more precise information in the health context. Another interesting finding is that over 10% more females in Taiwan preferred EL than their Australian counterparts. If we associate EL with uncertainty and vagueness, and non-EL with assertiveness, then this result reinforces the cultural masculinity/femininity distinction (Hofstede et al., 2010). Taiwan is more feminine than masculine in cultural terms, while Australia is more masculine than feminine. One significant implication is that when information about a health condition is delivered, where possible, relatively precise language would be needed more in Australia than in Taiwan. This is also reinforced by the survey result that a relatively higher percentage of participants preferred non-EL in Australia than in Taiwan.

Because our participants in Taiwan and Australia were university students, their age range is not vast and the number of participants in each of the age groups is not equal. As such, it is challenging to claim a definite correlation between age and perceptions of or attitudes towards EL. Nevertheless, two observations can be made across cultures. First, our results show that Taiwan and Australia demonstrated two different patterns in terms of how age relates to Type A and Type B questions. In Taiwan, the order of the age groups from the highest to the lowest percentages of participants preferring EL completely matched the order of the groups from the highest to the lowest difficulty percentage. In Australia, a similar pattern was identified only in the two in-between groups (18–21- and 22–25 year-olds), while the other two groups had the opposite pattern. It is unsurprising that if one finds EL difficult, one naturally will prefer non-EL. What is interesting is the preference in the

Chinese data for EL despite its difficulty. It seems reasonable to interpret the tendency as embodying a somewhat collective or even cultural way of evincing the benefit of using EL as being weightier than its drawbacks. Second, the role that age plays is not necessarily a determinant factor that impacts the perceptions of and attitudes towards EL in health information. Instead, it represents a totality of age-related factors (e.g., maturity, critical thinking, health experience) that may contribute to influencing the use of EL to varying degrees (cf. Bol et al., 2018).

10 General Discussion

This study finds that EL use is context-driven and culturally motivated, findings that provide insight for the development of protocols of acceptable EL use for online medical information delivery. The data have revealed why some forms of EL delivery are better received than others, which opens the door for efficient medical communication. This chapter discusses the implications of the findings of this study for the following theoretical frameworks: elasticity and framing, pragmeme and pragmatic tolerance degree of fitness, and integrative pragmatics.

10.1 Elasticity and Its Framing

The elasticity theory (Zhang, 2015) has been strengthened by the findings drawn from the new data on online health information in this study. For example, the three principles of fluidity, stretchability and strategy are verified by the data, where EL featuring unspecific interpretations was stretched for strategic moves. The pragmatic functions found in the new data confirm the functions discussed in Zhang (2015). There are also new functions which have emerged, including the second-order functions, describing tendency, reporting, correcting, advising gently and supporting emotionally. These functions are closely linked with the nature of the new datasets: online health information. The new findings in this study widen the coverage of elasticity theory, increasing its explanatory power.

This study not only strengthens elasticity theory but also further develops it. The application of elasticity theory (Zhang, 2015) works on two levels. Level 1 is the basic pragmatic level with the actual use of EL in online health information. Level 2 is the metapragmatic level with participants' feedback on the use of EL. While the original theory conceptualises EL at Level 1, this study adds a new perspective to it, as observers' views on EL use are incorporated in this study, namely Level 2. This new dimension elevates the theory from the pragmatic level to the metapragmatic level, enriching the theory with greater depth. The participant feedback reveals that there is a mixture of positive and negative framing of EL, and the perception of and attitude towards EL vary depending on a number of factors, including language, cultural and personal experience and the nature of the disease in question. The new findings of EL at the metapragmatic level are that most participants had no cognitive problem understanding EL, so EL is suitable for delivering medical information online. Their attitude towards EL use is more or less neutral on average, indicating that it is unnecessary to deliberately use more or less EL – the key is to use EL appropriately when and where it is needed. Whilst in general there is no strong preference for either EL or non-EL, in specific cases some participants did prefer EL more than others for reasons of cultural influence, personal taste and expectation (among others).

Framing plays a crucial role in the metapragmatic interpretation of EL. It is a way of understanding social interactions. People's perception and interpretation of language and experience can be represented via frames (Fillmore, 1976). This study evaluates how EL is perceived, and the notion of frame is applicable in explaining the governing principles that underpin participants' reasons for preferences for EL or non-EL. A frame can be activated through positive or negative rhetoric or evaluation (Tseng and Zhang, 2020). This study confirms that when participants explained their preferences, they did it either positively or negatively. Positive-versus-negative thinking is an evaluation evoked by the questions, as participants were asked to make a choice and explain that choice. What has been demonstrated here is that, in the context of medical communication, the activation of positive feedback tends to involve a mention of desirable EL use while that of negative evaluation tends to refer to the undesirable aspects of EL use.

Vagueness in reference is often seen as an undesirable deviation from precision and clarity (Jucker et al., 2003: 1737). However, EL was seen by a group of participants as something with enormous expressive power in terms of its elasticity and stretchability. Rather than thinking of EL simply as exceptional asides, they should be recognised as essential aspects of communication. The feedback from the participants in this study supports the points raised in Tseng and Zhang (2018) relating to online medical consultation: EL in online medical information has to be elastic enough to serve several purposes: (1) without knowing the diagnoses of specific patients, the information provided must be broad enough to be helpful and cater to the needs of a vast and varied demographic; (2) the wording must not be so precise and technical as to cause potential problems to the online reader; and (3) it must not contradict, but supplement, face-to-face medical advice. As their study suggests, in high-rated online medical consultations, doctors' stretching of medical knowledge tends to run in parallel with the stretching of language.

10.2 Pragmeme and Pragmatic Tolerance Degree of Fitness

Taking a broad cross-cultural perspective, this study identifies some striking similarities and differences in the use of EL between the Chinese and English data. This section further explains the findings in light of pragmeme theory (Mey, 2001), with a particular focus on how EL is used to adapt to aspects of context when health professionals deliver medical information. Delivering health information online for the public exemplifies language use in context. Therefore, our health data are allopracts of a pragmeme – that is, actualised cases of the pragmeme of health professionals delivering health information on specific health conditions to the public online. The pragmeme instantiates the act of delivering health information from the health professional to the general public in the online context.

Adaptability is a central concept in pragmeme theory, which stresses the user's adaptability to the societal condition in which the act is performed (Mey, 2001, 2016b). In a general way, adaptability is also manifested in the use of EL because an elastic expression (e.g., *etc.*) allows the writer to adapt the given information to the general public, who are not health professionals and who do not anticipate the use of a writing style similar to that of research articles or technical reports. EL serves as a good resource for health professionals in their attempts to accommodate the general public. However, this explanation of EL in relation to the pragmeme is too general to elucidate why certain elastic/vague items are utilised to a large extent in Chinese but not so in English, or vice versa. A pragmeme 'is embedded in culture', its force 'is often tied to convention', and yet it allows for 'individual differences between one execution of the pragmeme and another' (Capone, 2016: xxiii). We need to address the aspects of the environment or situation that help us better understand why certain elastic terms are employed more in one language/culture but less in another, that is, 'the conditions that allow us' (Mey, 2016a: 242) or encourage us to use them or prevent us from using them.

We pay special attention to four interrelated aspects that have emerged as contributing factors to differences and similarities in the Chinese and English data (see Chapter 6). They are crucial to the explanation of why certain elastic expressions are used – or tolerated – much more frequently than others in a language: (1) sociocultural conventions concerning specific elastic terms, (2) genre-specific constraints, (3) writing about health conditions of differing severity and (4) formulaic expressions and textual practice. These four aspects constitute part of the environment in which a specific language is used and in which the pragmeme of delivering health information to the public is realised. They correspond to four types of context: context of culture, intertextual context, context of situation and intratextual context (Halliday and Hasan, 1989: 49). Because EL is embedded within health information in context, aspects of context may well motivate and constrain the overall landscape of EL in a specific language. In light of pragmeme theory, which owing to contextual differences is sensitive to potential differences in language use even for the same purpose, the discussion here aims to contribute to a better understanding of the landscape of EL in the data.

According to Halliday and Hasan (1989: 49), the context of culture refers to 'the institutional and ideological background that give value to the text and constrain its interpretation'. As our data were collected from the sites of hospitals and medical institutions in Taiwan and Australia, the use of EL in the data in Chinese and English is inevitably connected with their respective cultural contexts. For example, the category of epistemic stretchers (e.g., *may*) tops the distribution of EL in the English data, while the category of scalar stretchers (e.g., *chang* 'often', *hen* 'very', *geng* 'even more', *often*, *very*, *even more*) is the most-used type in the Chinese data. The difference may reveal a subtle aspect of medical communication in Taiwan and Australia. Specifically, Taiwanese health professionals use far more scalar stretchers than epistemic ones when delivering online health information, but their Australian counterparts utilise far more epistemic than scalar stretchers. We have called the two styles an *upward-looking*, *amplifying* style and an *inward-looking*, *attenuated* style in view of their respective uses of EL (see Chapter 6, Section 6.3). The underlying ideologies are different concerns: a preoccupation with comparisons and intensifications versus a concern with whether the information given can be considered as more a possibility than an absolute fact. The difference seems to evoke a contrast between more involving, people-oriented communication and more shield-like (Prince et al., 1982), evidence-oriented communication. Another difference is that while the sociocultural ideology concerning the general extender *etc.* constrains its use in scientific writing in English, *deng* in Chinese does not have a similar association but is conceived as a function word introducing one or more examples (He and Pan, 2015). Possibly because *deng* is more associated with giving examples and no list of examples can be complete, *deng* is not excluded from formal Chinese writing and, therefore, is tolerated much more in Chinese writing than *etc.* is in English writing. The frequencies of the two general extenders in the data are affected by the respective cultural contexts rather than being coincidental.

As has been revealed, the use of EL in the Chinese and English data is genre-specific to some extent, as similar elastic terms – *keneng* (可能 'possibly/may'), *chang* (常 'often'), and *tongchang* (通常 'usually') in Chinese and *may*, *often*, *usually* in English – are frequently used in both the Chinese and English data but are not shared on the lists of the most-used elastic items in previous studies (Chen, 2007; Zhang, 2015). The similarities may be motivated by the similar genre or genre family of health communication from which our data were collected. The genre constitutes the intertextual context, as a text echoes and relates to another text of the same type in form and function (Bauman, 1999). Intertextual links among practs (i.e., actualised discourse) instantiated by a pragmeme (i.e., a pragmatic act associated with a generalised situation), explain the similarity in the identified elastic items on the top-10 Chinese and English lists (see Figure 6.1). The epistemic stretchers (e.g., *keneng* and *may*) enable the health professional to grapple with the uncertainty of medicine, and scalar terms indicating high frequency (e.g., *chang, tongchang*, *often*, *usually*) allow for an account of the usual symptom, treatment, diagnosis and prognosis.

Some of the factors used to explain the forms, functions and distribution features of EL in Chapters 4 and 5 constitute the context of situation, which refers to 'the configuration of field, tenor and mode features that specify the register of the text' (Halliday and Hasan, 1989: 49). For example, the health topic, including its severity, is part of the field, that is., the activity engaged by language. The interacting roles of the participants – health professionals providing health information and readers looking for health information – are the tenor. The mode of written language precludes certain elastic terms widely used in conversations – for example, *shimede* ('or whatever') in Chinese and *and things like that* in English. We have identified possible correlations between EL and six health conditions with differing severity (e.g., more uses of *yue* and its English counterpart *about* in cancer datasets). The fact that the tenor and mode components are similar across the six datasets in Chinese and those in English but the field component (the health topic and disease severity) varies across the datasets means its impact on the use of EL is likely to be more visible.

Still another layer of context is the intratextual context, which, according to Halliday and Hasan (1989: 49), refers to coherence and cohesion. We extend the intratextual context beyond semantic relationships in the text to the linguistic context, which also covers language-specific features. For example, *duo* plus a verb phrase is used as a formulaic way of delivering advice in Chinese due to the established structure being a common practice in offering advice in Chinese. The top general stretcher in the English data, *things*, helps health professionals to articulate all manner of items and behaviours and to create cohesion in the text.

As language and culture are interconnected, so are the four types of context. Together they shape how health information is delivered, including the use of EL. Mey (2001: 227) states that 'a pragmatic act is an instance of adapting oneself to a context, as well as (on the basis of past situations and looking ahead to future situations) adapting the context to oneself'. In this study, we suggest that when performing the pragmatic act of delivering health information to the public, the health professional adapts the language to various layers of context, which affect and are shaped by the use of EL in the health information being delivered. In pragmeme theory, pragmatic acting exhibits 'contextualized adaptive behavior' (Mey, 2001: 227) and so does the use of EL. The respective overall landscape of EL use in the Chinese and English data evinces the contribution of EL to the adaptive process. The second-order functions of EL as analysed in Chapters 4 and 5 – describing a health tendency, reporting health research, correcting a health misconception, offering health advice leniently and supporting the target reader emotionally – constitute significant acts that contribute to the performance of the pragmatic act of delivering health information to the public inasmuch as they are all part and parcel of the act. The more frequently an elastic term is used, the more elasticity is tolerated and, at the same time, the more words are stretched. The landscape of the overall use of EL in a specific discourse type is connected with various layers of context and their interaction. EL is an 'interactional strategy' without which our range of communication strategies would be gravely restricted (Jucker et al., 2003: 1738) – an observation particularly applicable to health communication.

10.3 Integrated Pragmatic Explanation

Following Haugh and Culpeper's (2018) integrated pragmatic principles, this study examined the use of EL by the writers of medical websites. When the writers use EL, they assume that their intentions are shared by their readers. In other words, the readers should be able to interpret what is meant by EL. Therefore, any account of elasticity of language should address both the writer's and reader's pragmatic needs, by considering the EL use patterns of the writers and the evaluation of the readers on the use of EL by the writers. For the writer's part, authentic websites' corpora were used to provide actual uses of EL. For the reader's part, a questionnaire and an interview were conducted to obtain their feedback. These combined ways of collecting data allowed us to address EL behaviours and people's understanding of EL across groups of writers and readers. In this way, we can further develop the existing elasticity theory by addressing the complexity of EL use from different perspectives (see Section 10.1 for details).

Integrated pragmatics emphasises the interconnection between language form, function and context (Haugh and Culpeper, 2018: 221). The context is dynamic in that it shapes and is shaped using language itself. Metapragmatics refers to interactional meaning based on exchanges between users and observers. This study focuses on the interconnection between pragmatic form, function and context, and what interactional meanings they give rise to. The interactional meanings from both writer and reader are found in the data, including what the users write, how they write it and how and why the observers interpret the medical information.

In order to explore possible interconnections between form, function and health context, we have examined possible correlations between the four categories of EL and the six diseases/conditions in terms of whether more use of EL is exemplified in a more severe disease in each of the three disease clusters. More correlation is identified in the Chinese corpus than in the English corpus. Correlations are also identified between a disease-specific dataset and the highest or lowest frequency count of a specific elastic expression. From this perspective, the Chinese and English data show similarities as well as differences, suggesting that specific elastic expressions may be used frequently in condition-specific health information, but such correlations may be language-specific and are not necessarily spread across languages. When conducting a cross-cultural comparison of EL, we cannot rely only on one dimension of cultural variability (Gudykunst, 2003: 156–157). Instead, various aspects of health conditions, of health communication, of language, of rhetorical convention and of culture may all play a role in shaping the overall EL landscape.

The context of language use, as perceived in the spirit of integrated pragmatics, is partly embodied in cultural difference. EL is socioculturally grounded and co-constructed within a social group that has a shared sociohistoric reality (O'Keeffe, 2004). This study observes a cultural constraint or cultural pattern of reasoning, in that English participants relied on one category of EL considerably more than their Chinese counterparts. The epistemic-dominated tendency in English data can be called an *inward-looking*, *attenuated* style as it is based on the health professional's checking the given information against massive medical knowledge, resulting in a possible version of the health statement. By contrast, we can call the Chinese tendency an *upward-looking*, *amplifying* style, as most scalar stretchers used in the Chinese data are intensifiers and high-frequency adverbs. The two types are compatible with some previous studies of cross-cultural differences. For example, in Hofstede's (1979, 1980) cultural model, uncertainty avoidance is one of the dimensions that distinguish cultural differences. Higher uncertainty avoidance is characterised by a lower tolerance 'for uncertainty and ambiguity' (Hofstede, 1979: 395), while lower uncertainty avoidance is associated with a higher-level tolerance for uncertainty. If we compare the countries from which our Chinese and English data were collected, Australia has a lower score than Taiwan in terms of uncertainty avoidance, at 51 versus 69.[1] This contrast is reinforced by and compatible with the abovementioned two styles: the epistemic-dominated style of the (Australian) English data versus the low prevalence of epistemic stretchers in the Chinese data.

The highest use of scalar stretchers, especially high-end ones, also indirectly contributes to strengthening certainty as anticipated by the culture oriented towards higher uncertainty avoidance because expressions such as *chang* ('often') and *tongchang* ('usually') describe what is highly likely to happen or to be seen. Furthermore, Gudykunst and Kim (1984: 142) state that 'Asians tend to be concerned more with the overall emotional quality of the interaction than with the meaning of particular words or sentences.' Although scalar terms

[1] These scores were retrieved on 31 March 2020 from www.hofstede-insights.com/product/compare-countries/.

in Chinese such as *hen* ('very') and *geng* ('more') do not necessarily intensify aspects of emotion, they contribute to engaging the reader, thus enhancing the interpersonal and interactional dimension of language (Martin, 2000; Martin and White, 2005). As such, the *upward-looking*, *amplifying* style associated with the highest frequency in using scalar stretchers seems to echo Gudykunst and Kim's observation.

10.4 Concluding Remarks

The findings of this study can be explained by elasticity theory, frame theory, pragmeme theory and integrated pragmatics. For example, they show how language users carry out, adjust and adapt to the pragmeme of delivering online health information using EL in different and evolving contexts. This study supports the conceptualisations of these theories, and more importantly, it further develops the elasticity theory through adopting enriched perspectives of pragmatics as well as metapragmatics.

The results of this study indicate two suitable ways to communicate medical online information: elastic or non-elastic, depending on the context in question. The two are contrastive but can also be complementary, as they serve different purposes, and more significantly, they are preferred by different people or by the same person in different situations.

11 Conclusions and Implications

This study explores the pragmatics of EL through the lens of the linguistic and social practice of delivering online medical information. Moreover, an evaluative dimension that extends beyond the viewpoint of the analyst is incorporated into pragmatics – by investigating participants' feedback on the use of EL – which triangulates the findings of this study. This chapter first answers the research questions posed in the introduction to this book and then proposes an integrated model for the use of EL in online health information, before concluding with suggestions for future research.

11.1 Conclusions

In response to our first research question ('What are the pragmatic forms and frequencies of EL?'), we identify the forms of Chinese and English EL in our corpora. The distribution of Chinese elastic terms and that of their English counterparts show complex results. For example, similar expressions are found on the top-10 lists of both Chinese and English elastic terms. These cover three types of stretchers: epistemic (*keneng* 可能 and *may*), scalar (*duo* 多/*chang* 常/*tongchang* 通常 and *usually*/*often*, *hen* 很 and *very*, *geng* 更 and *more*) and approximate (*duo* 多/*xuduo* 許多 and *many*/*most*). Some very striking differences also exist. While the most frequently used stretcher in the Chinese corpus is the general extender *deng* 等, the top elastic term in the English corpus is the epistemic stretcher *may*, which occurred more than twice as frequently as the second-ranked term, *some*. This suggests that the Gricean Maxim of Quantity is most frequently utilised in the health information produced in Taiwan as *deng* assists in shortening a list of information items. By contrast, the Maxim of Quality is the top concern in the Australian health data as *may* modifies information by making it match the evidence the writer is aware of. Furthermore, as regards how the four categories of EL are distributed in decreasing order, the Chinese and English data demonstrate two different patterns, SC-AQ-GE-EP and EP-AQ-SC-GE, respectively. We characterise the Chinese pattern as an upward-looking, amplifying style and the English pattern is termed an inward-looking, attenuated style. The former highlights degree, extent and frequency while the latter is more concerned with reasoning over whether the information delivered accurately reflects current medical knowledge. The former is compatible with a culture that is more people-oriented and collectivistic (Hofstede, 2011), as high-end scalar stretchers enhance interpersonal function (Martin and Rose, 2003), while the latter seems to index a culture that prioritises evidence.

In response to our second research question ('How do these forms perform their pragmatic functions?'), we identify eleven pragmatic functions of EL in online health information. Six of them are first-order functions as they are interpreted based more on the propositional content of the elastic expression in the sentence: softening, avoiding, intensifying, deintensifying, approximating and shortening. Furthermore, five second-order functions are also identified: describing tendency, reporting research, correcting, advising gently and supporting emotionally. The first-order functions are more referential, while the second-order functions are more interpersonal and pertain particularly to the health context. A second-order function is performed especially when two or more elastic terms co-occur in the utterance. A first-order function (e.g., approximating) can have different second-order functions (e.g., reporting research, describing tendency, correcting) subject to the information of the sentence in which EL appears. All the eleven functions of EL are found in the Chinese and English data, and this may be due to the similar health information. Nevertheless, the ways a function is performed by EL vary in Chinese and English (see Table 6.1). In addition, it is possible that a particular pragmatic function of EL may be more prevalent in one language than in the other due to a wider occurrence of a particular type of EL in the corpus for that language.

In order to answer the third research question ('Are there any protocols concerning EL use? If so, what are they?') in the spirit of integrative pragmatics (see Section 2.2), this study conducted a survey in Taiwan and Australia. As regards whether EL is difficult to understand, it was found that in both Taiwan and Australia the large majority of participants did not find it difficult. A small proportion of participants reported difficulty. Their difficulty seems to derive from the key factors that affect discourse comprehension (cf. van Dijk and Kintsch, 1983). In the context of health information using EL, they concern the reader (e.g., episodic memories, intentions, expectations), the health topic (e.g., knowledge of the health condition) and the text (e.g., intensive use of EL, sentence length and other lexico-grammatical aspects). An interesting phenomenon has come to light from the analysis of participants' perceptions of and attitudes towards EL: those who do not find EL difficult do not necessarily prefer EL, and those who find EL difficult may still prefer EL. This study shows that participants' preferences over EL or non-EL in the health excerpts stem from a number of factors – for example, whether the health topic concerns the participant, whether the topic is deemed serious, whether the use of the elastic term may cause misunderstanding, and what frame is utilised when s/he reads the excerpt. Among the findings are similarities concealing differences in the frames activated by Taiwanese and Australian participants.

Among the most frequently used frames in both the Taiwanese and Australian questionnaire data are those that are communication-related, folk–idiosyncratic and voluntary–involuntary. The similarities are accompanied by differences, as the Taiwanese participants resort to the folk-oriented end of the frame much more frequently than the idiosyncratic end, while the Australian participants rely far more heavily on the individual-oriented end than the folk-oriented end. This reflects and reinforces a difference between a collectivistic versus individualistic culture (Hofstede, 1980, 1983). Furthermore, in the Taiwanese feedback, the voluntary and involuntary ends are about equally distributed, but in the Australian feedback, there is a much stronger presence of the voluntary end of the voluntary–involuntary frame. This phenomenon in the Australian dataset may relate to the accuracy frame, the most frequently used communication-related frame, as people are more willing to follow the given advice if the information is deemed accurate. The disease-related frame was identified only in the Australian data, and this is probably due to the presence of students studying health sciences among Australian participants only. By better understanding what shapes participants' attitudes towards EL, we are now in a better position to reveal protocols concerning EL and to make suggestions regarding the use of EL in online health communication (see Section 11.2).

Our fourth research question ('What are the impacts of context on the use of EL?') concerns the impact of context of different levels of generality and specificity on the use of EL. Our results have suggested that a mismatch of contexts affects the production and reception of EL in health communication. The severity of the health condition, the individual's knowledge, the online setting and the cultural context all have a role to play. By drawing on insights from integrative pragmatics, pragmeme theory, elasticity theory and frame theory, this study has attempted to discuss layers of context that may affect variability in the production and reception of EL in the Chinese and English data. We have also developed a fresh perspective from which to understand cross-linguistic and cross-cultural differences in the use of EL (see Chapter 10.)

11.2 Applications and Implications

Building on the insights of integrative pragmatics (see Chapter 2) and based on the key results of our analysis of participants' attitudes towards EL, this study develops a fresh perspective from which to analyse EL in public health information.[1] Bearing in mind the possible mismatch of the frames and potential generation of negative valence (e.g., being unclear, not accurate enough, unpersuasive and untrustworthy) owing to EL or non-EL, here we further extend the results of the survey to the development of a model for health communication, particularly concerning the use of EL. This lays a foundation for practical applications in the context of online health information. The model incorporates a set of salient frames, particularly in relation to EL (see Sections 7.2, 8.2 and 9.2) but recasts them as four considerations shaped by framing interactions, potential cultural tendencies and intersubjectivity manifested in production–reception interplay (i.e., 'the degree to which interlocutors in a shared communicative situation share a perspective'; Wertsch, 1998: 111). First and foremost, of primary significance are the positive communicative effects predicated on the communication frame. The largest proportion among the activated frames, both in the Chinese and the English data, relates to communication or language (e.g., truthfulness, informativeness, fluidity, accuracy and clarity). Nevertheless, a given use of EL might bring about two conflicting effects on different readers, and this phenomenon reveals that the communicative effect is produced by a combination of factors and an interaction of frames, as Figure 11.1 suggests.

Second, the folk-versus-idiosyncrasy/-individual framing also plays a role, as information may be needed or rejected as people see fit, based on idiosyncratic or individualised considerations. Our cross-cultural datasets suggest that Australians activate the individual-oriented end far more frequently than the folk-oriented end, while the Taiwanese show the opposite tendency. For example, as regards death rates, an approximate number is sufficient for most Taiwanese. By contrast, a death rate expressed using an exact figure is more necessary for Australians.

The third consideration concerns the reader's reactions – particularly in terms of trust–scepticism and/or attitude towards a specific disease. The health professional writes to the best of his/her knowledge, but studies show that perceptions of online health information vary (Thon and Jucks, 2017). The current study also confirms this, as the use of relatively precise figures may generate the trust–scepticism type of reaction among Taiwanese participants. Their Australian counterparts did not exhibit a similar tendency in their responses to precise figures. Instead, a number of their responses show that their experience or expectation of the disease under discussion may affect their attitudes towards EL. Indeed, the reader's knowledge about the disease being discussed and whether s/he prefers elasticity or precision may affect his/her perception of EL. Furthermore, this study shows that the use of EL varies in the

[1] Part of this section first appeared in Tseng and Zhang (2020).

disease-specific sub-corpora. Importantly, the reader's reaction, whether it be a sceptical reaction or a reaction motivated by his/her opinion of a disease, also impacts the second consideration – that is, what information is needed when a specific number is given or when a specific health issue is delivered. Indeed, as studies of risk communication have suggested, quantification expressions in health contexts are not always clear about how counting is conducted (Gigerenzer, 2003; Rifkin et al., 2006). One response to the Chinese excerpt containing a number (80%) (see Excerpt 4 in the Chinese questionnaire) provides a helpful suggestion: 'A statistical figure should not be expressed in such a simplified way but should be presented with additional information such as sample and sampling, otherwise it can be misleading' (統計值不應以如此概略方式表達, 應附註標記樣本和抽樣等資訊, 否則有誤導之嫌).

Finally, when advice is offered in health information, the action framing plays a role, and the other three considerations may all constrain the way advice is delivered and may affect the perceptions of advice giving. Our results show that the EL group tends to be motivated by the involuntary end of the action frame, while the non-EL group leans towards the voluntary end. This phenomenon is found across cultures. However, Australians show more responses involving non-EL and involuntary framing than those involving EL and voluntary framing (see Figure 8.4). By contrast, Taiwanese are rather divided between the two types of responses (see Figure 7.3). This may connect to the overall cultural tendency: most Australians prefer non-EL to EL, while most Taiwanese show the opposite tendency. Figure 11.1 summarises the key interconnected, mutually reinforcing and reinforced factors. Without generating any positive communication effect, providing the information needed, building trust and plugging the reader's knowledge gap about the disease, the given health information would be less likely to lead to the reader's acceptance of the advice being offered. This view explains why the use of EL may work in one case but may not in another and why views on its use may be divided in still another.

The two-way arrows in Figure 11.1 indicate interactions among the factors, reinforcing the multifaceted interplay between the production and reception of health communication. To use Bakhtin's (1981, 1984, 1986) terminology, the model also calls for a move from the seeming monologism of health professionals' authoritative delivery of specialised knowledge to a subtle level of dialogicality, where health professionals and health seekers converge to some extent in their perspectives.

As an increasing number of people find health information via the Internet (see Corrales, 2018; Lagan et al., 2010; McLaughlin, 2013; Neelapala et al., 2008), the demand for online health information makes the methods of communicating health information online all the more important. The model

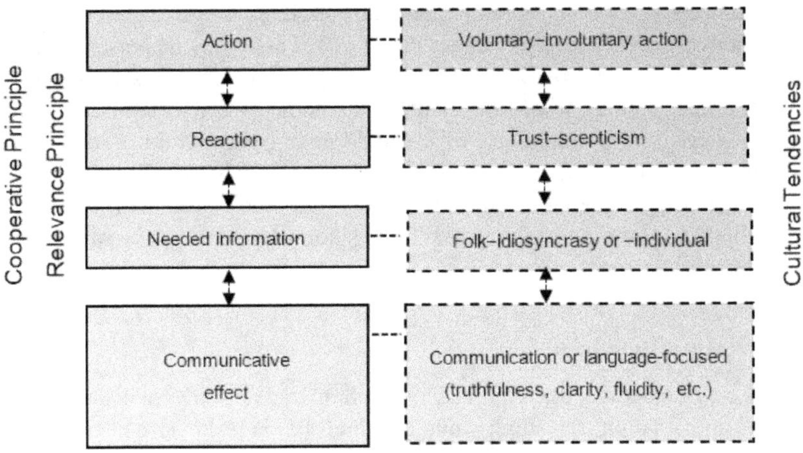

Figure 11.1 Key factors in the production and perception of EL

suggested by this study sheds light on the use of EL in the writing of online health information. Accordingly, this study has some implications. It not only contributes to the conceptualisation of EL but also informs communities, especially the medical community, of the various functions that EL can serve in health communication.

The fact that there are approximate correlations deriving from the data implies that research claims can accommodate some degree of fluidity because results are often not black and white. The feedback from our participants presents challenges to online health information providers in terms of how to handle elasticity in their wording, as too much or too little may cause problems in understanding. As Zhang (2020) points out, EL is a double-edged sword that can strengthen or break the communication chain; we need to learn how to use it skilfully.

It also sheds light on the need for guidelines on how to achieve an improved understanding and avoiding costly communicative mistakes. Raising the awareness that EL can occur anywhere across situations and cultures is useful to health communication trainers (cf. Adolphs et al., 2004) as mastering the skill of using EL appropriately is a key marker of a competent language user (Jucker et al., 2003: 1738). This study also suggests that language use should neither be completely prescribed to a 'correct' standard, nor should it be left entirely to the writer's discretion. A one-size-fits-all standard for language use does not exist; instead, there are multiple standards which guide our language use.

The current communication training in healthcare often neglects the component use of EL, despite the fact that EL 'is not merely a symptom of disfluency or communicative uncertainty but strategically motivated by the goal of interactional convergence' (Adolphs et al., 2007: 75). This study increases awareness of the effectiveness of EL by disseminating its evidence-based findings. One of the applications would be medical textbooks. Current textbooks and training materials often make use of invented examples, and these idealised, non-natural samples of language use fail to reproduce what really happens in everyday healthcare practice. The findings of this study offer real-life strategies, valuable in helping health professionals communicate in a sensitive and public-appropriate way.

11.3 Future Research

This research consitutes an unprecedented comparative study of EL used in healthcare information, revealing ways in which EL is used. The institutional goal for online medical information is to inform and educate the public, by different means from, for instance, a doctor's consultation report, where the goal is to inform a patient of a diagnosis. It is important to highlight the differences between spoken and written health communication and how that may affect the use of EL. Unlike most studies investigating medical discourse, which focus primarily on spoken data, this study examines written data. The data is the first written corpus of its kind. New findings regard shared and culture-specific features in terms of how and why language users stretch their words to play language 'games'. More research into EL in diverse health contexts will continue to illuminate the intricacy and complexity of this topic.

The hierarchical ordering derived from our surveys may have been shaped by the health excerpts used. It would be of interest to see more studies based on a wider diversity of health excerpts which feature different health conditions and are concerned with different aspects of health information. Furthermore, this study concentrates on Chinese/English as used in online health information from Taiwan-/Australia-based hospitals and on the perceptions of EL based on a survey of Taiwanese/Australian university students. It remains unknown whether the perceptions are culture-specific or relatively similar across languages and cultures. Further research taking a cross-cultural perspective will help shed more light on this issue. In particular, it remains to be further investigated whether the proposed model for analysing EL in online medical information (see Figure 11.1) is also applicable to its counterparts in other languages and societies and how it can be enriched to adapt to cultural idiosyncrasies.

The positive or negative framing might be examined in further research for possible correlations between EL/non-EL and positive/negative framing: when supporting EL or non-EL, is positive or negative framing used more? Because EL is also used in medical discourse mediated through other online instruments, further research into the use of EL in other forums such as blogs or social media may enable us to fathom the most accessible way to use EL in online health communication.

How health advice is best delivered using EL or non-EL, and with attention to cultural sensitivity, is also a highly relevant topic that requires further research. How emotional support to the patient may be enhanced through the use of language, including EL, remains to be further investigated (cf. Dean, 2016; Tseng, 2021; Tseng and Zhang, 2022; Veach et al., 2007). Finally, how elasticity in health communication may be further achieved through the use of elastic terms and EL in an even broader sense – for example, through metaphor and the stretching of pragmatic acts and of health options – remains an area for exploration.

Appendix 1: English Questionnaire Used in Perth, Australia

Participant Information Statement

HREC Project Number:	HRE2017-0590
Project Title:	**Elasticity of health communication in Taiwan and Australia: A cross-cultural perspective**
Chief Investigator:	Professor Grace Zhang
Version Number:	1
Version Date:	November 2017

What is the project about?

- Medical diagnoses and prognoses are often underspecified: they are not clear-cut 'facts'.
- There is little health communication research from elastic and cross-cultural perspectives; this project explores better ways to deliver medical information to the public.
- The aim of this project is to gather information regarding online language use in healthcare communication.
- This study will increase the awareness of the effectiveness of elastic language by disseminating its evidence-based findings to medical professionals and communities.
- There will be 300 questionnaires and 20 hours of follow-up interviews.
- Participants may be involved in two stages of the project, the initial questionnaire and a follow-up interview. Both are voluntary.

Who is doing the research?

- The project is being conducted by Professor Grace Zhang (Perth) and Professor Ming-Yu Tseng (Taiwan).
- This research project is funded by a grant from Chiang Ching-kuo Foundation for International Scholarly Exchange.

- There will be no costs to you, and you will not be paid for participating in this project.

Why am I being asked to take part and what will I have to do?

- We are looking for university students to participant in this project.
- You will be asked to complete a short one-off questionnaire about language used online. You may also be invited to take part in a voluntary interview to elaborate on the questionnaire you completed. The questionnaire and interview will take about 15 minutes each.
- The study will take place at a mutually convenient location.
- Please return a completed questionnaire to your lecturer or the researcher.
- For the follow-up interviews, we will make an audio recording so we can concentrate on what you have to say and not distract ourselves with taking notes. After the interview, we will make a full written copy of the recording.

Are there any benefits to being in the research project?

- This project may help make online medical information more useful to its users.
- Promote effective health communication.
- You will get a box of chocolates if you take part in an interview (about 5 mins).

Are there any risks from being in the research project?

- Apart from giving up your time, we do not expect that there will be any risks or inconveniences associated with taking part in this study.

Who will have access to my information?

- The information collected in this research will be non-identifiable (anonymous). This means that we do not need to collect individual names and that your information is anonymous and will not include a code number or name. No one, not even the research team will be able to identify your information. Any information we collect and use during this research will be treated as confidential. The following people will have access to the information we collect in this research: the research team and, in the event of an audit or investigation, staff from the Curtin University Office of Research and Development.

- Electronic data will be password-protected and hard copy data (including audio tapes) will be in locked storage.
- The information we collect in this study will be kept under secure conditions at Curtin University for 7 years after the research has ended and then it will be kept indefinitely.
- The results of this research may be presented at conferences and published academically. You will not be identified in any results that are published or presented.

Will you tell me the results of the research?

- We are not able to send you any results from this research, as we do not collect any personal information to be able to contact you.
- The results will be made available in our academic publications (e.g., journal article).

Do I have to take part in the research project?

Taking part in a research project is voluntary. If you decide to take part and then change your mind, that is okay, you can withdraw from the project. You do not have to give us a reason; just tell us that you want to stop. If you choose not to take part or start and then stop the study, it will not affect your relationship with the university, staff or colleagues. If you choose to leave the study, we will use any information collected unless you tell us not to. We will be unable to destroy your information because it has been collected in an anonymous way.

What happens next and whom can I contact about the research?

If you decide to take part in this research, we will ask you to sign the consent form. By signing, it is telling us that you understand what you have read and what has been discussed. Signing the consent indicates that you agree to be in the research project. Please take your time and ask any questions you have before you decide what to do. You will be given a copy of this information and the consent form to keep.

Our contact details are:

Professor Grace Zhang (Researcher in Australia)
School of Education
Curtin University, Australia
Tel: (+618) 9266 3478
Email: Grace.Zhang@exchange.curtin.edu.au

Professor Ming-Yu Tseng (Researcher in Taiwan)
Department of Foreign Languages and Literature
National Sun Yat-sun University, Taiwan
Tel. (+07) 52520003151
Email: mytseng@mail.nsysu.edu.tw

Curtin University Human Research Ethics Committee (HREC) has approved this study (HRE2017-0590). Should you wish to discuss the study with someone not directly involved, in particular, any matters concerning the conduct of the study or your rights as a participant, or you wish to make a confidential complaint, you may contact the Ethics Officer on (08) 9266 9223, or the Manager, Research Integrity, on (08) 9266 7093 or email hrec@curtin.edu.au.

Consent Form

HREC Project Number:	HRE2017-0590
Project Title:	**Elasticity of health communication in Taiwan and Australia: A cross-cultural perspective**
Chief Investigator:	Professor Grace Zhang
Version Number:	1
Version Date:	November 2017

- I have read the information statement version listed above and I understand its contents.
- I believe I understand the purpose, extent and possible risks of my involvement in this project.
- I voluntarily consent to take part in this research project.
- I have had an opportunity to ask questions and I am satisfied with the answers I have received.
- I understand that this project has been approved by Curtin University Human Research Ethics Committee and will be carried out in line with the National Statement on Ethical Conduct in Human Research (2007).
- I understand I will receive a copy of this Information Statement and Consent Form.

Participant Name
Participant Signature
Date

Declaration by researcher: I have supplied an Information Statement and Consent Form to the participant who has signed above and believe that they understand the purpose, extent and possible risks of their involvement in this project.

Researcher Name
Researcher Signature
Date

Curtin University Human Research Ethics Committee (HREC) has approved this study (HRE2017-0590). Should you wish to discuss the study with someone not directly involved, in particular, any matters concerning the conduct of the study or your rights as a participant, or you wish to make a confidential complaint, you may contact the Ethics Officer on (08) 9266 9223, or the Manager, Research Integrity, on (08) 9266 7093 or email hrec@curtin.edu.au.

Questionnaire

This questionnaire is about the language used in healthcare communication on the Internet. It has two sections, background information and excerpts. There are 6 excerpts, please answer the questions on the elastic expressions underlined. For example, many people, about 50%.

Thank you for your help!

Background Information

What is your age?

□ 18–21
□ 22–25
□ 26–29
Other (please specify)____________________

What is your gender?

□ Male
□ Female

First language:

□ English is my first language
□ English is not my first language; my first language is:____________________

How long have you been in Australia?

____________________year/s

What is your major?

□ I am an undergraduate, majoring in____________________
□ I am a postgraduate, majoring (researching) in____________________

A follow-up interview (about 5 minutes) may be arranged. On completing the interview, the research team would like to express our gratitude to you with a box of chocolates. Please leave contact details hereafter should you wish to participate further. Thank you!

Email:______________________________
Phone:______________________________
Social Media ID:____________________

Excerpts 1. In schizophrenia, these experiences last for **more than** a month – even for six months **or longer**. Other common symptoms of schizophrenia are problems with low mood and motivation, isolation from family and friends, and feeling cold or emotionless. People with schizophrenia **may** also have trouble with thoughts, concentration, speaking and memory.

1a. Do you have difficulty understanding the above paragraph due to the underlined expressions?
□ Yes
□ No

1b. Which of the following expressions do you prefer? (Multiple choices allowed).
□ In schizophrenia, these experiences last for a month.
□ In schizophrenia, these experiences last for **more than** a month.

Please briefly explain why you prefer such expression/s:

____

____

2. **Some** risk factors are modifiable, such as lifestyle or environmental risk factors, and others cannot be modified, such as inherited factors and whether **someone** in the family has had pancreatic cancer. Having 1 **or more** risk factors does not mean that you will develop cancer. **Many** people have at least 1 risk factor but will never develop cancer, while others with cancer **may** have had no known risk factors.
The age-standardised mortality rate remained relatively similar at 9.6 per 100,000 persons (13 for males and 7.2 for females) in 1968 to 9.3 per 100,000 persons in 2014.

2a. Do you have difficulty understanding the above paragraph due to the underlined expressions?
□ Yes
□ No

2b. Which of the following expressions do you prefer? (Multiple choices allowed).

- □ The age-standardised mortality rate remained relatively similar at 9.6 per 100,000 persons (13 for males and 7.2 for females) in 1968 to 9.3 per 100,000 persons in 2014.
- □ The age-standardised mortality rate remained relatively similar at 9.6 per 100,000 persons (13 for males and **about** 7 for females) in 1968 to 9.3 per 100,000 persons in 2014.

Please briefly explain why you prefer such expression/s:

____

____

3. **Many** people today have ultrasounds and other scans for totally unrelated health issues, and those tests **sometimes** end up picking up **very** small thyroid nodules. Even if they turn out to be cancerous, **many** of these are **so** tiny and slow-growing that they **might** not ever cause problems during your lifetime.
   3a. Do you have difficulty understanding the above paragraph due to the underlined expressions?
   - □ Yes
   - □ No

   3b. Which of the following expressions do you prefer? (Multiple choices allowed).
   - □ Many of these are so tiny and slow-growing that they **might** not ever cause problems during your lifetime.
   - □ Many of these are so tiny and slow-growing that they will never cause problems during your lifetime.

Please briefly explain why you prefer such expression/s:

____

____

4. Anxiety disorders are the most common mental disorders, affecting one in four Australians at **some** stage in their life. Women are **more likely** to develop anxiety than men, but it is not clear why. There are **many** forms of anxiety disorder, but the one thing they have in common is their impact on day-to-day activities.
   4a. Do you have difficulty understanding the above paragraph due to the underlined expressions?
   - □ Yes
   - □ No

   4b. Which of the following expressions do you prefer? (Multiple choices allowed).
   - □ There are **many** forms of anxiety disorder.
   - □ There are 10 forms of anxiety disorder.

Please briefly explain why you prefer such expression/s:

____

____

5. Influenza viruses can survive an hour **or more** in enclosed environments or surfaces, which means we can pick up the virus even without **someone** coughing or sneezing near us. Even before we display the virus symptoms, we can be spreading the influenza viruses, which **may** infect people around us. Influenza viruses are characterised by constant evolution, which can change their characteristics. Influenza type A, Influenza type B flu (**and so on**) are constantly changing.
   5a. Do you have difficulty understanding the above paragraph due to the underlined expressions?
      □ Yes
      □ No
   5b. Which of the following expressions do you prefer? (Multiple choices allowed).
      □ Influenza type A, Influenza type B flu are constantly changing.
      □ Influenza type A, Influenza type B flu (**and so on**) are constantly changing.

Please briefly explain why you prefer such expression/s:

____

____

6. There is no need for bed rest if your child has a cold – let the child decide **how much** activity they want to take part in. Although children are **unlikely** to be hungry, make sure they drink **lots of** fluids. Appetite will return as the child starts to feel better.
   6a. Do you have difficulty understanding the above paragraph due to the underlined expressions?
      □ Yes
      □ No
   6b. Which of the following expression/s do you prefer? (Multiple choices allowed).
      □ Although children are unlikely to be hungry, make sure they drink **lots of** fluids.
      □ Although children are unlikely to be hungry, make sure they drink 6 glasses of water daily.

Please briefly explain why you prefer such expression/s:

____

____

7. Do you have any additional comments about this questionnaire?

____

____

END OF QUESTIONNAIRE

THANK YOU!

Appendix 2: Chinese Questionnaire Used in Kaohsiung, Taiwan

(Note: In the Chinese questionnaire, information about 'participant information statement' and 'consent form' is the same as in the English questionnaire. Therefore, for an English translation of these two sections, please refer to the English questionnaire above. For the health excerpts used and all the questions in the Chinese questionnaire, an English translation is provided here.)

資訊說明頁 'Participant Information Statement'

HREC:	HRE2017-0590
計畫名稱:	台灣與澳洲醫療溝通所用的彈性語言: 跨文化視野
主持人:	張喬教授 (Professor Grace Zhang)
版本:	1 版
版本日期:	2017 年 11 月

這項計畫的內容為何?

醫療診斷與預後經常無法相當明確: 它們並非絕對的「事實」。
現存文獻少有從彈性語言及跨文化角度剖析醫療溝通的研究, 此計畫擬探討向大眾傳達醫療資訊的較佳方式。
計畫旨在收集網路醫療溝通的語言使用面面觀。
此研究取得之實證發現將傳達給醫療人員及機構, 使更了解彈性語言的功效。
會有 300 份的問卷及後續 20 的小時的訪談。
參加者可能參與計畫的兩個階段,一開始的問卷及後續的訪談, 皆是自願性質。

誰在執行這項研究?

此計畫研究員為張喬教授(澳洲伯斯)及曾銘裕教授(台灣高雄)。.
計畫由蔣經國國際學術交流基金會補助。
參與此項計畫您無須付費, 亦無酬勞。

為何要我參與以及我要做什麼呢?

我們正在找大學生參與此項計畫。
會請您填寫一份關於網路語言的簡短問卷調查, 亦可能會邀請您參與自願性的面談, 補充說明所填的問卷。問卷及面談分別花費 15 分鐘。
地點選在彼此都方便之處。
請將填完的問卷交給課堂的教師或研究人員。
後續的訪談我們會錄音, 以便專心聽您所言, 不必分心做筆記。面談之後, 我們會製作完整錄音稿。

參與此研究計畫有任何的好處嗎?

計畫可以提昇日後線上醫療資訊對使用者的助益。
促進有效的醫療溝通。
您將獲得一份巧克力禮物 (有參與訪談者)。

參與此研究計畫有任何的風險嗎?

除了花費您的時間, 我們預期參與此研究並無任何風險或不便

誰能取得我的資訊?

本研究收集之資訊不具個人辨識性 (匿名), 也就是說我們不會詢問您的姓名, 收集的係匿名資訊且不會註記代號或姓名。包含研究團隊在內, 不會有任何人得以辨識您的個人資訊, 且研究過程中所有取得的資訊將全程保密。以下人員將得以取得本研究計劃所收集之資訊: 研究團隊以及為查核及監管所必要之哥廷大學研究發展辦公室人員。
電子檔案將加密保護, 紙本檔案 (包含錄音帶) 將上鎖保存。
本研究計劃所收集之資訊將會安置於哥廷大學七年, 待研究結束後永久保存。
本研究計劃之成果可能會在學術會議中發表, 但足資辨識的個人資訊將不會出現其中。

我是否會被報告知研究成果?

由於我們不會收集任何個人資訊, 所以無法聯繫您並通知相關研究成果。
本研究計劃之成果可透過我們發表的學術刊物取得(例如期刊)。

本研究計劃及之資料收集是否為強制性質?

本計劃係自由參與, 您可以選擇參加但中途告知退出而不需任何理由。如果您決定不參加或是參加後退出, 您與哥廷大學及其人員之關係不會受任何影響。如果您決定退出, 除非您表示反對, 否則我們仍將繼續使用所收集之資訊。此外, 由於資訊係匿名取得, 我們也無法個別銷毀。

後續程序及聯絡窗口

如果您決定參與本研究計劃, 我們將請您簽署知情同意書, 簽署即代表您已了解所閱讀及討論之內容, 並且同意參與本研究計劃。在您做決定之前請儘管提問, 我們也將提供一份本資訊說明頁及知情同意書之副本以供您保存。
我們的聯絡方式如下:

(澳洲伯斯的研究人員)
Professor Grace Zhang (張喬教授)
School of Education
Curtin University
Australia
電話: (+618) 9266 3478
電子信箱: Grace.Zhang@exchange.curtin.edu.au

(台灣的研究人員)
台灣國立中山大學
外國語文學系
曾銘裕教授
電話: (+07) 5252000 #3151
電子信箱: mytseng@mail.nsysu.edu.tw

科廷大學人類研究倫理委員會(HREC)已審查通過此研究計畫(#HRE2017-0590)。若想諮詢參與研究的權益或提出申訴, 請聯絡該委員會負責人員, 電話: +61 (08) 9266 9223, 或聯絡研究誠信經理, 電話: +61 (08) 9266 7093 或以電子郵件聯絡: hrec@curtin.edu.au。

知情同意書 **'CONSENT FORM'**

HREC 計畫編號: HRE2017-0590
計畫名稱: 台灣與澳洲醫療溝通所用的彈性語言: 跨文化視野
主持人: 張喬教授 (Professor Grace Zhang)
版本: 1 版
版本日期: 2017 年 11 月

我已閱讀上面提供的資訊並了解內容。
我相信我了解參與此計畫的目的、程度及可能的風險。
我出於自願參加此研究計畫。
我有機會提問, 並對回應感到滿意。
我理解該計畫業經澳洲科廷大學研究倫理委員會審查通過, 研究執行過程遵守澳洲的「人類研究的學術倫理規範」(2007)
我知悉有資訊說明頁及知情同意書。

參與者姓名
參與者簽名
日期(西元/月/日)

研究人員聲明: 本人已提供資訊說明頁及知情同意書給上面簽名的參與者, 相信他們了解參與此計畫的目的、程度及可能的風險。

研究人員姓名
研究人員簽名
日期

科廷大學人類研究倫理委員會(HREC)已審查通過此研究計畫(#HRE2017-0590)。若想諮詢參與研究的權益或提出申訴, 請聯絡該委員會負責人員, 電話: +61 (08) 9266 9223, 或聯絡研究誠信經理, 電話: +61 (08) 9266 92239266 或以電子郵件聯絡: hrec@curtin.edu.au。

說明 **'Explanation'**

這一份問卷是關於網路上醫療保健溝通所用的語言。以下將有6則文字節錄, 請針對底線部分的「彈性措辭」(如: 很多人、大約五成)提供您的意見。

'This questionnaire is about the language used in **healthcare communication on the Internet**. In the questionnaire, there are 6 excerpts. Please answer the questions on the elastic expressions underlined (e.g., many people, about 50%).'

感謝您寶貴的時間
'Thank you for your help.'

問卷 **'Questionnaire'**

年齡 'Age'
☐18–21
☐22–25
☐26–29
☐其他(請說明): 'Other (please specify):'

性别 'Gender'
☐男性 'Male'
☐女性 'Female'

第一語言 (不算台語、客語等鄉土語言的話)
'First language (excluding dialects such as Taiwanese, Hakka, etc.)'
☐中文是我的第一語言
'Chinese is my first language'
☐中文不是我的第一語言, 我的第一語言是: ______________
'Chinese is not my first language; my first language is ____'

在台時間 'Time living in Taiwan'
請問您已在台灣居住幾年: ____________年
'How long have you been in Taiwan: ___ years'

在中山大學主修科目:
'Your major at National Sun Yat-Sen University'
☐我是大學部學生, 主修______________
'I am an undergraduate, majoring in ___'
☐我是研究所學生, 主修______________
'I am a postgraduate, majoring in ___'

在問卷之後, 有一個後續訪談, 約佔用您5分鐘的時間, 訪談後您將獲得一份巧克力禮物。如果您願意接受訪談, 請留下電子郵件、電話或通訊軟體 ID (如 Line 或 WeChat):

'A follow-up interview (about 5 minutes) is anticipated. On completing the interview, the research team would like to express our gratitude to you with a chocolate gift. Should you wish to participate further, please leave your contact information (e.g., email, telephone or communication app):'

Email: ____________________________ 或 'or'
Phone: ____________________________ 或 'or'
Line ID: ____________________________ 或 'or'
WeChat ID: ________________________

1. 精神分裂症是精神科住院醫師在第一年就會不斷接觸到的住院病患，只要是精神科專科醫師，都累積了上百例精神分裂症病人的經驗，算是精神科醫師的基本功。藥物的副作用難測，有時藥物作用會比較慢，太急著換醫師，反而造成每次藥物都要重新來過一遍，醫師也得重新問診，病人也不好受。

'Schizophrenia is a common disease among hospitalised patients that psychiatrists would treat in their first year of residency training. During this period, they treat **over a hundred** cases of schizophrenia in patients, thus building up a basic skill set. The side effects of drugs are unpredictable. **Sometimes** a drug shows its effectiveness relatively slowly. If you are too eager to change doctors, you end up having to try a new drug again, and the doctor will have to conduct a new diagnosis, and to go through all these treatment processes again will not make the patient feel any better.'

1a. 上文中畫線的字詞是否構成您理解的困難?
'Do you have difficulty understanding the above paragraph due to the underlined expressions?'
☐是 'Yes'
☐否 'No'

1b. 您較喜歡下面哪一種表達? (可以兩個都選)
'Which of the following expressions do you prefer? (Multiple choices allowed)'
☐累積了一百例精神分裂症病人的經驗
'**treat a hundred** cases of schizophrenia in patients'
☐累積了上百例精神分裂症病人的經驗
'**treat over a hundred** cases of schizophrenia in patients'

可能的話, 請扼要說明原因:
'If possible, please briefly explain why you prefer such expression(s):'

2. 根據衛生署民國九十三年的統計, 民國九十二年台灣每十萬人口有四點九四人死於胰臟癌, 名列癌症十大死因的第十名(男性第九名, 女性第八名)。它的症狀往往不太明顯, 許多病人以輕微腹痛或背痛來表現, 因此如果腫瘤長在胰臟的頭部, 則可能有因阻塞膽管所導致的黃膽產生。

'According to statistics released in 2004 from the Bureau of Health in Taiwan, **4.94 people** per 100,000 died of pancreatic cancer in 2003, ranking 10th among the top ten causes of cancer (ninth for males, eighth for females). Its symptoms are **often** not obvious. **Many** patients **slightly** experience abdominal pain or back pain. Therefore, if the tumor grows on the head of the pancreas, the pain **may** be caused by the blockage of the duct which releases bile.'

2a. 上文中畫線的字詞是否構成您理解的困難?
'Do you have difficulty understanding the above paragraph due to the underlined expressions?'
□是 'Yes'
□否 'No'

2b. 您較喜歡下面哪一種表達? (可以兩個都選)
'Which of the following expressions do you prefer? (Multiple choices allowed)'.
□民國九十二年台灣每十萬人口有**四點九四人**死於胰臟癌
'According to statistics released in 2004 from the Bureau of Health in Taiwan,
4.94 people per 100,000 died of pancreatic cancer in 2003'
□民國九十二年台灣每十萬人口約有五人死於胰臟癌
'According to statistics released in 2004 from the Bureau of Health in Taiwan, **about 5 people** per 100,000 died of pancreatic cancer in 2003'

可能的話, 請扼要說明原因**:**
'If possible, please briefly explain why you prefer such expression(s):'

____

____

3. 甲狀腺癌的發生原因目前確認的包括遺傳因素和幼兒時期頸部輻射暴露, 其他包括飲食營養不均衡(例如碘過多及不足)與環境汙染或身心壓力也可能有關係。當腫瘤長大到壓迫臨近組織, 可能發生聲音沙啞(壓迫到喉返神經)、呼吸困難(壓迫到氣管)、吞嚥困難(壓迫到食道)等等。
'The causes of thyroid cancer are currently confirmed to include genetic factors and neck radiation exposure in early childhood, and other factors, including imbalances in diet (e.g., **too much** or insufficient iodine intake), environmental pollution, and physical and mental stress, **may** also be related. When the tumor grows to compress adjacent tissues, hoarseness (caused by compression to the recurrent laryngeal nerve), dyspnea (due to compression to the trachea), difficulty swallowing (owing to compression to the esophagus), **etc**. **may** occur.'

3a. 上文中畫線的字詞是否構成您理解的困難?
'Do you have difficulty understanding the above paragraph due to the underlined expressions?'
□是 'Yes'
□否 'No'

3b. 您較喜歡下面哪一種表達? (可以兩個都選)
'Which of the following expressions do you prefer? (Multiple choices allowed)'.
☐與環境汙染或身心壓力也有關係
'environmental pollution, and physical and mental stress, are also related'
☐與環境汙染或身心壓力也可能有關係
'environmental pollution, and physical and mental stress, may also be related'

可能的話, 請扼要說明原因:
'If possible, please briefly explain why you prefer such expression(s):'

____

____

4. 患有焦慮性精神官能症的個人會出現無法集中注意力、不能靜下來專心念書, 記憶力也受影響, 許多患者會有失眠的問題, 致使白天十分疲倦、頭昏腦脹, 念書效果當然會減低不少。 對一些焦慮精神官能症的患者而言, 家庭的一些問題 (如經濟問題、子女教育問題) 很可能帶給他們心理上的極大的壓力。

'Individuals with anxiety disorders are not able to concentrate, can't calm down or concentrate on their studies, and their memory is affected. **Many** patients suffer from insomnia, which makes them **very** tired and dizzy during the day. Of course, the effect of studying will be reduced **not by a little**. For **some** patients with anxiety disorders, **some** family issues (e.g., financial problems and children's educational problems) are **likely** to bring **considerable** psychological stress to them.'

4a. 上文中畫線的字詞是否構成您理解的困難?
'Do you have difficulty understanding the above paragraph due to the underlined expressions?'
☐是 'Yes'
☐否 'No'

4b. 您較喜歡下面哪一種表達? (可以兩個都選)
'Which of the following expressions do you prefer? (Multiple choices allowed)'.
☐許多患者會有失眠的問題
'**Many** patients suffer from insomnia'
☐**80%**的患者會有失眠的問題
'**Eighty percent of** patients suffer from insomnia'

可能的話, 請扼要說明原因:
'If possible, please briefly explain why you prefer such expression(s):'

____

____

5. 流感主要藉由咳嗽、打噴嚏等飛沫傳染方式, 將病毒傳播給周圍的人, 亦可能因接觸到污染物表面上的口沫或鼻涕等黏液, 再觸摸自己的口、鼻而傳染, 因此個人衛生及洗手是預防傳染的重要事項。
'The flu mainly spreads the virus to people around by means of droplet infection such as coughing, sneezing, **etc**. It **may** also be spread by touching mucus (e.g., mouth foam, nasal mucus, **etc**.) on the surface of pollutants and then touching one's own mouth and nose. Hygiene and hand washing are important to infection prevention.'

5a. 上文中畫線的字詞是否構成您理解的困難?
'Do you have difficulty understanding the above paragraph due to the underlined expressions?'
□是 'Yes'
□否 'No'

5b. 您較喜歡下面哪一種表達? (可以兩個都選)
'Which of the following expressions do you prefer? (Multiple choices allowed)'.
□流感主要藉由咳嗽、打噴嚏飛沫傳染方式, 將病毒傳播給周圍的人
'The flu mainly spreads the virus to people around by means of droplet infection such as coughing and **sneezing**'
□流感主要藉由咳嗽、打噴嚏等飛沫傳染方式, 將病毒傳播給周圍的人
'The flu mainly spreads the virus to people around by means of droplet infection such as coughing, **sneezing**, **etc**.'

可能的話, 請扼要說明原因:
'If possible, please briefly explain why you prefer such expression(s):'

---

6. 有感冒症狀時多休息, 多喝開水, 多進食些清淡好吸收的飲食, 少出入公共場所或空氣不流通的地方。
'When you have a cold, rest **frequently**, drink water **frequently**, eat light and easy-to-absorb food **regularly** while visiting public places **infrequently**.'

6a. 上文中畫線的字詞是否構成您理解的困難?
'Do you have difficulty understanding the above paragraph due to the underlined expressions?'
□是 'Yes'
□否 'No'

6b. 您較喜歡下面哪一種表達? (可以兩個都選)

'Which of the following expressions do you prefer? (Multiple choices allowed)'.

□有感冒症狀時多喝開水

'If you have a cold, rest frequently, drink water **frequently'**

□有感冒症狀時每天喝六杯開水

'If you have a cold, rest frequently, drink **six glasses** of water **every day'**

可能的話, 請扼要說明原因:

'If possible, please briefly explain why you prefer such expression(s):'

____

7. 其他評論:

'Any additional comments:'

____

____

再次感謝您寶貴的時間!

'Thank you again for your time.'

References

Adolphs, S., Atkins, S. & Harvey, K. (2007). Caught between professional requirements and interpersonal needs: Vague language in healthcare contexts. In J. Cutting, ed., *Vague Language Explored*. Hampshire and New York: Palgrave Macmillan, pp. 62–78.

Adolphs, S., Brown, B., Carter, R., Crawford, C. & Sahota, O. (2004). Applying corpus linguistics in a health care context. *Journal of Applied Linguistics*, 1(1), 9–28.

Aijmer, K. (1997). I think – an English modal particle. In T. Swan & O. J. Westvik, eds., *Modality in Germanic Languages: Historical and Comparative Perspectives*. Berlin: Mouton de Gruyter, pp. 1–47.

Aijmer, K. (2002). *English Discourse Particles: Evidence from a Corpus*. Amsterdam: John Benjamins.

Aijmer, K. (2013). *Understanding Pragmatic Markers: A Variational Pragmatic Approach*. Edinburgh: Edinburgh University Press.

Aijmer, K. (2015). General extenders in learner language. In N. Groom, M. Charles & S. John, eds., *Corpora, Grammar and Discourse*. Amsterdam: John Benjamins, pp. 211–233.

Ainsworth-Vaughn, N. (1998). *Claiming Power in Doctor-Patient Talk*. Oxford: Oxford University Press.

Akl, E. A., Oxman, A. D., Herrin, J., Vist, G. E., Terrenato, I., Sperati, F., Costiniuk, C., Blank, D. & Schünemann, H. (2011). Framing of health information messages. *Cochrane Database of Systematic Reviews*, 12, CD006777.

Allan, K. (2010). Referring as a pragmatic act. *Journal of Pragmatics*, 42(11), 2919–2931.

Allan, K. (2016). The pragmeme of insult and some allopracts. In K. Allan, A. Capone & I. Kecskes, eds., *Pragmemes and Theories of Language Use*. Springer: Cham, Switzerland, pp. 69–84.

Andersen, G. (2010). A contrastive approach to vague nouns. In G. Kaltenböck, W. Mihatsch & S. Schneider, eds., *New Approaches to Hedging*. Bingley: Emerald, pp. 35–48.

Arribas-Ayllon, M., Sarangi, S. & Clarke, A. (2011). Promissory accounts of personalisation in the commercialisation of genomic knowledge. *Communication & Medicine*, 8(1), 53–66.

Auerbach, C. F. & Silverstein, L. B. (2003). *Qualitative Data: An Introduction to Coding and Analysis*. New York: New York University Press.

Austin, J. L. (1962). *How to Do Things with Words*. Cambridge: Harvard University Press.

Babrow, A. S. & Mattson, M. (2011). Building health communication theories in the 21st Century. In T. L. Thompson, R. Parrott & J. Nussbaum, eds., *The Routledge Handbook of Health Communication*. New York: Routledge, pp. 18–35.

Babrow, A. S., Kasch, C. R. & Ford, L. A. (1998). The many meanings of 'uncertainty' in illness: Toward a systematic accounting. *Health Communication*, 10(1), 1–23.

Bakhtin, M. M. (1981). *The Dialogic Imagination: Four Essays* (translated by C. Emerson & edited by M. Holquist). Austin: University of Texas Press.

Bakhtin, M. M. (1984). *Problems of Dostoevsky's Poetics* (translated and edited by C. Emerson). Minneapolis: University of Minnesota Press.

Bakhtin, M. M. (1986). *Speech Genres and Other Late Essays* (translated by V. W. McGee). Austin: University of Texas Press.

Barry, C., Brescoll, V. L. & Gollust, S. E. (2013). Framing childhood obesity: How individualizing the problem affects public support for prevention. *Political Psychology*, 34(3), 327–349.

Basnyat, I., Nekmat, E., Jiang, S. h. & Lin, J. (2018). Applying the modified comprehensive model of information seeking to online health information seeking in the context of India. *Journal of Health Communication*, 23(6), 563–572.

Bauman, R. (1999). Genre. *Journal of Linguistic Anthropology*, 9(1/2), 84–87.

Beach, W. (2002). Between dad and son: Initiating, delivering, and assimilating bad cancer news. *Health Communication*, 14(3), 271–298.

Beck, S. J., Paskewitz, E. A., Anderson, W. A., Bourdeaux, R. & Currie-Mueller, J. (2017). The task and relational dimensions of online social support. *Health Communication*, 32(3), 347–355.

Bennett, G. G. & Glasgow, R. E. (2009). The delivery of public health interventions via the Internet: Actualizing their potential. *Annual Review of Public Health*, 30, 273–292.

Bernard, H. R. (2011). *Research Methods in Anthropology: Qualitative and Quantitative Approaches* (5th ed.). Plymouth: AltaMira Press.

Biber, D., Johansson, S., Leech, G., Conrad, S. & Finegan, E. (1999). *Longman Grammar of Spoken and Written English*. London: Longman.

Biber, D., Johansson, S., Leech, G., Conrad, S. & Finegan, E. (2010). *Longman Grammar of Spoken and Written English* (8th ed.). London: Longman.

Bigi, S. (2011). The persuasive role of ethos in doctor-patient interactions. *Medicine & Communication*, 8(1), 67–76.

Blackwell, S. E. (2010). Evaluation as a pragmatic act in Spanish film narratives. *Journal of Pragmatics*, 42(11), 2945–2963.

Blank, T. O. & Adams-Blodnieks, M. (2007). The who and the what of usage of two cancer online communities. *Computers in Human Behavior*, 23, 1249–1257.

Bol, N., Smets, E. M. A., Burgers, J. A., Samii, S. M., De Haes, H. C. J. M. & Van Weert, J. C. M. (2018). Older patients' recall of online cancer information: Do ability and motivation matter more than chronological age? *Journal of Health Communication*, 23(1), 9–19.

Borah, P. & Xiao, X. (2018). The importance of 'likes': The interplay of message framing, source, and social endorsement on credibility perceptions of health information on Facebook. *Journal of Health Communication*, 23(4), 399–411.

Bradac, J. J., Mulac, A. & Thompson, S. A. (1995). Men's and women's use of intensifiers and hedges in problem-solving interaction: Molar and molecular analyses. *Research on Language & Social Interaction*, 28(2), 93–116.

Britt, R. K. (2017). Online social support for participants of Crohn's and Ulcerative Colitis Groups. *Health Communication*, 32(12), 1529–1538.

Brown, P. & Levinson, S. C. (1987). *Politeness: Some Universals in Language Usage*. Cambridge: Cambridge University Press.

Bryant, A. & Norman, G. R. (1979). The communication of uncertainty. In D. L. C. Jones, ed., *Eighteenth Annual Conference on Research in Medical Education*. Washington, DC: Association of American Medical Colleges, pp. 205–213.

Bryman, A. (2012). *Social Research Methods* (4th ed.). Oxford: Oxford University Press.

Bursztajn, H. J., Brodsky, A., Feinbloom, R. I. & Hamm, R. M. (1990). *Medical Choices, Medical Chances: How Patients, Families, and Physicians Can Cope with Uncertainty*. New York: Routledge.

Bylund, C. L., Fisher, C. L., Brashers, D., Edgerson, S., Glogowski, E. A., Boyar, S. R., Kemel, Y., Spencer, S. & Kissane, D. (2012). Sources of uncertainty about daughters' breast cancer risk that emerge during genetic counseling consultations. *Journal of Genetic Counseling*, 21(2), 292–304.

Caffi, C. (1999). On mitigation. *Journal of Pragmatics*, 31, 881–909.

Caffi, C. (2009). Metapragmatics. In J. L. Mey, ed., *Concise Encyclopedia of Pragmatics* (2nd ed.). Oxford: Elsevier, pp. 625–630.

Candlin, C. N. & Candlin, S. (2003). Health care communication: A problematic site for applied linguistics research. *Annual Review of Applied Linguistics*, 23, 134–154.

Capone, A. (2005). Pragmemes. *Journal of Pragmatics*, 37(9), 1355–1371.

Capone, A. (2016). Introducing the notion of the pragmeme. In K. Allan, A. Capone & I. Kecskes, eds., *Pragmemes and the Theories of Language Use*. Cham, Switzerland: Springer, pp. xv–xxiv.

Capone, A. (2018). Pragmemes (again). *Lingua*, 209, 89–104.

Capone, A. & Bucca, A. (2018). Why did Trump say 'I hope you will let Flynn go' to Comey? *Pragmatics & Society*, 9(2), 208–231.

Carter, R. (1980). The language of sisterhood. In Michaels, L. and Ricks, C., eds., *The State of the Language*. Berkeley: University of California Press, pp. 226–234.

Carter, R. (2003). The grammar of talk: Spoken English, grammar and the classroom. In *New Perspectives on English in the Classroom*. London: Qualifications and Curriculum Authority, pp. 5–13.

Carter, R. & McCarthy, M. (2006). *Cambridge Grammar of English: A Comprehensive Guide*. Cambridge: Cambridge University Press.

Channell, J. (1994). *Vague Language*. Oxford: Oxford University Press.

Chen, C. (2008). A case study on the grammaticalization of adverbs of quantification in Mandarin Chinese. Paper presented at the conference *New Reflections on Grammaticalization 4*, Leuven, July. http://wwwling.arts.kuleuven.be/nrg4/_pdf/chencj .pdf.

Cheng, W. (2007). The use of vague language across spoken genres in an intercultural Hong Kong corpus. In J. Cutting, ed., *Vague Language Explored*. Basingstoke: Palgrave Macmillan, pp. 161–181.

Cheng, W. & O'Keeffe, A. (2015). Vagueness. In C. Rühlemann & K. Aijmer, eds., *Corpus Pragmatics: A Handbook*. Cambridge: Cambridge University Press, pp. 360–378.

Cheng,W. & Warren, M. (2001). The use of vague language in intercultural conversations in Hong Kong. *English World-Wide*, 22(1), 81–104.

Cheng, W. & Warren, M. (2003). Indirectness, inexplicitness and vagueness made clearer. *Pragmatics*, 13(3), 381–400.

Cheshire, J. (2007). Discourse variation, grammaticalisation and stuff like that. *Journal of Sociolinguistics*, 11(2), 155–193.

Cho, H. Y. & Sands, L. (2011). Gain- and loss-frame sun safety messages and psychological reactance of adolescents. *Communication Research Reports*, 28, 308–317.

Clark, H. H. (1996). *Using Language*. Cambridge: Cambridge University Press.

Clark, H. H. & Wilkes-Gibbs, D. (1986). Referring as a collaborative process. In H. H. Clark, ed., *Arenas of Language Use*. Chicago: University of Chicago Press, pp. 107–143.

Clerehan, R. (2014). Quality and usefulness of written communication for patients. In W.-Y. Chou & H. Hamilton, eds, *The Routledge Handbook of Language and Health Communication*. London: Routledge, pp. 212–217.

Clerehan, R. & Buchbinder, R. (2006). Towards a more valid account of functional text quality: The case of the patient information leaflet. *Text & Talk*, 26, 37–68.

Clerehan, R., Buchbinder, R. & Moodie, J. A. (2005). Linguistic framework for assessing the quality of written patient information: Its use in assessing methotrexate information for rheumatoid arthritis. *Health Education Research*, 20, 334–344.

Clerehan, R., Hirsh, D. & Buchbinder, R. (2009). Medication information leaflets for patients: The further validation of an analytic linguistic framework. *Communication and Medicine*, 6(2), 117–127.

Cocco, A. M., Zordan, R., Taylor, D. M., Weiland, T. J., Dilley, S. J., Kant, J., Dombagolla, M., Hendarto, A., Lai, F. & Hutton, J. (2018). Dr. Google in the ED: Searching for online health information by adult emergency department patients. *The Medical Journal of Australia*, 209(8), 342–347.

Conrad, S. & Biber, D. (2000). Adverbial marking of stance in speech and writing. In S. Hunston & G. Thompson, eds., *Evaluation in Text: Authorial Stance and the Construction of Discourse*. Oxford: Oxford University Press, pp. 56–73.

Corrales, D. M., Wells, A. E., Breitkopf, C. R., Pena, G., Kaplan A. L., King, L. S., Robazetti, S. C. & Dinh, T. A. (2018). Internet use by gynecologic oncology patients and its relationship with anxiety. *Journal of Health Communication*, 23 (3), 299–305.

Craig, R. T. (1999). Communication theory as a field. *Communication Theory*, 9(2), 119–161.

Crawford, T., Roger P. & Candlin S. (2018). The consequences of diverse empathic responses in nurse-patient interactions: A discourse analysis. *Journal of Communication in Healthcare*, 11(2), 87–94.

Creswell, J. W. (2009). *Research Design: Qualitative, Quantitative and Mixed Methods Approaches* (3rd ed.). Los Angeles: Sage.

Creswell, J. W. & Plano Clark, V. L. (2011). *Designing and Conducting Mixed Methods Research*. Los Angeles: Sage.

Crouch, M. A., Davis, T. C., Miller, S. & Wills, G. (1990). The gap between patient reading comprehension and the readability of patient education materials. *Journal of Family Practice*, 31(5), 533–538.

Cruse, A. (2006). *A Glossary of Semantics and Pragmatics*. Edinburgh: Edinburgh University Press.

Crystal, D. & Davy, D. (1979). *Advanced Conversational English* (8th ed.). London: Longman.

Culpeper, J. & Haugh, M. (2014). *Pragmatics and the English Language*. Basingstoke: Palgrave Macmillan.

Cutting, J. (2000). *Analysing the Language of Discourse Communities*. Oxford: Elsevier Science.

Cutting, J. (2007). *Vague Language Explored*. Basingstoke: Palgrave Macmillan.

Cutting, J. (2012). Vague language in conference abstracts. *Journal of English for Academic Purposes*, 11, 283–293.

Cutting, J. (2015). Dingsbums und so: Beliefs about German vague language. *Journal of Pragmatics*, 85, 108–121.

Cutting, J. (2019). German, Spanish and Mandarin speakers' attitudes to vague language compared. *Journal of Pragmatics*, 151, 128–140.

Danisch, R. & Mudry, J. (2008). Is it safe to eat that? Raw oysters, risk assessment and the rhetoric of science. *Social Epistemology*, 22(2), 129–143.

Davies, P., Peacock, C. & Scullard, P. (2010). Googling children's health: Reliability of medical advice on the Internet. *Archives of Disease in Childhood*, 95, 580–582.

De Pablos-Ortega, C. & Pounds, G. (2015). Patient-centred communication in British, Italian and Spanish 'Ask-the-Expert' healthcare websites. *Communication & Medicine*, 12(2–3), 225–241.

Dean, M. (2016). 'It's not if I get cancer, it's when I get cancer': BRCA positive patients' (un)certain health experiences regarding hereditary breast and ovarian cancer risk. *Social Science & Medicine*, 163, 21–27.

Delorme, D. E., Huh, J. & Reid, L. N. (2006). Age differences in how consumers behave following exposure to DTC advertising. *Health Communication*, 20(3), 255–265.

des Bordes, J. K. A., Suarez-Almazor, M. E., Volk, R. J., Lu, H., Edwards, B. & Lopez-Olivo, M. A. (2017). Online educational tool to promote bone health in cancer survivors. *Journal of Health Communication*, 22(10), 808–817.

Dines, E. R. (1980). Variation in discourse – 'and stuff like that'. *Language in Society*, 9, 13–31.

Ediger, A. (1995). Joanna Channell: *Vague language* [Review of the book *Vague Language* by J. Channell]. *Applied Linguistics*, 16(1), 127.

Evison, J., McCarthy, M. & O'Keeffe, A. (2007). 'Looking out for love and all the rest of it': Vague category markers as shared social space. In J. Cutting, ed., *Vague Language Explored*. Basingstoke: Palgrave Macmillan, pp. 138–157.

Fele, G. (2014). Requesting help with null or limited knowledge entitlements and responsibility in emergency calls. In A. Zuczkowski, R. Bongelli, I. Riccioni & C. Canestrari, eds., *Communicating Certainty and Uncertainty in Medical, Supportive and Scientific Contexts*. Amsterdam: John Benjamins, pp. 139–156.

Fiksdal, A. S., Kumbamu, A., Jadhav, A. S., Cocos, C., Nelsen, L. A., Pathak, J. & McCormick, J. B. (2014). Evaluating the process of online health information searching: A qualitative approach to exploring consumer perspectives. *Journal of Medical Internet Research*, 16(10), e224.

Fillmore, C. (1976). Frame Semantics and the nature of language. *Annals of the New York Academy of Sciences*, 280, 20–32.

Folkman, S., Schaefer, C. & Lazarus, R. S. (1979). Cognitive processes as mediators of stress and coping. In V. Hamilton & D. M. Warburton, eds., *Human Stress and Cognition. An Information Processing Approach*. New York: Wiley, pp. 265–298.

Fox, S. & Duggan, M. (2013). Health online 2013. [Internet]. *Pew Research Center's Internet & American Life Project*. www.pewresearch.org/internet/2013/01/15/health-online-2013/.

Fraser, B. (1980). Conversational mitigation. *Journal of Pragmatics*, 4(4), 341–350.

Gamson, W. A. & Modigliani, A. (1989). Media discourse and public opinion on nuclear power: A constructionist approach. *American Journal of Sociology*, 95(1), 1–37.

Gibson, J. J. (1986). The theory of affordances. In J. J. Gibson, ed., *The Ecological Approach to Visual Perception*. Hillsdale: Lawrence Erlbaum Associates, pp. 127–137.

Gigerenzer, G. (2003). *Reckoning with Risk: Learning to Live with Uncertainty*. London: Penguin Books.

Glinert, L. (2010). Apologizing to China: Elastic apologies and the meta-discourse of American diplomats. *Intercultural Pragmatics*, 7(1), 47–74.

Goffman, E. (1974). *Frame Analysis*. New York: Harper & Row.

Gooden, R. J. & Winefield, H. R. (2007). Breast and prostate cancer online discussion boards: A thematic analysis of gender differences and similarities. *Journal of Health Psychology*, 12(1), 103–114.

Grice, H. P. (1975). Logic and conversation. In P. Cole & J. L. Morgan, eds., *Syntax and Semantics*, vol. 3, *Speech Acts*. New York: Academic Press, pp. 41–58.

Guan, B. (2010). Collective behaviour and gender difference: Examples from vague language (in Chinese). *Contemporary Language Studies*, 12, 35–38.

Gudykunst, W. B. (2003). Issues in cross-cultural communication research. In W. B. Gudykunst, ed., *Cross-Cultural and Intercultural Communication*. Thousand Oaks, CA: Sage, pp. 149–161.

Gudykunst, W. B. & Kim, Y. Y. (1984). *Communicating with Strangers: An Approach to Intercultural Communication*. Reading: Addison-Wesley.

Gudykunst, W. B. & Matsumoto, Y. (1996). Cross-cultural variability in communication in personal relationships. In W. B. Gudykunst, S. Ting-Toomey & T. Nishida, eds., *Communication in Personal Relationships Across Cultures*. Thousand Oaks: Sage, pp. 19–56.

Gumperz, J. (1982). *Discourse Strategies*. Cambridge: Cambridge University Press.

Hall, E. T. (1976). *Beyond Culture*. New York: Anchor Books.

Halliday, M. A. K. & Hasan, R. (1976). *Cohesion in English*. London: Longman.

Halliday, M. A. K. & Hasan, R. (1989). *Language, Context and Text: Aspects of Language in A Social-Semiotic Perspective* (2nd ed.). Oxford: Oxford University Press.

Haluza, D., Naszay, M., Stockinger, A. & Jungwirth, D. (2017). Digital natives versus digital immigrants: Influence of online health information seeking on the doctor–patient relationship. *Health Communication*, 32(11), 1342–1349.

Hamilton, H. E. & Chou, W.-Y. S. (2014a). Introduction: Health communication as applied linguistics. In H. E. Hamilton & W.-Y. S. Chou, eds., *The Routledge Handbook of Language and Health Communication*. London: Routledge, pp. 1–12.

Hamilton, H. E. & Chou, W.-Y. S. (2014b). *The Routledge Handbook of Language and Health Communication*. London: Routledge.

Han, J. Y., Hawkins, R., Baker, T., Shah, D. V., Pingree, S. & Gustafson, D. H. (2017). How cancer patients use and benefit from an interactive cancer communication system. *Journal of Health Communication*, 22(10), 792–799.

Han, P. K. J., Zikmund-Fisher, B., Duarte, C. W., Knaus, M., Black, A., Scherer, A. M. & Fagerlin, A. (2018). Communication of scientific uncertainty about a novel pandemic health threat: Ambiguity aversion and its mechanisms. *Journal of Health Communication*, 23(8), 1–10.

Haugh, M. (2016). Prompting social action as a higher-order pragmatic act. In: K. Allan, A. Capone & I. Kecskes, eds., *Pragmemes and Theories of Language Use*. Cham, Switzerland: Springer, pp. 167–90.

Haugh, M. & Culpeper, J. (2018). Integrative pragmatics and (im)politeness theory. In C. Ilie & N. R. Norrick, eds., *Pragmatics and Its Interfaces*. Pragmatics and Beyond, New Series 294. Amsterdam: John Benjamins, pp. 213–239.

He, W. & Pan, X.-D. (2015). A functional study of the Chinese function word *deng* from the perspective of the Cardiff Grammar. *Foreign Language Research*, 184(3), 22–28.

Heath, C. (1986). *Body Movement and Speech in Medical Interaction*. Cambridge: Cambridge University Press.

Hennemann, S., Beutel, M. E. & Zwerenz, R. (2017). Ready for eHealth? Health professionals' acceptance and adoption of eHealth interventions in inpatient routine care. *Journal of Health Communication*, 22(3), 274–284.

Heritage, J. & Maynard, D. W. (2006a). *Communication in Medical Care: Interactions between Primary Care Physicians and Patients*. Cambridge: Cambridge University Press.

Heritage, J. & Maynard, D. W. (2006b). Problems and prospects in the study of doctor–patient interaction: 30 years of research in primary care. *Annual Review of Sociology*, 32, 351–374.

Heritage, J. & Raymond, G. (2005). The terms of agreement: Indexing epistemic authority and subordination in talk-in-interaction. *Social Psychology Quarterly*, 68, 15–38.

Hofstede, G. (1979). Value systems in forty countries: Interpretation, validation, and consequences for theory. In L. H. Eckensberger, W. J. Lonner & Y. H. Poortinga, eds., *Cross-Cultural Contributions to Psychology*. Lisse: Swets and Zeitlinger, pp. 389–407.

Hofstede, G. (1980). *Culture's Consequences: International Differences in Work-Related Values*. Beverley Hills: Sage.

Hofstede, G. (1983). National culture revisited. *Behavior Science Research*, 18(4), 285–305.

Hofstede, G. (2011). Dimensionalizing cultures: The Hofstede model in context. *Online Readings in Psychology and Culture*, 2(1). https://doi.org/10.9707/2307-0919.1014.

Hofstede, G., Hofstede, J. G. & Minkov, M. (2010). *Cultures and Organizations: Software of the Mind: Intercultural Cooperation and Its Importance for Survival* (3rd ed.). New York: McGraw-Hill.

Holmes, J. (1984). Modifying illocutionary force. *Journal of Pragmatics*, 8(3), 345–365.

Holmes, J. (1988). *Sort of* in New Zealand women's and men's speech. *Studia Linguistica*, 42(2), 85–121.
Holmes, J. (1990). Hedges and boosters in women's and men's speech. *Language and Communication*, 10(3), 185–205.
Holmes, J. (1995). *Women, Men and Politeness*. London: Longman.
Hong, T. (2012). Examining the role of exposure to incongruent messages on the effect of message framing in an internet health search. *Communication Research*, 41(2), 159–179.
Hsieh, C.-Y. C. (2019). Linguistic typology, language modality, and stuff like that: A corpus-based study on the general extender *zhilei(de)* 'of that kind' in spoken and written Chinese. *Studies in Language*, 43(1), 92–119.
Hwang, Y., Cho, H. Y., Sands, L. & Jeong, S. H. (2012). Effects of gain- and loss-framed messages on the sun safety behavior of adolescents: The moderating role of risk perceptions. *Journal of Health Psychology*, 17(6), 929–940.
Hyland, K. (1996). Nurturing hedges in the ESP curriculum. *System*, 24(4), 477–490.
Hyland, K. (1998a). Boosting, hedging and the negotiation of academic knowledge. *Text*, 18(3), 349–382.
Hyland, K. (1998b). *Hedging in Scientific Research Articles*. Amsterdam: John Benjamins.
Hyland, K. (2000). Hedges, boosters and lexical invisibility: Noticing modifiers in academic texts. *Language Awareness*, 9(4), 179–197.
Hyland, K. (2005). Stance and engagement: A model of interaction in academic discourse. *Discourse Studies*, 7, 173–192.
Hymes, D. (1962). The ethnography of speaking. In T. Gladwin & W. C. Sturtevant, eds., *Anthropology and Human Behavior*. Washington, DC: Anthropology Society of Washington, pp. 13–53.
Jaffe, A. (2009). *Stance: Sociolinguistic Perspectives*. Oxford: Oxford University Press.
Jefferson, G. (1990). List construction as a task and resource. In G. Psathas, ed., *Interaction Competence*. Lanham, MD: University Press of America, pp. 63–92.
Jensen, T. W. (2014). Emotion in languaging: Languaging as affective, adaptive, and flexible behavior in social interaction. *Frontiers in Psychology*, 5(720), 1–14.
Jick, T. D. (1979). Mixing qualitative and quantitative methods: Triangulation in action. *Administrative Science Quarterly*, 24, 602–611.
Johnstone, B. (2018). *Discourse Analysis* (3rd ed.). Oxford: Blackwell.
Jones, R. H. (2013). *Health and Risk Communication: An Applied Linguistic Perspective*. London: Routledge.
Jucker, A. H., Smith, S. W. & Lüdge, T. (2003). Interactional strategy: Interactive aspects of vagueness in conversation. *Journal of Pragmatics*, 35(12), 1737–1769.
Kahneman, D. & Tversky, A. (1979). Prospect theory: An analysis of decision under risk. *Econometrica*, 47, 263–291.
Kärkkäinnen, E. (2003). *Epistemic Stance in English Conversation. A Description of Its Interactional Functions, with a Focus on 'I think'*. Amsterdam: John Benjamins.
Kärkkäinnen, E. (2006). Stance taking in conversation: From subjectivity to intersubjectivity. *Text & Talk*, 26, 699–731.
Kay, P. (2004). Pragmatic aspects of grammatical constructions. In L. R. Horn & G. Ward, eds., *The Handbook of Pragmatics*. Malden: Blackwell, pp. 675–700.

Kecskes, I. (2010). Situation-bound utterances as pragmatic acts. *Journal of Pragmatics*, 42, 2889–2897.

Kline, K. N. (2007). Cultural sensitivity and health promotion: Assessing breast cancer education pamphlets designed for African American women. *Health Communication*, 21(1), 85–96.

Koehly, L. M., Peters, J. A., Kenen, R., Hoskins, L. M., Ersig, A. L., Kuhn, N. R., Loud, J. T. & Greene, M. H. (2009). Characteristics of health information gatherers, disseminators, and blockers within families at risk of hereditary cancer: Implications for family health communication interventions. *American Journal of Public Health*, 99(12), 2203–2209.

Koester, A. (2007). 'About twelve thousand or so': Vagueness in North American and UK offices. In J. Cutting, ed., *Vague Language Explored*. Basingstoke: Palgrave Macmillan, pp. 40–61.

Krosnick, J. A. & Presser, S. (2010). Questionnaire design. In J. D. Wright & P. V. Marsden, eds., *Handbook of Survey Research* (2nd ed.). Bingley: Emerald, pp. 263–314.

Lagan, B. M., Sinclair, M. & Kernohan, W. (2010). Internet use in pregnancy informs women's decision making: A web-based survey. *Birth*, 37(2), 106–115.

Lakoff, G. & Johnson, M. (1980). *Metaphors We Live By*. Chicago: Chicago University Press.

Lavrakas, P. (2008). *Encyclopedia of Survey Research Methods*. Thousand Oaks: Sage.

Layder, D. (2013). *Doing Excellent Small-Scale Research*. London: Sage.

Le, N. & Zhang, G. (2018). *Vague Language, Elasticity Theory and the Use of 'Some'*. London: Bloomsbury.

Lee, S. A. & Zuercher, R. J. (2017). A current review of doctor–patient computer-mediated communication. *Journal of Communication in Healthcare*, 10(1), 22–30.

Leech, G. (2000). Grammars of spoken English: New outcomes of corpus-oriented research. *Language Learning*, 50(4), 675–724.

Levey, S. (2012). General extenders and grammaticalization: Insights from London preadolescents. *Applied Linguistics*, 33(3), 257–281.

Li, C. & Thompson, S. (1979). Third-person pronouns and zero anaphora in Chinese discourse. In T. Givón, ed., *Syntax and Semantics*, vol. 12, *Discourse and Syntax*. New York: Academic Press, pp. 311–355.

Li, C. & Thompson, S. (1981). *Mandarin Chinese: A Functional Reference Grammar*, Berkeley: University of California Press.

Lim, N.-E. (2011). From subjectivity to intersubjectivity: Epistemic marker *wo juede* in Chinese. In Y. Xiao, L. Tao & H. L. Soh, eds., *Current Issues in Chinese Linguistics*. Newcastle: Cambridge Scholars Press, pp. 265–300.

Lim, N.-E. & Hong, H. Q. (2012). Intensifiers as stance markers: A corpus study on genre variations in Mandarin Chinese. *Chinese Language & Discourse*, 3(2), 129–166.

Lippincott, G. (2004). Gray matters: Where are the technical communicators in research and design for aging audiences? *IEEE Transactions on Professional Communication*, 47(3), 157–170.

Locher, M. A. (2010). Health Internet sites: A linguistic perspective on health advice columns. *Social Semiotics*, 20(1), 43–59.

Lombardi Vallauri, E. (2016). Implicits as evolved persuaders. In In K. Allan, A. Capone & I. Kecskes, eds., *Pragmemes and Theories of Language Use*. Cham, Switzerland: Springer, pp. 724–748.

Lumpkins, C. Y., Mabachi, N., Lee, J., Pacheco, C., Greiner, K. A. & Geana, M. (2017). A prescription for Internet access: Appealing to middle-aged and older racial and ethnic minorities through social network sites to combat colorectal cancer. *Health Communication*, 32(7), 916–920.

Lyons, J. (1977). *Semantics*, vol. 2. Cambridge: Cambridge University Press.

Maertens, J. A., Jimenez-Zambrano, A. M., Albright, K. & Dempsey, A. F. (2017). Using community engagement to develop a web-based intervention for Latinos about the HPV vaccine. *Journal of Health Communication*, 22(4), 285–293.

Major, L. H. (2009). Break it to me harshly: The effects of intersecting news frames on lung cancer and obesity coverage. *Journal of Health Communication*, 14(2), 174–188.

Major, L. H. (2018). Mental health news: How frames influence support for policy and civic engagement intentions. *Journal of Health Communication*, 23(1), 52–60.

Martin, J. R. (2000). Beyond exchange: Appraisal systems in English. In S. Hunston & G. Thompson, eds., *Evaluation in Text*. Oxford: Oxford University Press, pp. 142–175.

Martin, J. R. & Rose, D. (2003). *Working with Discourse: Meaning Beyond the Clause*. London: Continuum.

Martin, J. R. & White, P. (2005). *The Language of Evaluation: Appraisal in English*. New York: Palgrave Macmillan.

Mashiach, R., Seidman, G. I. & Seidman, D. S. (2002). Use of mifepristone as an example of conflicting and misleading medical information on the Internet. *BJOG: An International Journal of Obstetrics and Gynaecology*, 109(4), 437–442.

Matthews, P. H. (1997). *The Concise Dictionary of Linguistics*. Oxford: Oxford University Press.

McCarthy, M. (1998). *Spoken Language and Applied Linguistics*. Cambridge: Cambridge University Press.

McLaughlin, A. (2013). Why social media matters in your medical practice. www.physicianspractice.com/view/why-social-media-matters-your-medical-practice.

Metsä-Ketelä, M. (2016). Pragmatic vagueness: Exploring general extenders in English as a lingua franca. *Intercultural Pragmatics*, 13(3), 325–351.

Mey, J. L. (2001). *Pragmatics: An Introduction* (2nd ed.). Malden, MA: Blackwell.

Mey, J. L. (2013). The well-timed speech act: Bourrée for Bache, *RASK: International Journal of Language and Communication*, 38, 265–278.

Mey, J. L. (2016a). Practs and facts. In K. Allan, A. Capone & I. Kecskes, eds., *Pragmemes and Theories of Language Use*. Cham. Switzerland: Springer, pp. 239–248.

Mey, J. L. (2016b). Pragmatics seen through the prism of society. In K. Allan, A. Capone & I. Kecskese, eds., *Pragmemes and Theories of Language Use*. Cham Switzerland: Springer, pp. 105–132.

Mey, J. L. (2016c). Why we need the pragmeme, or: Speech acting and its peripeties. In K. Allan, A. Capone & I. Kecskes, eds., *Pragmemes and Theories of Language Use*. Cham, Switzerland: Springer, pp. 133–140.

Miller, S. M. (1987). Monitoring and blunting: Validation of a questionnaire to assess styles of information seeking under threat. *Journal of Personality and Social Psychology*, 52(2), 345–353.

Miller, S. M. & Mangan, C. E. (1983). Interacting effects of information and coping style in adapting to gynecologic stress: Should the doctor tell all? *Journal of Personality and Social Psychology*, 45(1), 223–236.

Mo, P. K. H., Malik, S. H. & Coulson, N. S., (2009). Gender differences in computer-mediated communication: A systematic literature review of online health-related support groups. *Patient Education and Counseling*, 75(1), 16–24.

Morse, J. M. (2003). Principles of mixed methods and multi-method research design. In A. Tashakkori & C. Teddlie, eds., *Handbook of Mixed Methods in Social and Behavioral Research*. Thousand Oaks, CA: Sage, pp. 189–208.

Moxey, L. & Sanford, A. (1993). *Communicating Quantities – A Psychological Perspective*. Hove: Lawrence Erlbaum.

Muijs, D. (2011). *Doing Quantitative Research in Education with SPSS* (2nd ed.). Los Angeles, CA: Sage.

Munné, F. (2013). The fuzzy complexity of language. In A. Massip-Bonet & A. Bastardas-Boada, eds., *Complexity Perspectives on Language, Communication and Society*. Heidelberg: Springer, pp. 175–196.

Murphy, B. (2010). *Corpus and Sociolinguistics: Investigating Age and Gender in Female Talk*. Amsterdam: John Benjamins.

Musambira, G. W., Hastings, S. O. & Hoover, J. D. (2006). Bereavement, gender, and cyberspace: A content analysis of parents' memorials to their children. Omega: *Journal of Death and Dying*, 54(4), 263–279.

Myers, G. (1996). Strategic vagueness in academic writing. In E. Ventola & A. Mauranen, eds., *Academic Writing: Intercultural and Textual Issues*. Pragmatics & Beyond, New Series 41. Amsterdam: John Benjamins, pp. 3–18.

Neelapala, P., Duvvi, S. K., Kumar, G. & Kumar, B. N. (2008). Do gynaecology outpatients use the Internet to seek health information? A questionnaire survey. *Journal of Evaluation in Clinical Practice*, 14(2), 300–304.

Neely, L. (2014). Risk communication in social media. In J. Arvai & L. Riveres, eds., *Effective Risk Communication*. London: Routledge, pp. 143–164.

Nguyen, M. H., Smets, E. M. A., Bol, N., Loos, E. F. & Van Weert, J. C. M. (2018). How tailoring the mode of information presentation influences younger and older adults' satisfaction with health websites. *Journal of Health Communication*, 23(2), 170–180.

Nicholson-Perry, K. & Burgess, M. (2002). *Communication and Cancer Care*. Malden: BPS Blackwell.

O'Keefe, D. J. & Jensen, J. D. (2007). The relative persuasiveness of gain-framed and loss-framed messages for encouraging disease prevention behaviors: A meta-analytic review. *Journal of Health Communication*, 12, 623–644.

O'Keeffe, A. (2004). Like the wise virgins and all that jazz: Using a corpus to examine vague language and shared knowledge. *Language and Computers*, 52(1), 1–20.

Odebunmi, A. (2006). A pragmatic reading of Ahmed Yerima's proberbs in Yemoja, Attahiru, and Dry Leaves on Ukan Trees. *Intercultural Pragmatics*, 3(2), 153–169.

Oppenheim, A. N. (1992). *Questionnaire Design, Interviewing and Attitude Measurement*. London: Pinter.

Ordóñez-López, P. & Edo-Marzá, N. (2016). *Medical Discourse in Professional, Academic and Popular Settings*. Bristol: Multilingual Matters.

Overstreet, M. (1999). *Whales, Candlelight, and Stuff Like That: General Extenders in English Discourse*. Oxford: Oxford University Press.

Overstreet, M. (2005). And stuff *und so*: Investigating pragmatic expressions in English and German. *Journal of Pragmatics*, 37, 1845–1864.

Overstreet, M. (2011). Vagueness and hedging. In G. Andersen & K. Aijmer, eds., *Handbook of Pragmatics: Pragmatics of Society.* Berlin: Mouton de Gruyter, pp. 293–318.

Overstreet, M. (2014). The role of pragmatic function in the grammaticalization of English general extenders. *Pragmatics*, 24(1), 105–129.

Overstreet, M. & Yule, G. (1997). Locally contingent categorization in discourse. *Discourse Processes*, 23, 83–97.

Paige, S. R., Krieger, J. L. & Stellefson, M. L. (2017). The Influence of eHealth literacy on perceived trust in online health communication channels and sources. *Journal of Health Communication*, 22(1), 53–65.

Palacios Martínez, I. (2011). 'I might, I might go I mean it depends on money things and stuff'. A preliminary analysis of general extenders in British teenagers' discourse. *Journal of Pragmatics*, 43, 2452–2470.

Palmer, F. R. (1986). *Mood and Modality.* Cambridge: Cambridge University Press.

Pan, Z. & Kosicki, G. M. (1993). Framing analysis: An approach to news discourse. *Political Communication*, 10, 55–75.

Parvaresh, V. (2015). Vague language that is vague in both L1 and L2: A comment on Gassner (2012). *International Review of Pragmatics*, 7(1), 129–143.

Parvaresh, V. (2017a). Introduction: Death, dying and the pragmeme. In V. Parvaresh V. & A. Capone, eds., *The Pragmeme of Accommodation: The Case of Interaction around the Event of Death.* Perspectives in Pragmatics, Philosophy & Psychology 13. Cham, Switzerland: Springer, pp. 1–13.

Parvaresh, V. (2017b). Book review: Grace Q Zhang, Elastic language: How and why we stretch our words. *Discourse Studies*, 19(1), 115–117.

Parvaresh, V. (2018). 'We are going to do a lot of things for college tuition': Vague language in the 2016 US presidential debates. *Corpus Pragmatics*, 2(2), 167–192.

Parvaresh, V. & Capone, A. (2017). *The Pragmeme of Accommodation: The Case of Interaction around the Event of Death*. Cham, Switzerland: Springer.

Parvaresh, V. & Tayebi, T. (2014). Vaguely speaking in Persian. *Discourse Processes*, 51(7), 565–600.

Parvaresh, V. & Zhang, G., eds., (2019). *Vagueness and Elasticity of 'Sort of' in TV Discussion Discourse in the Asian Pacific. Special issue of Journal of Asian Pacific Communication*, 29(1). https://doi.org/10.1075/japc.29.1.

Parvaresh, V., Tavanger, M., Eslami, A. & Izadi, D. (2012). About his friend, how good she is and this and that: General extenders in native Persian and non-native English discourse. *Journal of Pragmatics*, 44, 261–279.

Patton, M. Q. (1990). *Qualitative Evaluation and Research Methods* (2nd ed.). Newbury Park: Sage.

Paugh, A. & Izquierdo, C. (2009). Why is this a battle every night? Negotiating food and eating in American dinnertime interaction. *Journal of Linguistic Anthropology*, 19(2), 185–204.

Payne, S., Large, S., Jarrett, N. & Turner, P. (2000). Written information given to patients and families by palliative care units: A national survey. *The Lancet*, 355, 1792.

Peräkylä, A., Antaki, C., Vehviläinen, S. & Leudar, I. (2008). *Conversation Analysis and Psychotherapy.* Cambridge: Cambridge University Press.

Pichler, H. & Levey, S. (2011). In search of grammaticalization in synchronic dialect data: General extenders in north-east England. *English Language and Linguistics*, 14(3), 441–471.

Potter, J., Wetherell, M. & Chitty, A. (1991). Quantification rhetoric: Cancer on television. *Discourse and Society*, 2, 333–365.

Pounds, G. (2018). Patient-centred communication in ask-the-expert healthcare websites. *Applied Linguist*, 39(2), 117–134.

Powell, M. J. (1985). Purposive vagueness: An evaluative dimension of vague quantifying expressions. *Journal of Linguistics*, 21(1), 31–50.

Preacher, K. J. (2001). Calculation for the chi-square test: An interactive calculation tool for chi-square tests of goodness of fit and independence [Computer software]. http://quantpsy.org.

Prince, E. F., Frader, J. & Bosk, C. (1982). On hedging in physician–physician discourse. In R. D. Pietro, ed., *Linguistics and the Professions: Proceedings of the Second Annual Delaware Symposium on Language Studies*. Norwood, NJ: Ablex, pp. 83–97.

Pullen, S., Golden, M. A. & Cacciatore, J. (2012). 'I'll never forget those cold words as long as I live': Parent perceptions of death notification for stillbirth. *Journal of Social Work in End-of-Life & Palliative Care*, 8(4), 339–55.

Quirk, R., Greenbaum, S., Leech, J. & Svartvik, J. (1985). *A Comprehensive Grammar of the English Language*. New York: Longman.

Ran, Y. P. (2010). Approximative expressions and their loose uses in Chinese. In G. Kaltenböck, W. Mihatsch & S. Schneider, eds., *New Approaches to Hedging*. Bingley, UK: Emerald, pp. 165–180.

Rauscher, E. A. (2017). Investigating uncertainty in genetic counseling encounters: Managing information about genetic cancer risk. *Journal of Health Communication*, 22(11), 896–904.

Ravert, R. D., Hancock, M. D. & Ingersoll, G. M. (2004). Online forum messages posted by adolescents with type 1 diabetes. *The Diabetes Educator*, 30(5), 827–834.

Rifkin, E., Bouwer, E. & Sheff, B. (2006). *The Illusion of Certainty: Health Benefits and Risks*. New York: Springer.

Rising, C. J., Bol, N., Burke-Garcia, A., Rains, S. & Wright, K. B. (2017). Perceived stress in online prostate cancer community participants: Examining relationships with stigmatization, social support network preference, and social support seeking. *Journal of Health Communication*, 22(6), 469–476.

Ritterband, L. M., Gonder-Frederick, L. A., Cox, D. J., Clifton, A. D., West, R. W. & Borowitz, S. M. (2003). Internet interventions: In review, in use, and into the future. *Professional Psychology: Research & Practice*, 34(5), 527–534.

Rothman, A. J. & Salovey, P. (1997). Shaping perceptions to motivate healthy behavior: The role of message framing. *Psychological Bulletin*, 121(1), 3–19.

Rothman, A. J., Bartels, R. D., Wlaschin, J. & Salovey, P. (2006). The strategic use of gain- and loss-framed messages to promote healthy behavior: How theory can inform practice. *Journal of Communication*, 56, 202–220.

Rowland, T. (2007). Well maybe not exactly, but it's around fifty basically? Vague language in mathematics classrooms. In J. Cutting, ed., *Vague Language Explored*. Basingstoke: Palgrave Macmillan, pp. 79–96.

Ruck, K., Cooper, A., Hurley, A., Ashton, K., Lines, C. & Willson, A. (2017). Effective messages and media for employee health campaigns. *Journal of Communication in Healthcare*, 10(3), 180–187.

Russell, B. J. & Ward, A. M. (2011). Deciding what information is necessary: Do patients with advanced cancer want to know all the details? *Cancer Management and Research*, 3, 191–199.

Ruzaitė, J. (2004). Academic precision reconsidered: A corpus-based account. *SKY Journal of Linguistics*, 17, 217–247.

Ruzaitė, J. (2007). *Vague Language in Educational Settings: Quantifiers and Approximators in British and American English*. Frankfurt am Main: Peter Lang.

Sadock, J. M. (1977). Truth and approximations. *Berkeley Linguistic Society Papers*, 3, 430–439.

Salager-Meyer, F. (1994). Hedges and textual communicative function in medical English written discourse. *English for Specific Purposes*, 13(2), 149–170.

Samuelsson, C., Plejert, C. & Anward, J. (2014). Defusing practices as mitigation in speech and language intervention. *Communication & Medicine*, 11(3), 299–312.

Sarangi, S. (2004). Towards a communicative mentality in medical and healthcare practice. *Communication & Medicine*, 1(1), 1–11.

Sarangi, S. & Clarke. A. (2002). Zones of expertise and the management of uncertainty in genetics risk communication. *Research on Language and Social Interaction*, 35, 139–171.

Scherr, C. L., Dean, M., Clayton, M. F., Hesse, B. W., Silk, K., Street Jr., R. L. & Krieger, J. (2017). A research agenda for communication scholars in the precision medicine era. *Journal of Health Communication*, 22(10), 839–848.

Schwartz, S. H. (1990). Individualism-collectivism: Critique and proposed refinements. *Journal of Cross-Cultural Psychology*, 21, 139–157.

Schwarz-Friesel, M. & Consten, M. (2011). Reference and anaphora. In W. Bublitz & N. R. Norrick, eds., *Handbooks of Pragmatics*, vol.1, *Foundations of Pragmatics*. Berlin: Mouton de Gruyter, pp. 347–372.

Searle, J. R. (1975). Indirect speech acts. In P. Cole & J. Morgan, eds., *Syntax and Semantics*, vol. 3, *Speech Acts*. Academic Press, New York, pp. 59–82.

Segal, J. Z. (2005). *Health and The Rhetoric of Medicine*. Carbondale: Southern Illinois University Press.

Sharkey, S., Smithson, J., Hewis, E., Jones, R. B., Emmens, T., Ford, T. J. & Owens, C. (2012). Supportive interchanges and face-work as 'protective talk' in an online self-harm support forum. *Communication & Medicine*, 9(1), 71–82.

Shirato J. & Stapleton, P. (2007). Comparing English vocabulary in a spoken learner corpus with a native speaker corpus: Pedagogical implications arising from an empirical study in Japan. *Language Teaching Research*, 11(4), 393–412.

Sigurd, B. (1988). Round numbers. *Language in Society*, 17, 243–252.

Silverstein, M. (1976). Shifters, linguistic categories and cultural description. In K. H. Basso & H. A. Selby, eds., *Meaning in Anthropology*. Albuquerque: University of New Mexico Press, pp. 11–55.

Silverstein, M. (1993). Metapragmatic discourse and metapragmatic function. In J. A. Lucy, ed., *Reflexive Language: Reported Speech and Metapragmatics*. New York: Cambridge University Press, pp. 33–58.

Simpson R. C. (2004). Formulaic expressions in academic speech. In U. Connor & T. A. Upton, eds. *Discourse in the Professions*. Amsterdam: John Benjamins, pp. 37–64.

Smith,J. A., Flowers, P. & Larkin, M. (2009). *Interpretative Phenomenological Analysis: Theory, Method and Research*. Los Angeles: Sage.

Sontag, S. (1991). *Illness as Metaphor: AIDS and Its Metaphors*. London: Penguin.

Southwell, B. G. (2010). On the need for a life-span approach to health campaign evaluation. *Health Communication*, 25(6–7), 525–528.

Spencer-Oatey, H. (2000). Rapport management: A framework for analysis. In H. Spencer-Oatey, ed., *Culturally Speaking: Managing Rapport through Talk across Cultures*. London: Continuum, pp. 11–46.

Sperber, D. & Wilson, D. (1995 [1986]). *Relevance: Communication and Cognition* (2nd ed.). Oxford: Blackwell.

Staples, S. (2015). *The Discourse of Nurse-Patient Interactions: Contrasting the Communicative Styles of US and International Nurses*. Amsterdam: John Benjamins.

Stenström, A. B., Andersen, G. & Hasund, I. K. (2002). *Trends in Teenage Talk: Corpus Compilation, Analysis and Findings*. Amsterdam: John Benjamins.

Strekalova, Y. A. & Krieger, J. L. (2017). Beyond words: Amplification of cancer risk communication on social media. *Journal of Health Communication*, 22(10), 849–857.

Stubbs, M. (1981). *Language and Literacy: The Sociolinguistics of Reading and Writing*. London: Routledge Kegan & Paul.

Stubbs, M. (1986). A matter of prolonged fieldwork: Notes towards a modal grammar of English. *Applied Linguistics*, 7(1), 1–25.

Sunderland, J. (2004). *Gendered Discourses*. New York, NY: Palgrave Macmillan. Switzerland.

Tagliamonte, S. A. & Denis, D. (2010). The stuff of change: General extenders in Toronto, Canada. *Journal of English Linguistics*, 38, 335–368.

Tashakkori, A. & Teddlie, C. (2009). *Foundations of Mixed Methods Research: Integrating Quantitative and Qualitative Approaches in the Social and Behavioral Sciences*. Los Angeles, CA: Sage.

Terraschke, A. & Holmes, J. (2007). 'Und Tralala': Vagueness and general extenders in German and New Zealand English. In J. Cutting, ed., *Vague Language Explored*. Basingstoke: Palgrave Macmillan, pp. 198–220.

Thibault, P. J. (2011). First-order languaging dynamics and second-order language: The distributed language view. *Ecological Psychology*, 23, 210–245.

Thompson, T. L., Parrott, R. & Nussbaum, J. F., eds., (2011). *The Routledge Handbook of Health Communication*. London: Routledge.

Thon, F. M. & Jucks, R. (2017). Believing in expertise: How authors' credentials and language use influence the credibility of online health information. *Health Communication*, 32(7), 828–836.

Trappes-Lomax, H. (2007). Vague language as a means of self-protective avoidance: Tension management in conference talks. In J. Cutting, ed., *Vague Language Explored*. Basingstoke: Palgrave Macmillan, pp. 117–137.

Triandis, H. C. (1989). Cross-cultural studies of individualism and collectivism. In J. Berman, ed., *Nebraska Symposium on Motivation*. Lincoln: University of Nebraska Press, pp. 41–133.

Tsai, W.-T. D. (2003). Three types of existential quantification in Chinese. In A. Li & A. Simpson, eds., *Functional Structure(s), Form and Interpretation: Perspectives from East Asian Languages*. London and New York: Routledge, pp. 161–179.

Tseng, M.-Y. (2010). The pragmatic act of fishing for personal details: From choice to performance. *Journal of Pragmatics*, 42(7), 1982–1996.

Tseng, M.-Y. (2021). Toward a cognitive-pragmatic account of metonymic schemes of thought: Examples from online medical consultation. *Journal of Pragmatics*, 173, 177–188.

Tseng, M.-Y. & Zhang, G. (2018). Pragmeme, adaptability, and elasticity in online medical consultations. *Journal of Pragmatics*, 137, 40–56.

Tseng, M.-Y. & Zhang, G. (2020). Perceptions of and attitudes toward elastic language in online health communication in Chinese. *Lingua*, 233, 1–24.

Tseng, M.-Y. & Zhang, G. (2022). Conceptual metonymy and emotive-affective meaning at the interface: Examples from online medical consultations. *Lingua*, 268, article no. 103192, 1–17. https://doi.org/10.1016/j.lingua.2021.103192.

Tversky, A. & Kahneman, D. (1981). The framing of decisions and the psychology of choice. *Science*, 211, 453–458.

Uhlirovà, L. (1994). E-mail as a new subvariety of medium and its effects upon the message. In S. Čmejrková & F. Štícha, eds., *The Syntax of Sentence and Text: A Festschrift for František Daneš*. Amsterdam: John Benjamins, pp. 273–282.

van Dijk, T. A. (1988). *News as Discourse*. Hillsdale: Lawrence Erlbaum.

van Dijk, T. A. & Kintsch, W. (1983). *Strategies of Discourse Comprehension*. New York: Academic Press.

Varttala, T. (1999). Remarks on the communicative functions of hedging in popular scientific and specialist research articles on medicine. *English for Specific Purposes*, 18(2), 177–200.

Vasilescu, A. (2016). Towards a 'theory of everything' in human communication. In K. Allan, A. Capone & I. Kecskes, eds., *Pragmemes and Theories of Language Use*. Cham, Switzerland: Springer, pp. 305–333.

Veach, P. M., Bartels, D. M. & LeRoy, B. S. (2007). Coming full circle: A reciprocal-engagement model of genetic counseling practice. *Journal of Genetic Counseling*, 16(6), 713–728.

Verschueren, J. (1999). *Understanding Pragmatics*. London: Arnold.

Verschueren, J. (2017). The pragmatics of humor in a serious story. *ELUA: Estudios de Lingüística Universidad de Alicante*, 31, 311–326.

Verschueren, J. & Brisard, F. (2009). Adaptability. In J. Verschueren & J.-O. Östman, eds., *Handbook of Pragmatics Highlights*, vol. 1, *Key Notions for Pragmatics*. Amsterdam: John Benjamins, pp. 28–47.

Walther, J. B., Jang, J. W. & Edwards, A. A. H. (2018). Evaluating health advice in a web 2.0 environment: The impact of multiple user-generated factors on HIV advice perceptions. *Health Communication*, 33(1), 57–67.

Wang, H. (2003). On fuzzy language and its pragmatic functions. *Foreign Language Education*, 3(2), 9–12.

Wertsch, J. V. (1998). *Mind as Action*. Oxford & New York: Oxford University Press.

Westerman, D., Spence, P. R. & Van Der Heide, B. (2012). A social network as information: The effect of system generated reports of connectedness on credibility on Twitter. *Computers in Human Behavior*, 28(1), 199–206.

Williamson, T. (1994). Vagueness. In R. Asher & S. Simpson, eds., *The Encyclopedia of Language and Linguistics*. Oxford: Pergamon Press, pp. 4869–4871.

Willis, E. & Royne, M. B. (2017). Online health communities and chronic disease self-management. *Health Communication*, 32(3), 269–278.

Wong, T. P. (2010). The pure way to create lean and excellent organizations. *International Journal of Existential Psychology & Psychotherapy*, 3(2), 1–21.

Wright II, J. W. & Hosman, L. A. (1983). Language style and sex bias in the courtroom: The effects of male and female use of hedges and intensifiers on impression information. *Southern Speech Communication Journal*, 48(2), 137–152.

Wu, Y., Wang, J. & Zhou, C. (2010). The use of 'I think' by Chinese EFL learners: A study revisited. *Chinese Journal of Applied Linguistics*, 33(1), 3–23.

Yan, J., Wei, J., Zhao, D., Vinnikova, A., Li, L. & Wang, S. (2018). Communicating online diet-nutrition information and influencing health behavioral intention: The role of risk perceptions, problem recognition, and situational motivation. *Journal of Health Communication*, 23(7), 624–633.

Yule, G. (1996). *Pragmatics*. Oxford: Oxford University Press.

Zayts, O., Sarangi, S. & Schnurr, S. (2016). The management of diagnostic uncertainty and decision-making in genetics case conferences. *Communication & Medicine*, 13(1), 37–50.

Zhang, G. (2011). Elasticity of vague language. *Intercultural Pragmatics*, 8, 571–599.

Zhang, G. (2013). The impact of touchy topics on vague language use. *Journal of Asian Pacific Communication*, 23(1), 87–118.

Zhang, G. (2015). *Elastic Language: How and Why We Stretch Our Words*. Cambridge: Cambridge University Press.

Zhang, G. (2016). How elastic a little can be and how much a little can do in Chinese. *Chinese Language and Discourse*, 7(1), 1–22.

Zhang, G. (2019). The pragmatic use of 'sort of' in TV forums: A Chinese perspective. *Journal of Asian Pacific Communication*, 29(1), 62–85.

Zhang, G. (2020). Vague language challenged: Australian customs encounters. *International Review of Pragmatics*, 12(1), 1–28.

Zhang, G. & Feng, H. (2013). The sensitivity of conversational topics and vague language in Mandarin Chinese. *Contemporary Linguistics*, 15(1), 45–61.

Zhang, G. & Sabet, P. G. P. (2016). Elastic 'I think': Stretching over L1 and L2. *Applied Linguistics*, 37(3), 334–353.

Zhang, G. & Tseng, M.-Y. (2020). Attitudes towards elastic language in Australian online healthcare communication. *Internet Pragmatics*, 3(1), 34–63.

Zhang, R. H. (2010). The development of fuzzy linguistics in China over the past 30 years. *Journal of Tianjin Foreign Studies University*, 17(1), 1–9.

Zhao, X. (2010). *Investigating the Use of Vague Language as a Communicative Strategy in Chinese Business Negotiations*. Unpublished PhD Dissertation, Curtin University, Australia.

Zhou, F. F. & Zhang, Y. J. (2018). Wǎngluò huìhuà jiāojì zhōng móhú wēi yǔyán shèhuì yǔ yòng gōngnéng yánjiū (in Chinese) [Research on the social pragmatic function of fuzzy micro-language in Internet conversational communication]. *Meiji Wenhua [Media Culture]*, 23, 60–64.

Zimmerman, D. H. (1992). The interactional organization of calls for emergency assistance. In P. Drew & J. Heritage, eds., *Talk at Work*. Cambridge: Cambridge University Press, pp. 359–469.

Zummo, M. L. (2015). Exploring web-mediated communication: A genre-based linguistic study for new patterns of doctor–patient interaction in online environment. *Communication & Medicine*, 12(2–3), 187–198.

Author Index

Adolphs, S., 1, 2, 4, 11, 14, 15, 59, 90, 101, 108, 217, 218
Adolphs, S., Atkins, S. and Harvey, K., 33
Aijmer, K., 18, 20, 44, 97, 183, 184
Ainsworth-Vaughn, N., 1, 25
Akl, E. A., 13
Allan, K., 8
Andersen, G., 19
Arribas-Ayllon, M., 27
Auerbach, C. F. and Silverstein, L. B., 37
Austin, J. L., 7

Babrow, A. S., 28, 29, 30, 174
Babrow, A. S. and Mattson, M., 30
Bakhtin, M. M., 216
Barry, C., 165, 178
Basnyat. I., 26
Beach, W., 25
Beck, S. J., 27
Bennett, G. G. and Glasgow, R. E., 27
Bernard, H. R., 37
Biber, D., 19, 45
Bigi, S., 29
Blackwell, S. E., 8
Blank, T. O. and Adams-Blodnieks, M., 154
Bol, N., 200, 203
Borah, P. and Xiao, X., 26, 137, 175
Bradac, J. J., 88
Britt, R. K., 27
Brown, P. and Levinson, S. C., 20, 90
Bryant, A., 16
Bryant, A. and Norman, G. R., 101
Bryman, A., 33
Bursztajn, H. J., 28
Bylund, C. L., 2

Caffi, C., 20, 125
Candlin, C. N. and Candlin, S., 29
Capone, A., 7, 22, 30, 158, 206
Capone, A. and Bucca, A., 8
Carter, R., 19, 90, 183, 184, 185
Carter, R. and McCarthy, M., 1, 16, 20, 56, 90
Channell, J., 1, 4, 11, 14, 16, 17, 18, 20, 21, 22, 94, 161, 180, 182, 184, 185, 198
Chen, C., 3, 16, 17, 18, 21, 22, 111, 115, 207
Cheng, W., 3, 16, 17, 18
Cheng, W. and O'Keeffe, A., 34, 93
Cheng, W. and Warren, M., 16, 21, 22
Cheshire, J., 18, 89, 157, 183, 184
Cho, H. Y. and Sands, L., 13
Clark, H. H., 17, 59, 101, 163
Clark, H. H. and Wilkes-Gibbs, D., 17
Clerehan, R., 25
Clerehan, R. and Buchbinder, R., 26
Cocco, C., 26
Conrad, S. and Biber, D., 69
Corrales, D. M., 2, 26, 216
Craig, R. T., 29
Crawford, T., 29
Creswell, J. W., 33, 35
Creswell, J. W. and Plano Clark, V. L., 33
Cruse, A., 18
Crystal, D. and Davy, D., 17, 89
Culpeper, J. and Haugh, M., 4, 11, 12, 125
Cutting, J., 4, 16, 17, 18, 20, 22, 23, 56, 90, 91, 97, 100, 160, 180, 185, 191

Davis, T. C., 26
Dean, M., 219
Delorme, D. E., 10
des Bordes, J. K., 26
Dines, E. R., 18, 115, 161

Ediger, A., 1, 16
Evison, J., 21, 56

Fele, G., 25
Fiksdal, A. S., 26
Fillmore, C., 205
Folkman, S., 16
Fox and Duggan, M., 35
Fraser, B., 20

Gamson, W. A., 13
Gibson, J. J., 9
Gigerenzer, G., 216
Glinert, L., 24
Goffman, E., 13
Gooden, R. J. and Winefield, H. R., 154
Grice, H. P., 12, 18, 20, 52, 119, 133, 170, 171, 172, 174, 212
Guan, B., 154
Gudykunst, W. B., 194, 210
Gudykunst, W. B. and Kim, Y. Y., 210
Gudykunst, W. B. and Matsumoto, Y., 194
Gumperz, J., 112

Hall, E. T., 4, 194, 207
Halliday, M. A. K. and Hasan, R., 115, 118, 206, 208
Haluza, D., 26
Hamilton, H. E. and Chou, W.-Y., 29
Han, J. Y., 27, 28
Haugh, M., 8
Haugh, M. and Culpeper, J., 3, 11, 12, 32, 108, 150, 209
He, W. and Pan, X.-d., 207
Heath, C., 1
Hennemann, S., 27
Heritage, J. and Maynard, D. W., 25
Heritage, J. and Raymond, G., 25
Hofstede, G., 194, 198, 202, 210, 213, 214
Holmes, J., 14, 19, 101
Hong, T., 13, 111
Hsieh, C-Y., 44
Hwang, Y., 13
Hyland, K., 4, 14, 16, 19, 21, 89
Hymes, D., 114

Jaffe, A., 69
Jefferson, G., 115
Jensen, J. D., 57
Jick, T. D., 33
Johnson, M., 175
Johnstone, B., 10
Jones, R. H., 29, 138
Jucker, A. H., 14, 16, 17, 19, 20, 22, 43, 89, 161, 163, 180, 187, 205, 209

Kahneman, D. and Tversky, A., 13
Kärkkäinnen, E., 72
Kay, P., 19
Kecskes, I., 8, 32
Kline, K. N., 30
Koehly, L. M., 2
Koester, A., 17, 21
Krosnick, J. A. and Presser, S., 33

Lagan, B. M., 187, 216
Lakoff, G. and Johnson, M., 146
Lavrakas, P., 37
Layder, D., 33
Le, N. and Zhang, G., 66, 97
Lee, S. A. and Zuercher, R. J., 26
Leech, G., 89
Li, C. and Thompson, S., 71
Lim, N.-E., 44, 45, 51, 62
Lim, N.-E. and Hong, H. Q., 44
Lippincott, G., 200
Locher, M. A., 90
Lombardi Vallauri, E., 100
Lumpkins, A., 26
Lyons, J., 69

Maertens, J. A., 27
Major, L. H., 29, 165, 178
Martin, J. R., 44, 68, 211
Martin, J. R. and Rose, D., 44, 213
Martin, J. R. and White, P., 68, 211
Mashiach, R., 2
Matthews, P. H., 21
McCarthy, M., 21
McLaughlin, A., 216
Metsä-Ketelä, M., 22
Mey, J. L., 4, 7, 8, 9, 12, 106, 125, 206, 208
Miller, S. M., 2
Miller, S. M. and Mangan, C. E., 2
Mo, P. K. H., 154
Modigliani, A., 13
Morse, J. M., 35
Moxey, L. and Sanford, A., 17, 89, 170
Muijs, D., 33
Munné, F., 3
Murphy, B., 183
Musambira, G. W., 154
Myers, G., 91

Neelapala, P., 33, 187, 216
Neely, L., 2, 5
Nguyen, M. H., 26
Nicholson-Perry, K. and Burgess, M., 11, 14
Norman, G. R., 16

O'Keefe, D. J. and Jensen, J. D., 13
O'Keeffe, A., 210
Odebunmi, A., 8
Ordóñez-López, P. and Edo-Marzá, N., 1, 2, 4
Overstreet, M., 18, 44, 89, 113, 115, 176
Overstreet, M. and Yule, G., 18, 44

Paige, S. R., 26, 137, 175
Palacios Martínez, I., 183, 188
Palmer, F. R., 46, 69

Pan, Z. and Kosicki, G. M., 14
Parvaresh, V., 8, 16, 21, 23, 38, 44, 161, 183, 186
Parvaresh, V. and Capone, A., 8
Parvaresh, V. and Tayebi, T., 38
Parvaresh, V. and Zhang, G., 21
Patton, M. Q., 32, 34, 35, 36
Paugh, A. and Izquierdo, C., 29
Payne, S., 26
Peräkylä, A., 25
Pichler, H. and Levey, S., 183, 188
Potter, J., 50, 138
Pounds, G., 29, 90
Pounds, G. and De Pablos-Ortega, C., 29
Preacher, K. J., 163
Prince, E. F., 10, 16, 25, 43, 148, 207
Pullen, S., 59

Quirk, R., 18, 44

Ran, Y. P., 23, 104
Rauscher, E. A., 27
Ravert, R. D., 154
Rising, C. J., 27, 216
Ritterband, L. M., 27
Rothman, A. J., 13
Rothman, A. J. and Salovey, P., 13
Rowland, T., 19
Ruck, K., 26
Russell, B. J. and Ward, A. M., 35
Ruzaitė, J., 4, 14, 15, 16, 17, 20, 21, 22, 23, 43, 94

Sadock, J. M., 16
Salager-Meyer, F., 91
Samuelsson, C., 28
Sarangi, S., 29
Sarangi, S. and Clarke, A., 59, 101
Scherr, C. L., 28
Schwartz, S. H., 194
Schwarz-Friesel, M. and Consten, M., 93
Scullard, P., 2
Searle, J. R., 7
Segal, J. Z., 30
Shirato, J. and Stapleton, P., 17
Sigurd, B., 17
Silverstein, M., 114, 125
Simpson, S. A., 18
Smith, S. W., 163
Southwell, B. G., 10, 200
Spencer-Oatey, H., 21
Sperber, D. and Wilson, D., 12, 136, 171
Staples, S., 2, 15, 25
Stenström, A-B., 183, 187
Strekalova, Y. A. and Krieger, J. L., 26
Stubbs, M., 14, 20
Sunderland, J., 183

Tagliamonte, S. A. and Denis, D., 183, 187
Tashakkori, A. and Teddlie, C., 33
Terraschke, A. and Holmes, J., 20, 21, 56, 101, 118
Thompson, T. L., 29, 69
Thon, F. M. and Jucks, R., 26, 137, 175, 215
Trappes-Lomax, H., 20, 50, 97
Triandis, H. C., 194
Tsai, W.-T., 44
Tseng, M.-Y., 8, 219, 220, 223
Tseng, M.-Y. and Zhang, G., 4, 7, 8, 10, 11, 12, 13, 14, 33, 43, 57, 125, 160, 169, 170, 175, 176, 177, 185, 187, 205, 215, 219
Tversky, A. and Kahneman, D., 13

Uhlirovà, L., 34

van Dijk, T. A., 14
van Dijk, T. A. and Kintsch, W., 193, 201, 213
Varttala, T., 14
Vasilescu, A., 9, 38
Veach, P. M., 219
Verschueren, J., 9, 12, 22
Verschueren, J. and Brisard, F., 9

Walther, J. B., 2, 27, 32
Wang, H., 46
Wertsch, J. V., 215
Westerman, D., 33
Williamson, T., 14
Willis, E. and Royne, M. B., 27
Wong, T. P., 22
Wright II, J. W. and Hosman, L. A., 185

Yan, J., 26, 55
Yule, G., 17

Zayts, O., 27
Zhang, G., 1, 3, 10, 11, 14, 15, 16, 17, 18, 19, 20, 21, 22, 23, 24, 25, 38, 43, 47, 48, 56, 87, 89, 90, 104, 111, 125, 148, 164, 171, 184, 199, 204, 207, 217, 220, 222, 223, 231, 232
Zhang, G. and Feng, H., 43, 125
Zhang, G. and Sabet, P. G. P., 21, 25, 72
Zhang, G. and Tseng, M.-Y., 20, 160
Zhao, X., 125
Zhou, F. F. and Zhang, Y. J., 46
Zimmerman, D. H., 25
Zummo, M. L., 26

Subject Index

adaptability, 8, 9, 10, 11, 206
affordance, 8, 9, 10
age factor, 155, 159, 186, 189, 199, 202
allopract, 206
approximate stretcher, 17, 39, 40, 43, 49, 59, 82, 100, 112
approximator, 17, 20, 43, 63, 101, 138, 145, 175
assertive, 19, 20, 21, 69, 72, 90, 198, 202

certainty, 19, 21, 40, 69, 71, 89, 97, 106, 180, 190, 210
Chi-square test, 152, 153, 154, 163, 168, 185, 188, 197, 198
conversation analysis, 25
conversational maxims, 18, 20, 119, 133, 134, 137, 170, 171, 172, 212
cooperation, 19
Cooperative Principle, 12, 133, 189
correlation, 12, 21, 43, 73, 75, 80, 84, 104, 105, 106, 120, 126, 164, 165, 186, 200, 201, 202, 205, 208, 209, 217, 218
credibility, 2, 26, 42, 137, 144, 174
cross-cultural comparison, 59, 114, 210
  differences, 109, 114, 117
  patterns, 117, 120
  similarity, 20, 109, 114, 117, 118, 119, 121, 196, 207
cultural sensitivity, 219

data-driven, 37, 42, 46, 89
degree of fitness, 205

elastic language, 1, 2, 3, 4, 5, 8, 9, 10, 12, 13, 15, 16, 17, 19, 20, 21, 22, 23, 24, 25, 26, 30, 31, 32, 33, 34, 35, 36, 37, 38, 39, 40, 41, 42, 43, 45, 46, 47, 48, 50, 52, 54, 55, 56, 57, 58, 59, 63, 67, 73, 74, 75, 79, 80, 82, 83, 84, 85, 87, 89, 90, 91, 92, 94, 95, 99, 100, 103, 104, 106, 109, 111, 113, 114, 115, 116, 117, 119, 120, 121, 122, 123, 125, 126, 127, 128, 129, 130, 131, 132, 133, 134, 136, 137, 138, 141, 142, 144, 145, 146, 147, 148, 149, 150, 151, 152, 153, 154, 155, 156, 157, 158, 159, 160, 161, 162, 163, 165, 166, 167, 168, 169, 170, 171, 172, 173, 174, 175, 176, 177, 178, 179, 180, 181, 182, 183, 184, 185, 186, 187, 188, 190, 191, 192, 193, 194, 195, 196, 197, 198, 199, 200, 201, 202, 203, 204, 205, 206, 208, 209, 211, 212, 213, 214, 215, 216, 217, 218, 219
elasticity theory, 7, 14, 15, 23, 24, 30, 191, 204, 209, 211, 214
  fluidity principle, 3, 24, 204
  strategy principle, 3, 24, 204
  stretchability principle, 3, 24, 204, 205
empathy, 29, 99
epistemic stretcher, 19, 39, 40, 45, 69, 74, 83, 112
evasiveness, 19, 199

first-order function, 38, 46, 59, 83, 89, 123, 213
formulaic, 18, 115, 116, 123, 138, 139, 140, 206, 208
frame/framing
  accuracy frame, 133, 169, 170, 172, 173, 180, 181, 189, 196, 197, 215
  clarity frame, 170, 173, 181, 182, 189, 196, 197, 215
  communication frame, 42, 133, 134, 136, 145, 146, 148, 149, 151, 158, 196, 201, 215
  definition, 13
  difference–indifference frame, 42, 142, 145, 158
  discourse management frame, 169, 170, 173, 174, 180, 181, 182
  disease-focused frame, 42, 169, 180, 181, 182, 190
  fluidity frame, 169, 170, 180, 181, 182, 189, 196, 202, 215

frame/framing (cont.)
folk–idiosyncratic frame, 42, 138, 146, 158, 196
folk–individual frame, 169, 173, 175, 180, 181, 182, 190, 215, 217
gain-framed, 13
informativeness frame, 133, 169, 170, 181, 189, 215
lay–professional frame, 42, 140, 158
loss-framed, 13
relevance frame, 169, 170, 171, 181, 189
trust–scepticism frame, 137, 138, 144, 145, 158, 202
voluntary–involuntary action frame, 141, 145, 158, 196
function of elastic language
advising gently, 41, 55, 83, 89, 98, 105, 113, 123, 204, 213
approximating, 40, 49, 63, 83, 89, 93, 105, 112, 123, 213
avoiding, 18, 22, 40, 50, 51, 83, 89, 90, 93, 99, 123, 213
correcting, 11, 41, 54, 63, 67, 80, 83, 84, 89, 97, 98, 105, 113, 114, 116, 123, 204, 209, 213
deintensifying, 40, 48, 49, 59, 83, 89, 92, 105, 112, 123, 213
describing tendency, 52, 57, 63, 65, 67, 83, 84, 89, 114, 213
intensifying, 25, 40, 47, 59, 67, 92, 105, 112, 151, 213
reporting, 41, 53, 83, 89, 96, 105, 113, 123, 131, 204, 208, 213
shortening, 40, 64, 83, 89, 94, 105, 112, 114, 115, 123, 212, 213
softening, 15, 40, 46, 59, 70, 83, 89, 105, 112, 114, 123, 213
supporting emotionally, 41, 56, 67, 83, 84, 89, 99, 105, 113, 114, 123, 204, 209, 213

gender factor, 92, 152, 159, 184, 197, 202
general stretcher, 17, 39, 40, 44, 63, 74, 82, 108, 112, 117

healthcare communication, 4, 7, 15, 33, 108, 220, 224, 232
healthcare discourse, 25, 32, 42
hedge, 45
hedging, 4, 22, 23, 28, 90
Hofstede's model of culture
collectivism, 202
collectivist, 194, 213, 214
direct, 5, 14, 90
directness, 5
feminine, 198, 202
femininity, 198, 199, 202
indirect, 106
indirectness, 5, 90
individualism, 202
individualist, 194, 214
masculine, 198, 199, 202
masculinity, 198, 199, 202

implicature, 17, 18, 89, 150
integrative pragmatics, 11, 12, 30, 32, 125, 150, 191, 204, 213, 214
intensification, 59, 83, 117, 119, 207
intensifier, 43, 44, 59, 67, 69, 84, 123, 185, 210
interpersonal, 11, 12, 14, 15, 20, 21, 46, 48, 52, 68, 84, 113, 115, 123, 211, 213
intimacy, 12, 20
power, 12, 18, 22, 100, 182, 185, 198, 204, 205
intersubjectivity, 215
inward-looking, attenuated style, 123, 207, 210, 212

medical discourse, 10, 14, 25, 30, 42, 190, 218
medical language, 2, 4
metaphor, 3, 7, 13, 23, 146, 199, 219
metapragmatics, 12, 31, 125, 133, 204, 205, 211
miscommunication, 22, 42

non-elastic language, 1, 31, 36, 37, 93, 125, 132, 133, 134, 137, 138, 142, 143, 144, 145, 147, 148, 149, 150, 151, 152, 153, 154, 156, 157, 158, 159, 160, 167, 168, 169, 170, 171, 172, 173, 175, 176, 177, 178, 180, 181, 182, 183, 185, 187, 188, 190, 194, 195, 196, 198, 199, 201, 202, 205, 211, 213, 215, 216, 218, 219

online discourse, 26
Internet intervention, 27
online community, 27
persuasive strategy, 29
tension, 29
online health communication, 10, 11, 13, 46, 55, 57, 67, 123, 214, 219
online health information, 9, 26, 30, 31, 32, 38, 46, 49, 63, 67, 115, 118, 119, 123, 125, 161, 189, 198, 202, 204, 207, 211, 212, 213, 215, 216, 217, 218
online medical data, 2
over-directness, 20

pragmatic act, 7, 9, 12, 150, 207, 219
pragmatic function, 4, 11, 12, 19, 25, 38, 46, 54, 83, 89, 105, 111, 112, 123, 204, 213

pragmeme, 7, 8, 9, 30, 204, 206, 207, 208, 211, 214
precise language, 2, 14, 15, 16, 21, 24, 96, 158, 166, 196, 202
presupposition, 130, 158, 194
prolific information, 2

quantifier, 17, 21, 23, 43, 93, 101, 108, 115

relevance theory, 136, 171, 189
reliability, 16, 19, 37, 175
rhetoric, 29, 67, 109, 118, 122, 124, 138, 205, 210
rhetorical, 29, 67, 109, 122, 124, 138, 210

scalar stretcher, 18, 39, 40, 44, 59, 66, 74, 82, 83
second-order function, 39, 46, 59, 63, 80, 83, 89, 112, 113, 114, 123, 208, 213
speech act, 7, 8, 9, 11, 12
stance, 29, 45, 69, 72, 86, 124, 138, 175, 195

tendency, 2, 41, 52, 74, 79, 80, 95, 96, 102, 105, 108, 113, 121, 123, 139, 187, 195, 197, 201, 203, 204, 208, 210, 213, 215, 216
tentativeness, 20, 91
tolerance for uncertainty, 210

uncertainty, 2, 5, 10, 14, 15, 16, 19, 27, 28, 29, 30, 59, 66, 69, 71, 101, 108, 119, 131, 148, 158, 167, 174, 194, 202, 208, 210, 218
upward-looking, amplifying style, 123, 207, 210, 211, 212

vague expression, 15, 24, 43, 66, 89, 128, 137, 149, 183, 186
vague language, 4, 7, 10, 11, 14, 15, 16, 17, 19, 20, 21, 22, 23, 25, 33, 43, 46, 48, 50, 56, 90, 111, 125, 129, 130, 132, 154, 155, 157, 160, 161, 163, 164, 165, 166, 180, 182, 183, 184, 185, 187, 188, 190, 191, 193, 198, 201, 202
vague language function
  mitigation, 19, 21, 22, 29, 48, 199
  rapport-building, 21
  right amount of information, 20, 23, 24, 46
  self-protection, 19, 21, 22, 25, 50, 89, 97, 101
  solidarity, 14, 17, 20, 21, 23, 27, 57, 115
  strengthening, 21, 23, 210
  withholding information, 22, 23
vagueness, 11, 14, 16, 20, 22, 30, 100, 130, 132, 158, 165, 166, 184, 189, 193, 198, 199, 202, 205

written health discourse, 25, 111
  consent form, 25, 222, 229
  dietary information, 25
  medication information, 25
  patient decision aid, 25
  patient education brochure, 25
  prescription, 26
  referral letter, 26
  sickness proof, 26

For EU product safety concerns, contact us at Calle de José Abascal, 56–1°, 28003 Madrid, Spain or eugpsr@cambridge.org.

www.ingramcontent.com/pod-product-compliance
Lightning Source LLC
LaVergne TN
LVHW011811200926
848484LV00005B/1147

* 9 7 8 1 1 0 8 8 4 2 3 9 6 *